Respiratory System

Adam Myers, PhD

Professor and Director of Graduate Studies
Department of Physiology and Biophysics
Georgetown University School of Medicine
Washington, DC

UK edition authors:

Pippa McGowan, Angus Jeffries, and Andrew Turley

UK series editor
Daniel Horton-Szar

ELSEVIER
MOSBY

ELSEVIER
MOSBY

1600 John F. Kennedy Blvd.
Ste 1800
Philadelphia, PA 19103-2899

CRASH COURSE: RESPIRATORY SYSTEMS
Copyright 2006, Elsevier, Inc. All rights reserved.

ISBN-13: 978-1-4160-2991-5
ISBN-10: 1-4160-2991-5

Notice

Adapted from Crash Course Respiratory System 2e by Pippa McGowan, ISBN 0-7234-3293-7. © 2002, Elsevier Science Limited. All rights reserved.

The rights of Pippa McGowan to be identified as the author of this work have been asserted by her in accordance with the Copyright, Designs and Patents Act, 1988.

Library of Congress Cataloging-in-Publication Data
Myers, Adam K.
    Respiratory system / Adam Myers.—1st ed.
      p. ; cm.—(Crash course)
    ISBN 1-4160-2991-5
    1. Respiratory organs. 2. Respiration. I. Title. II. Series.
    [DNLM: 1. Respiratory System. 2. Respiratory Physiology. 3. Respiratory Tract Diseases.
WF 100M996r 2006]
    QP121.M94 2006
    612.2—dc22

2005052203

Commissioning Editor: *Alex Stibbe*
Project Development Manager: *Stan Ward*
Project Manager: *David Saltzberg*
Designer: *Andy Chapman*
Cover Design: *Antbits Illustration*
Illustration Manager: *Mick Ruddy*

Printed in China

Last digit is the print number:
9 8 7 6 5 4 3 2 1

Preface

Respiratory physiology and medicine are considered difficult by many students because of the integrative nature of the field. A full understanding of the respiratory system entails integration of concepts from basic physics, chemistry, and biology as well as multiple biomedical disciplines. Furthermore, respiratory diseases are complex, often life-threatening conditions that require not only an understanding of the respiratory system but also comprehension and knowledge from many fields, including acid–base physiology, cardiovascular function, fluid and electrolyte balance, cell physiology, emergency medicine, clinical chemistry, pharmacology, and medical imaging.

This text presents the respiratory system in an integrative context and includes not only basic respiratory physiology but also essential components of respiratory pathophysiology, pharmacology, and medicine. Basic science and clinical concepts are presented in an easy-to-follow progression, with key concepts reinforced in tables, diagrams, and bulleted highlights.

Because of its integrative format, this text should be suitable for any of the diverse methods now used in medical education, ranging from traditional lectures to small-group teaching, problem-based learning, and systems approaches. For example, for students in the traditional curriculum, the fundamentals of respiratory physiology are clearly and concisely presented, and such students will find the text useful in subsequent courses in pathology and pharmacology. In a systems-based or problem-based curriculum, all major aspects of the respiratory system are presented in this book. All students should find the book useful as they progress through clinical clerkships as well.

Respiratory physiology and medicine are an integral part of the practice of most physicians. Despite the complexity of the field, the respiratory system is a fascinating one, and future physicians will benefit greatly from an understanding of basic science and clinical concepts. This text is aimed at providing a concise and readable gateway to that understanding. I wish you well in your voyage toward becoming a skilled and compassionate physician and hope that this book aids you in that journey.

Adam Myers, PhD

Acknowledgments

My thanks to Adriane Fugh-Berman, MD, for her helpful comments and review of this manuscript. I gratefully acknowledge the original hard work of the authors of the UK edition of this book.

Contents

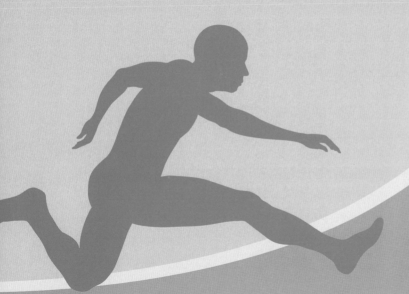

BASIC MEDICAL SCIENCE OF
THE RESPIRATORY SYSTEM

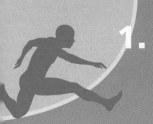

1. Overview of the Respiratory System

Overall structure and function

Respiration

Respiration refers to the processes involved in oxygen transport from the atmosphere to the body tissues and the release and transportation of carbon dioxide produced in the tissues to the atmosphere.

This book will not discuss cellular respiration, in which oxygen is used by the cell to liberate energy; this is also known as internal respiration and is covered in *Crash Course: Metabolism and Nutrition*. The focus of this book is external respiration, or the exchange of gases between the environment and the blood.

Microorganisms rely solely on diffusion to and from their environment for the supply of oxygen and removal of carbon dioxide. Humans, however, are unable to rely on diffusion alone because:

- Their surface area:volume ratio is too small.
- The diffusion distance from the surface of the body to the cells is too large, and the process would be far too slow to be compatible with life.

Remember that diffusion time increases with the square of the distance and as a result, the human body has had to develop a specialized respiratory system to overcome these problems. This system has two components:

- A gas-exchange system that provides a large surface area for the uptake of oxygen from, and the release of carbon dioxide to, the environment. This function is performed by the lungs.
- A transport system that delivers oxygen to the tissues from the lungs and carbon dioxide to the lungs from the tissues. This function is carried out by the cardiovascular system.

Structure

The respiratory system can be neatly divided into upper respiratory tract (nasal and oral cavities, pharynx, larynx, and trachea) and lower respiratory tract (main bronchi and lungs) (Fig. 1.1).

Upper respiratory tract

The upper respiratory tract has a large surface area, a rich blood supply, and its epithelium (respiratory epithelium) is covered by a mucous secretion. Within the nose, hairs are present, which act as a filter. The function of the upper respiratory tract is to warm, moisten, and filter the air so that it is in a suitable condition for gaseous exchange in the distal part of the lower respiratory tract.

Lower respiratory tract

The lower respiratory tract consists of the lower part of the trachea, the two primary bronchi and the lungs. These structures are contained within the thoracic cavity.

Lungs

The lungs are the organs of gas exchange and act as both a conduit for air flow (the airway) and a surface for movement of oxygen into the blood and carbon dioxide out of the blood (the alveolar capillary membrane).

The lungs consist of airways, blood vessels, nerves, and lymphatics, supported by parenchymal tissue. Inside the lungs, the two main bronchi divide into smaller and smaller airways until the end respiratory unit (acinus) is reached (Fig. 1.2).

Acinus

The acinus is that part of the airway that is involved in gaseous exchange (i.e., the passage of oxygen from the lungs to the blood and carbon dioxide from the blood to the lungs). The structure of the acinus is considered in detail in Chapter 3.

Pleurae

The lung, chest wall, and mediastinum are covered by two continuous layers of epithelium known as the pleurae. The inner pleura covering the lung is the visceral pleura and the outer pleura covering the chest wall and mediastinum is the parietal pleura. These two pleurae are closely apposed and are separated by only a thin layer of liquid. The liquid

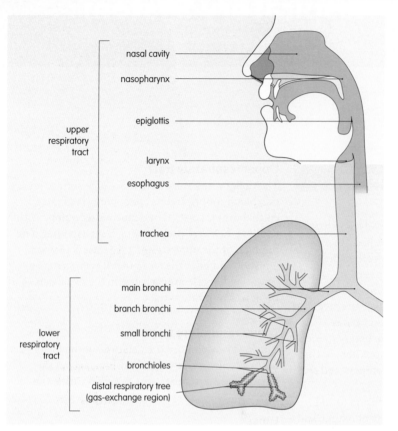

Fig. 1.1 A schematic diagram of the respiratory tract.

upper respiratory tract
- nasal cavity
- nasopharynx
- epiglottis
- larynx
- esophagus
- trachea

lower respiratory tract
- main bronchi
- branch bronchi
- small bronchi
- bronchioles
- distal respiratory tree (gas-exchange region)

acts as a lubricant and allows the two surfaces to slip over each other during breathing.

Basic concepts in respiration

The supply of oxygen to body tissues is essential for life; after only a brief period without oxygen, cells undergo irreversible change and eventually death. The respiratory system plays an essential role in preventing tissue hypoxia by optimizing the oxygen content of arterial blood through efficient gas exchange. The three key steps involved in gas exchange are:
- Ventilation
- Perfusion
- Diffusion.

Together these processes ensure that oxygen is available for transport to the body tissues and that carbon dioxide is eliminated (Fig. 1.3). If any of the three steps are compromised, for example through lung disease, then the oxygen content of the blood will fall below normal (hypoxemia) and levels of

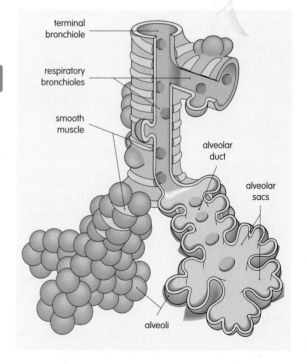

terminal bronchiole
respiratory bronchioles
smooth muscle
alveolar duct
alveolar sacs
alveoli

Fig. 1.2 The acinus, or respiratory unit. This part of the airway is involved in gas exchange.

4

Fig 1.3 Key steps involved in respiration. (Adapted with permission from *Physiology of Respiration* by M.P. Hlastala and A.J. Berger. Oxford University Press, 2001.)

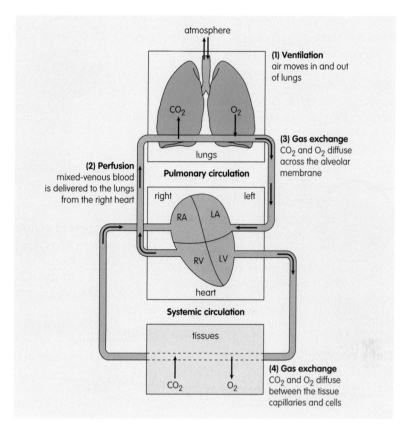

carbon dioxide may rise (hypercapnia) (Fig. 1.4). In clinical practice, we do not directly test for tissue hypoxia but look for:

- Symptoms and signs of impaired gas exchange (e.g., breathlessness or central cyanosis)
- Abnormal results from arterial blood gas tests (see Chapter 10).

Severe hypoxemia, with or without hypercapnia, is known as respiratory failure (see Chapter 8).

Ventilation

Ventilation is the movement of air in and out of the respiratory system. It is determined by both:

- The respiratory rate (i.e. number of breaths per minute, normally 12–20)
- The volume of each breath, also known as the tidal volume.

A change in ventilation, in response to the metabolic needs of the body, can therefore be brought about by either:

Common respiratory terms	
Hypocapnia	Decreased carbon dioxide tension in arterial blood ($P_aCO_2 < 40$ mmHg or 5.3 kPa)
Hypercapnia	Increased carbon dioxide tension in arterial blood ($P_aCO_2 > 45$ mmHg or 6 kPa)
Hypoxemia	Deficient oxygenation of the arterial blood
Hypoxia	Deficient oxygenation of the tissues
Hyperventilation	Ventilation that is in excess of metabolic requirements (results in hypocapnia)
Hypoventilation	Ventilation that is too low for metabolic requirements (results in hypercapnia)

Fig. 1.4 Definitions of common respiratory terms.

5

- Altering the number of breaths per minute
- Adjusting the amount of air that enters the lungs with each breath.

In practice, the most common response to hypoxemia is rapid, shallow breathing which increases the elimination of carbon dioxide and often leads to hypocapnia.

A raised respiratory rate, or tachypnea, is not the same as hyperventilation. The term hyperventilation refers to a situation where ventilation exceeds the body's metabolic needs (see Chapter 5).

The mechanisms of ventilation

The movement of air into and out of the lungs takes place because of pressure differences caused by changes in lung volumes. Air flows from a high-pressure area to a low-pressure area. We cannot change the local atmospheric pressure around us to a level higher than that inside our lungs; the only obvious alternative is to lower the pressure within the lungs. We achieve this pressure reduction by expanding the size of the chest.

The main muscle of inspiration is the diaphragm, upon which the two lungs sit. The diaphragm is dome-shaped; contraction flattens the dome, increasing intrathoracic volume. This is aided by the external intercostal muscles, which raise the rib cage; this results in a lowered pressure within the thoracic cavity and hence the lungs, supplying the driving force for air flow into the lungs. Inspiration is responsible for most of the work of breathing; diseases of the lungs or chest wall may increase the work load so that accessory muscles are also required to maintain adequate ventilation.

Expiration is largely a result of elastic recoil of the lung tissue. However, in forced expiration (e.g., during coughing), the abdominal muscles increase intra-abdominal pressure, forcing the contents of the abdomen against the diaphragm. In addition, the internal intercostal muscles lower the rib cage. These actions greatly increase intrathoracic pressure and enhance expiration.

Relating the physiology to clinical practice can make it more memorable. Ventilation is brought about by altering lung volumes and this can be affected by disease. That is why measurement of lung volumes, and knowing their normal values, is so important in assessing lung function (see Chapter 10).

Impaired ventilation

There are two main types of disorder which impair ventilation. These are:
- Obstructive disorders in which the airways become narrowed, increasing the resistance to airflow
- Restrictive disorders in which expansion of the lungs is compromised and the volume of gas in the lungs is limited.

Obstructive and restrictive disorders have characteristic patterns of lung function, measured by pulmonary function tests (see Chapter 3).

Ventilatory failure occurs if the work of breathing becomes excessive and muscles fail. In this situation, or to prevent it from occurring, mechanical ventilation is required. Respiratory support is discussed in Chapter 6.

Perfusion

The walls of the alveoli contain a dense network of capillaries bringing mixed-venous blood from the right heart. The barrier separating blood in the capillaries and air in the alveoli is extremely thin. Perfusion of blood through these pulmonary capillaries allows diffusion, and therefore gas exchange, to take place.

Ventilation:perfusion inequality

To achieve efficient gaseous exchange, it is essential that the flow of gas (ventilation: V) and the flow of blood (perfusion: Q) are closely matched. The V:Q ratio in a normal, healthy lung is approximately 1:1. Two extreme scenarios illustrate mismatching of ventilation and perfusion. These are:
- Normal alveolar ventilation but no perfusion (e.g., due to a blood clot obstructing flow). This is called dead space ventilation

- Normal perfusion but no air reaching the lung unit (e.g., due to a mucus plug occluding an airway). Flow through such a region is called shunt flow.

Ventilation:perfusion inequality is the most common cause of hypoxemia and underlies many respiratory diseases.

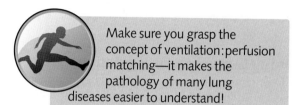

Make sure you grasp the concept of ventilation:perfusion matching—it makes the pathology of many lung diseases easier to understand!

Diffusion

At the gas exchange surface, diffusion occurs across the alveolar capillary membrane.

Molecules of CO_2 and O_2 diffuse along their partial pressure gradient.

Partial pressures

Air in the atmosphere, before it is inhaled and moistened, contains 21% oxygen. This means that:

- 21% of the total molecules in air are oxygen molecules
- Oxygen is responsible for 21% of the total air pressure; this is its partial pressure, measured in mmHg or kPa and abbreviated as PO_2 (Fig. 1.5).

Partial pressure also determines the gas content of liquids, but it is not the only factor. Gas enters the liquid as a solution, and the amount that enters depends on its solubility. The more soluble a gas the more molecules that will enter solution for a given partial pressure. The partial pressure of a gas in a liquid is sometimes referred to as its tension (i.e., arterial oxygen tension is the same as P_aO_2).

PO_2	Oxygen tension
P_aO_2	Arterial oxygen tension
P_vO_2	Oxygen tension in mixed-venous blood
P_AO_2	Alveolar oxygen tension

Carbon dioxide tensions follow the same format (PCO_2 etc)

Fig. 1.5 Abbreviations used in denoting partial pressures.

Because blood perfusing the pulmonary capillaries is mixed-venous blood:

- Oxygen will diffuse from the higher PO_2 environment of the alveoli into the capillaries
- Carbon dioxide will diffuse from the blood towards the alveoli, where PCO_2 is lower.

Blood and gas equilibrate as the partial pressures become the same in each and gas exchange then stops.

Oxygen transport

Once oxygen has diffused into the capillaries, it must be transported to the body tissues. The solubility of oxygen in the blood is low, and only a small percentage of the body's requirement can be carried in dissolved form. Therefore, most of the oxygen is combined with hemoglobin in red blood cells. Hemoglobin has four binding sites, and the amount of oxygen carried by hemoglobin in the blood depends on how many of these sites are occupied. If they are all occupied by oxygen, the molecule is said to be saturated. The arterial oxygen saturation (S_aO_2) tells us the relative percentage of the maximum possible sites that are bound. Note that anemia will not reduce S_aO_2; lower hemoglobin means there are fewer available sites but the relative percentage of possible sites that are saturated stays the same.

The relationship between the partial pressure of oxygen and % saturation of hemoglobin is represented by the oxygen dissociation curve (see Chapter 5).

Diffusion defects

If the blood–gas barrier becomes thickened through disease then the diffusion of O_2 and CO_2 will be impaired. Any impairment is particularly noticeable during exercise, when pulmonary flow increases and blood spends an even shorter time in the capillaries, exposed to alveolar oxygen. Impaired diffusion is, however, a much less common cause of hypoxemia than ventilation/perfusion mismatching.

Control of respiration

Respiration must respond to the metabolic demands of the body. This is achieved by a control system within the brainstem (the respiratory centers—see Chapter 6) which receives information from various sources in the body where sensors monitor:

- Partial pressures of oxygen and carbon dioxide in the blood
- pH of the extracellular fluid within the brain
- Mechanical changes in the chest wall.

On the basis of information they receive, the respiratory centers modify ventilation to ensure that oxygen supply and carbon dioxide removal from the tissues matches their metabolic requirements. The actual mechanical change to ventilation is carried out by the respiratory muscles: these are known as the effectors of the control system.

Respiration can also be modified by higher centers (e.g., during speech, anxiety, emotion).

It is easy to get confused about P_aO_2, S_aO_2 and oxygen content. P_aO_2 tells us the pressure of the oxygen molecules dissolved in arterial plasma, not those bound to hemoglobin. It is not a measure of how much oxygen is in the arterial blood. S_aO_2 tells us the percentage of the possible hemoglobin binding sites occupied by oxygen. To calculate the amount of oxygen you would also need to know hemoglobin levels and how much oxygen is dissolved. Oxygen content (C_aO_2) is the only value that actually tells us how much oxygen is in the blood and, unlike P_aO_2 or S_aO_2, it is given in units which denote quantity (ml O_2/dl).

Other functions of the respiratory system

Respiration is also concerned with a number of other functions, including metabolism, excretion, hormonal activity, and, most importantly:
- Regulation of the pH of body fluids
- Regulation of body temperature.

Acid–base regulation

Carbon dioxide forms carbonic acid in the blood, which dissociates to form hydrogen ions, lowering pH. By controlling the partial pressure of carbon dioxide, the respiratory system plays an important role in regulating the body's acid–base status (see Chapter 5); lung disease can therefore lead to acid–base disturbance. In acute disease it is important to test for blood pH and bicarbonate levels and these are included in the standard arterial blood gas results.

Body temperature regulation

Body temperature is greatly affected by insensible heat loss. Thus, by altering ventilation, body temperature may be regulated.

Metabolism

The lungs have a huge vascular supply and thus a large number of endothelial cells. Hormones such as noradrenaline (norepinephrine), prostaglandins and 5-hydroxytryptamine are taken up by these cells and destroyed. Some exogenous compounds are also taken up by the lungs and destroyed (e.g., amphetamine and imipramine).

Excretion

Carbon dioxide and some drugs (notably those administered through the lungs; e.g., general anesthetics) are excreted by the lungs.

Hormonal activity

Hormones (e.g., steroids) act on the lungs. Insulin enhances glucose utilization and protein synthesis. Angiotensin II is formed in the lungs from angiotensin I (by angiotensin-converting enzyme). Damage to the lung tissue causes the release of prostacyclin PG I_2, which prevents platelet aggregation.

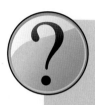

- Why have humans developed a respiratory system?
- Describe how breathing is brought about.
- What is the difference between the partial pressure of a gas and its concentration?
- How can defects in ventilation, perfusion, and diffusion cause hypoxemia?
- What effect will anemia have on P_aO_2, S_aO_2, and on the total oxygen content of the blood?
- Which structures are involved in gas exchange and how does it occur?
- What is the difference between restrictive and obstructive disorders?
- What happens if lung disease increases the work of breathing to excessive levels?
- Describe how respiration is controlled.
- List the main functions of the respiratory system.

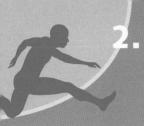

2. The Upper Respiratory Tract

Structure of the upper respiratory tract

Nose

The nose consists of an external part (the external nose) and an internal part (the nasal cavities, including the nasal septum). These structures are adapted to the main functions of the nose, which are olfaction (smelling) and breathing. This book will be concerned only with the internal nose and its function in breathing.

Nasal cavities and paranasal sinuses

The lateral wall of the nasal cavity consists of bony ridges called conchae or turbinates (Figs 2.1 and 2.2). These provide a large surface area covered in highly vascularized mucous membrane, which warms and humidifies inspired air.

The important role of the nasal cavities in warming and humidifying air is illustrated by patients who have had tracheostomies or endotracheal intubation for long periods. Without nose breathing, the mucosa of the trachea can become dry and crusted.

Under each turbinate there is a groove or meatus. The paranasal air sinuses (frontal, sphenoid, ethmoid, and maxillary) drain into these meatuses via small ostia, or openings. The drainage sites of each of the sinuses are shown in Fig. 2.2.

The anatomy of the paranasal sinuses is important clinically. If the mucosa of the meatuses becomes inflamed (e.g., through a common cold or allergic rhinitis) then the ostia may be blocked. This prevents mucus from draining from the sinuses, leading to increased pressure and infection: sinusitis. It is common clinically for sinusitis to occur in the maxillary, frontal, and anterior ethmoidal sinuses; this is because they all drain into a single, small area in the middle meatus. Inflammation here will obstruct all three sinuses.

Blood and nerve supply and lymphatic drainage

The terminal branches of the internal and external carotid arteries provide the rich blood supply for the internal nose. The sphenopalatine artery (from the maxillary artery) and the anterior ethmoidal artery (from the ophthalmic) are the two most important branches. Sensation to the area is provided mainly by the maxillary branch of the trigeminal nerve. Lymphatic vessels drain into the submandibular node, then drain into deep cervical nodes.

Pharynx

The pharynx extends from the base of the skull to the inferior border of the cricoid cartilage where it is continuous anteriorly with the trachea and posteriorly with the esophagus. It is described as being divided into three parts: the nasopharynx, oropharynx, and the laryngopharynx, which open anteriorly into the nose, the mouth, and the larynx, respectively (Fig. 2.3).

The nasopharynx is situated above the soft palate and opens anteriorly into the nasal cavities at the

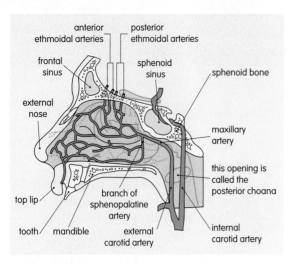

Fig. 2.1 Lateral view of the nasal cavity showing the rich blood supply.

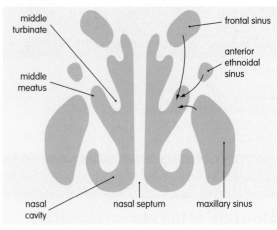

Fig. 2.2 Frontal view of the nasal cavity drainage sites of the paranasal sinuses.

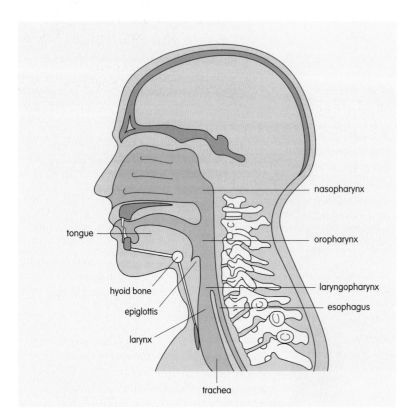

Fig. 2.3 Schematic diagram showing midline structures of the head and neck.

choanae (posterior nares). During swallowing, the nasopharynx is cut off from the oropharynx by the soft palate. The nasopharynx contains the opening of the eustachian canal (pharyngotympanic or auditory tube) and the adenoids, which lie beneath the epithelium of its posterior wall.

Detailed discussion of the oropharynx and laryngopharynx is beyond the scope of this book.

Musculature, blood and nerve supply, and lymphatic drainage

Three muscles surround the fascial tube of the pharynx: the superior, middle, and inferior constrictor muscles (Fig. 2.4).

> Muscle tone of the pharynx, particularly at the level of the soft palate, is important in maintaining airway patency. During sleep, the upper airway dilating muscles relax and in some individuals the airway may be partially or completely occluded. This leads to recurrent episodes of sleep apnea.

The arterial blood supply of the pharynx is from the external carotid through the superior thyroid, ascending pharyngeal, facial, and lingual arteries. Venous drainage is by a plexus of veins on the outer surface of the pharynx to the internal jugular vein.

Both sensory and motor nerve supplies are from the pharyngeal plexus (cranial nerves IX and X); the maxillary nerve (cranial nerve V) supplies the nasopharynx with sensory fibers.

Lymphatic vessels drain directly into the deep cervical lymph nodes.

Larynx

At its inferior end, the larynx is continuous with the trachea. At its superior end, it is attached to the U-shaped hyoid bone and lies below the epiglottis of the tongue. The larynx is made up of a cartilaginous skeleton linked by a number of membranes. This cartilaginous skeleton consists of the epiglottis, thyroid, arytenoid, and cricoid cartilages. Fig. 2.5 shows an external view and a median section through the larynx.

The larynx has three main functions:
- As an open valve, to allow air to pass when breathing

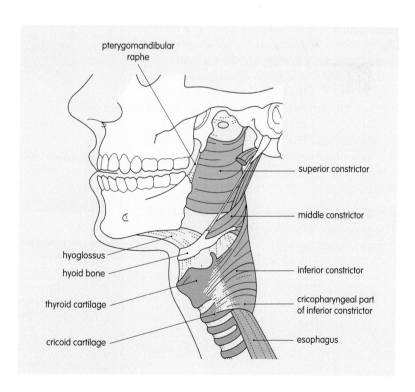

Fig. 2.4 The pharynx, showing the superior, middle, and inferior constrictors.

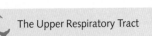

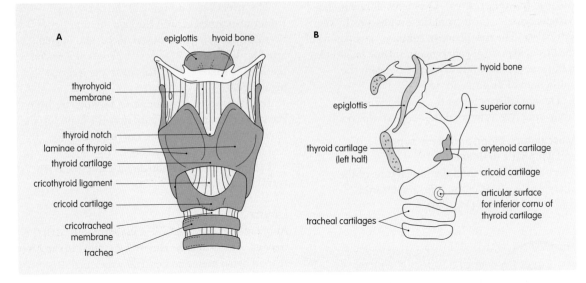

Fig. 2.5 The larynx. (A) External view—anterior aspect. (B) Median section through the larynx, hyoid bone, and trachea.

- Protection of the trachea and bronchi during swallowing. The vocal cords close, the epiglottis folds back covering the opening to the larynx, and the larynx is pulled upward and forward beneath the tongue
- Speech production (phonation).

Musculature

The muscles of the larynx are split into external and internal muscles. There is only one external muscle of the larynx (cricothyroid), although many other muscles attach to the thyroid membrane and cartilage. Cricothyroid has its origin at the arch of the cricoid and attaches to the lower border of the thyroid cartilage. The internal muscles may change the shape of the larynx; they protect the lungs by a sphincter action and adjust the vocal cords in phonation.

Blood and nerve supply and lymphatic drainage

The blood supply of the larynx is from superior and inferior laryngeal arteries, which are accompanied by the superior and recurrent laryngeal branches of the vagus nerve (cranial nerve X). The internal branch of the superior laryngeal nerve supplies the mucosa of the larynx above the vocal cords, the external branch supplies the cricothyroid muscle. The recurrent laryngeal nerve supplies the mucosa below the vocal cords and all the intrinsic muscles apart from cricothyroid.

The left recurrent laryngeal nerve has a long path through the thorax from the aortic arch, where it leaves the vagus, to the larynx. It is therefore vulnerable to compression by neoplasms, including those of the lung. Hoarseness, loss of voice power and a "bovine" cough are all signs of left recurrent nerve paralysis.

Lymph vessels above the vocal cords drain into the upper deep cervical lymph nodes; below the vocal cords lymphatic vessels drain into the lower cervical lymph nodes.

Trachea

The trachea is a cartilaginous and membranous tube of about 10 cm in length. It extends from the larynx to its bifurcation at the carina (at the level of the fourth or fifth thoracic vertebra). The trachea is approximately 2.5 cm in diameter and is supported by C-shaped rings of hyaline cartilage. The rings are completed posteriorly by the trachealis muscle. Important relations of the trachea within the neck are:

- The thyroid gland, which straddles the trachea, its two lobes sitting laterally, and its isthmus anteriorly with the inferior thyroid veins
- The common carotid arteries, which lie lateral to the trachea
- The esophagus, which lies directly behind the trachea, and the recurrent laryngeal nerve, which lies between these two structures.

Tissues of the upper respiratory tract
Nose and nasopharynx
The upper one-third of the nasal cavity is the olfactory area and is covered in yellowish olfactory epithelium. The lower two-thirds of the nasal cavity, the nasal sinuses and the nasopharynx comprise the respiratory area, which is adapted to its main functions of filtering, warming, and humidifying inspired air. These areas are lined with pseudostratified ciliated columnar epithelium (Fig. 2.6), also known as respiratory epithelium. With the exception of a few areas, this pattern of epithelium lines the whole of the respiratory tract down to the terminal bronchioles. Throughout these cells are numerous mucus-secreting goblet cells with microvilli on their luminal surface. Coordinated beating of the cilia propels mucus and entrapped particles to the pharynx where it is swallowed.

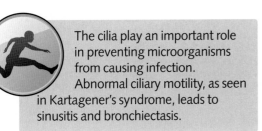

The cilia play an important role in preventing microorganisms from causing infection. Abnormal ciliary motility, as seen in Kartagener's syndrome, leads to sinusitis and bronchiectasis.

Adenoids
The nasopharyngeal tonsil is a collection of mucosa-associated lymphoid tissue (MALT) that lies behind epithelium of the roof and the posterior surface of the nasopharynx. Together with the palatine tonsils and the lymphoid tissue on the dorsum of the tongue these form Waldeyer's ring.

Oropharynx and laryngopharynx
The oropharynx and laryngopharynx have two functions as parts of both the respiratory and alimentary tracts. They are lined with nonkeratinized

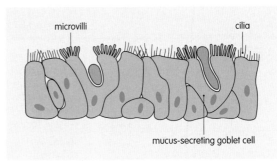

Fig. 2.6 Respiratory epithelium.

stratified squamous (NKSS) epithelium several layers thick and are kept moist by numerous salivary glands.

Larynx and trachea
The epithelium of the larynx is made up of two types: NKSS epithelium and respiratory epithelium. NKKS epithelium covers the vocal folds, vestibular fold, and larynx above this level. Below the level of the vestibular fold (with the exception of the vocal folds, which are lined with keratinized stratified squamous epithelium), the larynx and trachea are covered with respiratory epithelium.

Development of the upper respiratory tract

Branchial arches and pharyngeal pouches
During week 4 of development, the branchial arches are formed; these are gill-like pairs of folds at the cranial (head) end of the embryo. Eventually, six pairs of branchial arches are formed, which are numbered craniocaudally (head to tail) from first to sixth arches. Not all arches are present at once; the first two branchial arches degenerate before the sixth arch is formed. The branchial arches form the major part of the branchial apparatus, which consists of:
- Branchial arches
- Pharyngeal pouches: evaginations of endodermal tissue, situated inside the primitive pharynx
- Branchial grooves: located between the branchial arches
- Branchial membrane: bilaminar layer of ectodermal and endodermal tissue between the branchial arches.

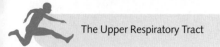

A	Branchial arch derivatives			
Arch No.	Bones and cartilage	Muscles	Nerves	Ligaments
1	incus and malleus	tensor tympani tensor veli palatini muscles of mastication mylohyoid anterior belly of digastric	cranial nerve V (trigeminal nerve)	anterior ligament of malleus sphenomandibular ligament
2	stapes styloid process lesser coruna of the hyoid bone superior part of hyoid	stapedius stylohyoid posterior belly of digastric muscles of facial expression	cranial nerve VII (facial nerve)	stylohyoid ligament
3	inferior part of body of hyoid greater coruna of hyoid	stylopharyngeus	cranial nerve IX (glossopharyngeal nerve)	
4/6	thyroid cartilage cricoid cartilage arytenoid cartilage corniculate and cuneiform cartilage	cricothyroid levator veli palatini pharyngeal constrictors intrinsic laryngeal muscles striated esophageal muscle	cranial nerve X recurrent laryngeal nerve superior laryngeal nerve branches of the vagus nerve	

B	Pharyngeal pouch derivatives		
Pouch No.	Development		
1	tubotympanic recess	→	auditory tube and tympanic cavity
2	mostly obliterate endoderm	→ →	intratonsillar cleft epithelium of tonsil and crypts
3	endoderm (dorsal) endoderm (ventral)	→ →	inferior parathyroids thymus
4	endoderm (dorsal) endoderm (ventral)	→ →	superior parathyroid ultimobranchial bodies, which fuse with the thyroid gland to form the parafollicular cells

Fig. 2.7 Derivatives of (A) branchial arches and (B) pharyngeal pouches.

The branchial arches form the skeletal and muscular components of the head and neck. Mesenchymal cells group together within the arches to form clusters called branchial arch cartilages, which form skeletal structures. Mesenchymal cells also form myoblasts (primitive muscle cells), which migrate to form the musculature of the head and neck.

Figure 2.7 shows the formation of structures from the branchial arches and pharyngeal pouches.

The nerve supply of the branchial arches is derived from the cranial nerves. The first and second branchial arches receive sensory fibers from cranial nerve V and motor fibers from cranial nerve VII.

The nerve supply to the third branchial arch is from cranial nerve IX, which also supplies the stylopharyngeus. The fourth and sixth branchial arches are supplied by two branches of the vagus nerve (cranial nerve X): the superior laryngeal and recurrent laryngeal nerves.

Primitive mouth, nasal, and oral cavities

The primitive mouth is formed by a depression in the ectoderm at the cranial end of the embryo called the stomodeum, initially separated from the primitive pharynx by a bilaminar membrane called the

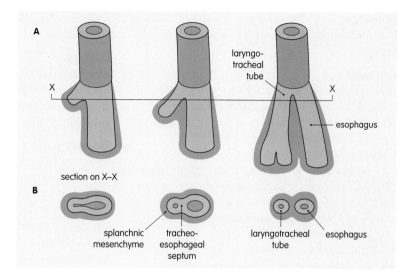

Fig. 2.8 Formation of the trachea and larynx: (A) lateral view; (B) cross-section on X–X. Note how defects in formation of the septum can lead to a fistula between trachea and esophagus.

oropharyngeal membrane. This membrane ruptures at about day 24–26, by which time the ectoderm of the cranial end of the embryo has already invaginated, forming the nasal and oral cavities.

Respiratory tract: larynx and trachea

The respiratory tract starts as a groove in the median plane of the primitive pharynx, the laryngotracheal groove. This groove deepens to form the laryngotracheal diverticulum and continues caudally (towards the tail) into the splanchnic mesenchyme, its distal end forming the lung bud. The cartilage and smooth muscle of the larynx are formed from the mesenchyme surrounding the diverticulum (Fig. 2.8). The foregut is separated from the diverticulum by the tracheoesophageal septum; when the diverticulum lengthens this is called the laryngotracheal tube. Defects in development may result in a tracheoesophageal fistula.

The connective tissue, cartilages and smooth muscle of trachea develop from the splanchnic mesenchyme, the glandular tissue developing from the endoderm.

Disorders of the nose

Inflammatory conditions
Infectious rhinitis (acute coryza or common cold)

The term "rhinitis" indicates that the mucosal membrane lining the nose is inflamed. Inflammation in the common cold is caused by a number of viral infections:

- Rhinovirus
- Coronavirus
- Adenovirus
- Parainfluenza virus
- Respiratory syncytial virus.

The common cold is a highly contagious self-limiting condition, with the highest incidence in children. Symptoms are nasal obstruction, rhinorrhea (runny nose), and sneezing. Complications include sinusitis, otitis media, and lower respiratory tract infections such as bronchitis.

Many different disorders affecting the upper respiratory tract are described here; some are much more common than others. The most common disorders of the upper respiratory tract are those that involve inflammation of the lining of the nose (rhinitis), particularly when associated with infection (e.g., the common cold). Another important condition associated with the upper respiratory tract is sleep apnea. In contrast, many of the nasal neoplasms are very rare.

Pathology

Acute inflammation with edema, glandular hypersecretion, and loss of surface epithelium.

Treatment

Treat symptomatically with decongestants and analgesics. Unless bacterial complications ensue, antibiotics are useless because of viral etiology.

Chronic rhinitis

Chronic rhinitis may follow an acute inflammatory episode. Predisposing factors include inadequate drainage of sinuses, nasal obstruction caused by polyps, and enlargement of the adenoids.

Allergic rhinitis

Allergic rhinitis is a common condition, affecting up to 30% of the Western population (Fig. 2.9). It is classified as either seasonal rhinitis (hayfever) or perennial rhinitis.

Seasonal rhinitis

Seasonal rhinitis has maximum prevalence in patients aged 10–20 years. It occurs during summer months. Approximately 20% of patients with allergic rhinitis also suffer from asthma.

Perennial rhinitis

The incidence of perennial rhinitis decreases with age. It is most common in patients aged 10–30 years.

There is no seasonal variation in symptoms which are mainly caused by Der p1 allergen in fecal particles of the housedust mite. Proteins from the urine and saliva of domestic pets, especially cats, also cause problems.

In some cases the pathology of perennial rhinitis is nonallergic and is due to abnormalities of the autonomic nervous system; this is termed vasomotor, or intrinsic, rhinitis. Nasal polyps may also present with perennial rhinitis secondary to nasal obstruction.

Etiology

Rhinitis is caused by hypersensitivity to allergens; the most common allergens are highly soluble proteins or glycoproteins (e.g., from pollens, molds, cat dander, and dustmite).

Pathology

Symptoms are caused by a type I IgE-mediated hypersensitivity reaction. IgE fixes onto mast cells in nasal mucous membranes. Upon re-exposure to allergen, cross-linking of the IgE receptor occurs on the surface of the mast cells leading to mast cell degranulation, release of histamine, and synthesis of leukotrienes.

Investigations

Diagnosis of rhinitis is clinical. Skin prick tests, nasal smears, and provocation tests can be used. Blood tests are:
- PRIST (plasma radioimmunosorbent test)— measures total plasma IgE levels
- RAST (radioallergosorbent test)—measures specific serum IgE antibody.

Treatment

Treatment is by allergen avoidance and drug treatment with antihistamines, anti-inflammatory drugs (e.g., nasal corticosteroids), and sodium cromoglycate.

Acute sinusitis

Sinusitis is an inflammatory process involving the lining of paranasal sinuses. The maxillary sinus is most commonly clinically infected. The majority of infections are rhinogenic in origin and are classified as either acute or chronic.

Etiology

The causes of acute sinusitis are:
- Secondary bacterial infection (by *Streptococcus pneumoniae* or *Haemophilus influenzae*), often after upper respiratory tract viral infection
- Dental extraction or infection
- Swimming and diving
- Fractures involving sinuses.

Clinical features

Symptoms occur over several days with yellow-green nasal discharge, malaise, sinus tenderness, and disturbed sense of smell. There may be fullness and pain over the cheeks, maxillary toothache, or a

Clinical features of rhinitis	
Seasonal rhinitis	Perennial rhinitis
Sneezing	Sneezing
Watery nasal discharge	Watery nasal discharge
Nasal irritation	Nasal blockage
Watery eyes	

Fig. 2.9 Clinical features of rhinitis.

frontal headache. Pain is classically worse on leaning forward. Postnasal discharge may lead to cough.

Pathology
Hyperemia and edema of the mucosa occur. Blockage of sinus ostia and mucus production increase. Cilia stop beating; therefore, stasis of secretions leads to secondary infection.

Tests
The tests are:
- Blood—white cell count and erythrocyte sedimentation rate (may be raised but are often normal)
- Culture of pus from nose
- Radiology of paranasal sinuses—CT scan.

Treatment
Medical treatment is by analgesia, broad-acting antibiotic for 7 days, and a decongestant. Discourage smoking and alcohol consumption. If no response to two regimens of antibiotics, refer to ear, nose, and throat (ENT) specialist.

Chronic sinusitis
Chronic sinusitis is an inflammation of the sinuses which has been present for more than 3 months. It usually occurs after recurrent acute sinusitis and is common in patients who are heavy smokers and work in dusty environments (Fig. 2.10).

Clinical features
Clinical features are similar to those of acute sinusitis but are typically less severe.

Pathology
Prolonged infection leads to irreversible changes in the sinus cavity, including:

- An increase in vascular permeability
- Edema and hypertrophy of the mucosa
- Goblet-cell hyperplasia
- Chronic cellular infiltrate
- Ulceration of the epithelium, resulting in granulated tissue formation.

Tests
The investigations are through sinus radiographs, high-definition coronal-section CT, and diagnostic endoscopy.

Treatment
This condition is difficult to treat. Treatments are:
- Medical—broad-acting antibiotics and decongestant
- Surgical—antral lavage, inferior meatal intranasal antrostomy, and functional endoscopic sinus surgery.

Rarely, recurrent sinusitis may be caused by Kartagener's syndrome, a congenital mucociliary disorder due to the absence of the ciliary protein dynein. It is characterized by sinusitis, bronchiectasis, otitis media, dextrocardia, and infertility.

Necrotizing lesions
Mucormycotic infections
Mucormycosis (or zygomycosis) is a virulent fungal infection caused by *Rhizopus oryzae*. The organism rarely causes disease in immunocompetent hosts, but acidotic diabetics and patients with extensive burns, leukemia, or lymphoma are at risk of infection after inhalation of spores. The spores invade blood vessels causing thrombi and ischemic necrosis. The primary

Predisposing factors of sinusitis			
Acute factors		Chronic factors (same as for acute, plus the following)	
Local	General	Local	General
Pre-existing rhinitis	Debilitation		
Nasal polyps	Immunocompromised	Anatomical variants	Atmospheric irritants
Nasal foreign bodies	Mucociliary disorders	Dental disease	
URTI		Recurrent sinus infection	
Nasal tumors			

Fig. 2.10 Predisposing factors of sinusitis.

sites of infection are nasal turbinates; patients present with sinusitis, inflammation of the orbit with proptosis, and meningoencephalitis.

Treatment is by systemic amphotericin B. Prognosis is poor.

Wegener's granulomatosis

Wegener's granulomatosis is a rare, necrotizing vasculitis of unknown etiology affecting small arteries and veins. It classically involves the upper and lower respiratory tract and the kidneys (glomerulonephritis). Mucosal thickening and ulceration occur, producing the clinical features of rhinorrhea, cough, hemoptysis, and dyspnea.

If untreated, the mortality rate after 2 years is 93%, but the disease responds well to high-dose prednisolone and cyclophosphamide.

Lethal midline granuloma (lymphoma)

Malignant midline granuloma of the nose is a T-cell lymphoma that presents as an ulcerated lesion and which progressively destroys midfacial structures. The lesion consists of proliferating lymphocytes and macrophages. Treatment is by radiotherapy combined with surgical excision.

Neoplasms

Neoplasms of the nose and paranasal sinuses (Fig. 2.11) are rare, with malignant tumors accounting for only 1% of all malignancies. Known nasal carcinogens include hardwood dust, nickel dust, snuff, and radiation. Clinical features depend on the location and spread of the neoplasia; patients may present with unilateral nasal obstruction and epistaxis or symptoms may be predominantly dental, orbital, retroantral, or facial. Inverted papilloma is one of the more important benign tumors as it is associated with squamous carcinoma.

Neoplasms of the nose and paranasal sinuses	
Benign	**Malignant**
Papilloma (squamous cell, transitional cell)	Plastocytoma (lymphoma)
Osteomo	Olfactory neuroblastoma
	Adenocarcinoma
	Squamous cell carcinoma

Fig. 2.11 Neoplasms of the nose and paranasal sinuses.

Inverted papilloma (transitional cell papilloma)

Inverted papilloma is a benign epithelial tumor affecting men and women in the ratio of 5:1. The disease accounts for 5% of all nasal tumors. Etiology is unclear.

Pathology

A papilliferous exophytic mass arises from the lateral walls of the nose. The epithelium invaginates into underlying tissue, and microcyst formation occurs resembling nasal polyps. Approximately 10% of these tumors are associated with squamous carcinoma.

Disorders of the pharynx

Sleep apnea

Sleep apnea syndrome is characterized by recurrent upper airway obstruction during sleep. Predisposing factors include the male sex, middle-age, and obesity. A cycle is generated during sleep in which:
- The upper airway dilating muscles lose tone
- The airway is occluded
- The patient wakes
- The airway reopens.

As a consequence of this cycle, sleep is unrefreshing and daytime sleepiness is common, particularly during monotonous situations such as highway driving. Each arousal also causes a transient rise in blood pressure, which may lead to sustained hypertension, pulmonary hypertension and cor pulmonale, ischemic heart disease, and stroke.

Sleep apnea can markedly reduce a patient's quality of life. It is also a public health problem—patients with sleep apnea are at an increased risk of road accidents as they have difficulty concentrating when driving and may even fall asleep at the wheel.

Tests and treatment

Patients are referred to a sleep or respiratory specialist for overnight studies. Fifteen apneas/hypopneas (of 10 seconds or longer) per hour of sleep is diagnostic.

Some patients can be managed conservatively and are advised to lose weight and avoid alcohol and sedatives as these relax the upper airway dilating muscles. However, for most patients nightly continuous positive airway pressure (CPAP) is recommended.

Neoplasms
Nasopharyngeal carcinoma
Nasopharyngeal carcinoma is commonly a poorly differentiated squamous cell carcinoma. Men are more likely to suffer from the disease, which usually presents in patients aged 50–70 years. The disease is common in South-East Asia and is associated with the Epstein–Barr virus and salted preserved fish. Nasopharyngeal carcinoma presents with epistaxis, nasal obstruction, or a neck lump. Seventy per cent of patients have metastatic lymph node involvement at presentation. The overall 5-year survival rate is 35%. Treatment is by radiotherapy.

Nasopharyngeal angiofibroma
Nasopharyngeal angiofibroma is a benign neoplasm occurring in childhood, affecting boys more than girls. It arises unilaterally and frequently coincides with a pubertal growth spurt. The disease presents with epistaxis and nasal obstruction.

Pathology
An enlarging vascular tumor is present, which contains a fibrous component. The disease can cause bone erosion and destruction by pressure atrophy. The sphenopalatine foramen is always involved.

Tests and treatment
Investigate by MR imaging or CT scanning. Surgical treatment is possible, but vascularity may be a problem. Radiotherapy is used only in unresectable cases.

Disorders of the larynx

Inflammatory conditions
Acute laryngitis
Acute laryngitis is a common condition, usually caused by viral infection, although secondary infection with streptococci or staphylococci can occur. Patients typically present with a hoarse voice and feel unwell. Rarely, dysphagia and pain on phonation occur.

Acute laryngitis is usually a self-limiting condition. If symptoms persist, refer to an ENT specialist.

Chronic laryngitis
Chronic laryngitis is inflammation of the larynx and trachea associated with excessive smoking, continued vocal abuse, and excessive alcohol.

The mucous glands are swollen and the epithelium hypertrophied. Heavy smoking leads to squamous metaplasia of the larynx. Biopsy is mandatory to rule out malignancy. Management is directed at avoidance of etiologic factors.

Laryngotracheobronchitis (croup) and acute epiglottitis
The features of laryngotracheobronchitis (croup) and acute epiglottitis are described in Fig. 2.12.

Pathology
In laryngotracheobronchitis, there is necrosis of epithelium and formation of an extensive fibrous membrane on the trachea and main bronchi. Edema of the subglottic area occurs, with subsequent danger of laryngeal obstruction.

In acute epiglottitis, there is an acute inflammatory edema and infiltration by neutrophils. No mucosal ulceration occurs. Acute epiglottitis may also occur in adults, although it is much more common in children (see Fig. 2.12).

Treatment
To treat laryngotracheobronchitis, keep the patient calm and hydrated. Nurse in a warm room in an upright position. Drug treatment, if required, includes steroids, oxygen, and nebulized adrenaline (epinephrine).

Acute epiglottitis is a medical emergency. Call for the anesthesiologist, ENT surgeon, and, if appropriate, the pediatric team. Never attempt to visualize the epiglottis. Keep calm and reassure the patient. Never leave the patient alone.

Reactive nodules
Reactive nodules are common, small, inflammatory polyps usually measuring less than 10mm in diameter. They are also known as singer's nodules. They present in patients aged 40–50 years and are more common in men. Reactive nodules are caused

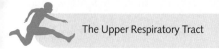

Laryngotracheobronchitis (croup) and acute epiglottitis		
	Croup	Epiglottitis
Etiology	Viral	Bacterial
Organism	Parainfluenza, respiratory syncytial virus	Group B *Haemophilus* influenza
Age range	6 months to 3 years	3–7 years
Onset	Gradual over days	Sudden over hours
Cough	Severe barking	Minimal
Temperature	Pyrexia <38.5°C	Pyrexia >38.5°C
Stridor	Harsh	Soft
Drooling	No	Yes
Voice	Hoarse	Reluctant to speak
Able to drink	Yes	No
Active	Yes	No, completely still
Mortality	Low	High

Fig. 2.12 Features of laryngotracheobronchitis (croup) and acute epiglottitis.

by excessive untrained use of vocal cords. Patients present with hoarseness of the voice.

Pathology
Keratosis develops at the junction of the anterior and middle thirds of the vocal cord on each side. Edematous myxoid connective tissue is covered by squamous epithelium. The reactive nodules may become painful because of ulceration.

> Some of these conditions may seem more relevant to an ENT specialist. However, a working knowledge is also important to the respiratory physician when considering differential diagnoses; for example, laryngeal disease may present as airway obstruction and hoarseness, and chronic sinusitis may present as a persistent cough.

Neoplasms
Squamous papilloma
Squamous papilloma is the most common benign tumor of the larynx; it usually occurs in children aged 0–5 years but can also affect adults.

Etiology
The disease is caused by infection of the epithelial cells with human papillomavirus (HPV) types 6 and 11 and can be acquired at birth from maternal genital warts.

Clinical features
Clinical features include hoarseness of the voice and an abnormal cry (Fig. 2.13).

Pathology
Tumors may be sessile or pedunculated. They can occur anywhere on the vocal cords. Lesions are more common at points of airway constriction (Fig. 2.14).

Tests and treatment
Tests include endoscopy, followed by histologic confirmation.

Surgical treatment is by removal with a carbon dioxide laser. Medical treatment is with alpha interferon.

Squamous cell carcinoma
Squamous cell carcinoma is the most common malignant tumor of the larynx, affecting men and women in the ratio of 5:1. The disease accounts for 1% of all male malignancies. Incidence increases with age, with peak incidence occurring in those aged 60–70 years. Patients present with

Fig. 2.13 Features of squamous papilloma.

Features of squamous papilloma		
	Adult	**Child**
Incidence	Rare	Common
Number of lesions	Single mass	Multiple masses
Outcome	Surgical removal	Regress spontaneously at puberty

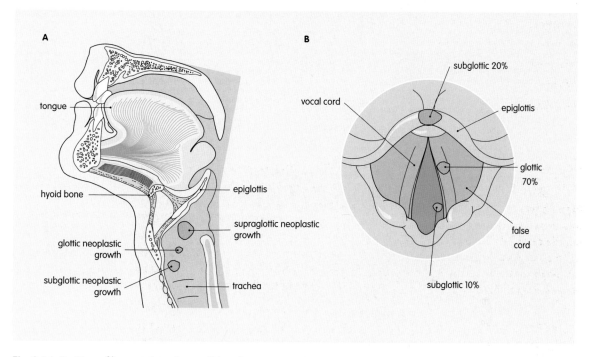

Fig. 2.14 Position of laryngeal carcinoma (A) and as seen on mirror examination (B).

hoarseness, although dyspnea and stridor are late signs.

Predisposing factors include alcohol and tobacco smoke (the condition is very rare in nonsmokers).

Pathology

Carcinoma of vocal cord appears first and subsequently ulcerates. Carcinoma of the larynx infiltrates and destroys surrounding tissue. Infection may follow ulceration.

Diagnostic tests and treatment

Investigations include chest radiography, complete blood count, serum analysis (liver function tests for metastatic disease), direct laryngoscopy under general anesthesia, and full paraendoscopy and bronchoscopy. Treatment is by radiotherapy and surgery.

Prognosis

Prognosis is poor if the tumor involves the upper part of the larynx or subglottic region.

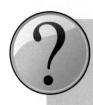

- Describe the anatomy of the upper respiratory tract, giving significant clinical details where appropriate.
- Where does the maxillary sinus open into the nasal cavity? What is the clinical significance of this position?
- Draw respiratory epithelium, indicating the functions of each cell type.
- List the derivatives of the branchial arches and pharyngeal pouches.
- Describe the pathology and management of allergic rhinitis.
- What are the different ways in which sinusitis can present?
- How does sleep apnea affect the patient? Why is it a public health issue?
- How do nasopharyngeal neoplasms commonly present?
- Describe the difference between croup and acute epiglottitis.
- List the causes of hoarseness of the voice.

3. The Lower Respiratory Tract

Organization of the lower respiratory tract

Organization of the lower respiratory tract

Structure of the lower respiratory tract

The lower respiratory tract consists of:

- The lower part of the trachea
- The two main bronchi
- Lobar bronchi, segmental bronchi, and smaller bronchi
- Bronchioles and terminal bronchioles
- The end respiratory unit.

These structures make up the tracheobronchial tree (Fig. 3.1). The structures distal to the two main

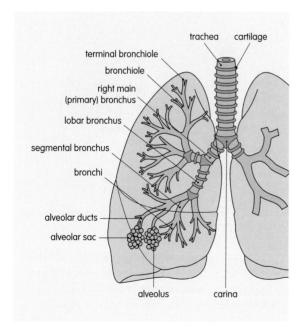

Fig. 3.1 Tracheobronchial tree. Schematic showing the divisions of the airway down to the end respiratory unit (acinus).

bronchi are contained within a tissue known as the lung parenchyma.

Thorax

The cone-shaped thoracic cavity is bounded superiorly by the first rib and inferiorly by the diaphragm. The thorax is narrow at the top (thoracic inlet) and wide at its base (thoracic outlet).

The thoracic wall is supported and protected by the bony thoracic cage consisting of:

- Thoracic vertebrae
- Manubrium
- Sternum
- Twelve pairs of ribs with associated costal cartilages (Fig. 3.2A).

Each rib makes an acute angle with the spine and:

- Articulates with the body and transverse process of its equivalent thoracic vertebra
- Articulates with the body of the vertebra above.

The upper seven ribs (true ribs) articulate anteriorly through their costal cartilages with the sternum. The eighth, ninth, and tenth ribs (false ribs) articulate with the costal cartilages of the next rib above. The eleventh and twelfth ribs (floating ribs) are smaller and their tips are covered with a cap of cartilage.

The space between each rib is known as the intercostal space. Lying obliquely between adjacent ribs are the internal and external intercostal muscles. The intercostal muscles support the thoracic cage; their other functions include:

- External intercostal muscles—raise the rib cage and increase intrathoracic volume
- Internal intercostal muscles—lower the rib cage and reduce intrathoracic volume.

The mechanics of breathing will be covered in detail in Chapter 4. Deep to the intercostal muscles and under cover of the costal groove lies a neurovascular bundle of vein, artery and nerve (see Fig. 3.2B). This anatomy is important during some procedures (e.g.,

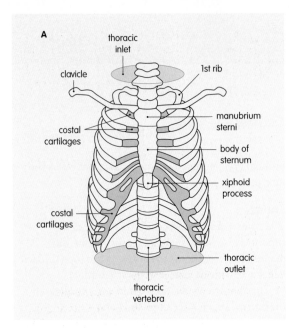

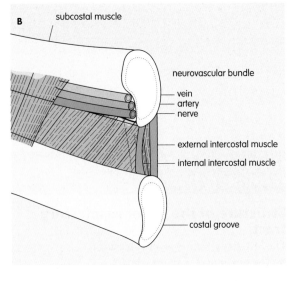

Fig. 3.2 The thoracic cage (A) and details of the subcostal neurovascular bundle (B).

when inserting a chest drain into a pneumothorax, the drain is inserted through the intercostal space just above the rib to avoid hitting the subcostal vessels).

The thorax contains:

- Lungs, heart, and major vessels
- Esophagus, lower part of the trachea, and main bronchi.

Mediastinum

The mediastinum is situated in the midline and lies between the two lungs. It contains the:

- Heart and great vessels
- Trachea and esophagus
- Phrenic and vagus nerves
- Lymph nodes.

Pleurae and pleural cavities

The pleurae consist of a continuous serous membrane, which covers the external surface of the lung and is then reflected to cover the inner surface of the thoracic cavity (Fig. 3.3).

The differences between the visceral and parietal pleurae are:

- The visceral pleura lines the surface of the lungs
- The parietal pleura lines the thoracic wall and the diaphragm.

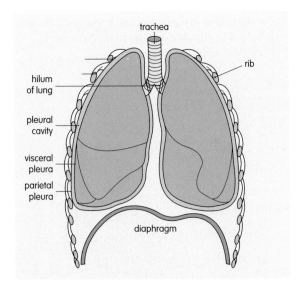

Fig. 3.3 The two pleurae form a potential space called the pleural cavity (shown in dark blue).

The pleurae form a double layer, creating a potential space known as the pleural cavity. The visceral and parietal pleurae are so closely apposed that only a thin film of fluid is contained within the pleural cavity. This allows the pleurae to slip over each other during breathing, thus reducing friction. Normally, no cavity is actually present, although in pathological states this potential space may expand.

Where the pleura is reflected off the diaphragm onto the thoracic wall, a small space is created which is not filled by the lung tissue; this space is known as the costodiaphragmatic recess. At the root of the lung (the hilum), the pleurae become continuous and form a double layer known as the pulmonary ligament.

The parietal pleura has a blood supply from intercostal arteries and branches of the internal thoracic artery. Venous and lymph drainage follow a return course similar to the arterial supply. Nerve supply is from the phrenic nerve; thus, if the pleura becomes inflamed this may cause ipsilateral (on the same side of the body) shoulder-tip pain.

The visceral pleura has a blood supply from bronchial arteries. Venous drainage is through the bronchial veins to the azygous and hemiazygous veins. Lymph vessels drain through the superficial plexus over the surface of the lung to bronchopulmonary nodes at the hilum. The visceral pleura has an autonomic nerve supply and therefore does not give rise to the sensation of pain.

Inflammation of the pleurae can cause an increase in fluid between the parietal and visceral pleurae. This inflammation may give rise to a pleural rub on auscultation, which is said to mimic the sound of a foot crunching through fresh snow. Excess liquid or air may be present within the pleural cavity caused by:

- Pneumothorax
- Hemothorax
- Pleurisy and pneumonia
- Malignancy.

Lungs

The two lungs are situated within the thoracic cavity and lie on either side of the mediastinum. During life, they appear pink and spongy, although carbon deposits give patchy discoloration. The lungs contain:

- Airways: bronchi, bronchioles, respiratory bronchioles, alveolar ducts, alveolar sacs, and alveoli
- Vessels: pulmonary artery and vein and bronchial artery and vein
- Lymphatics and lymph nodes
- Nerves
- Supportive connective tissue (lung parenchyma), which has elastic qualities.

Figures 3.4 and 3.5 show the lateral and medial surfaces of the lung.

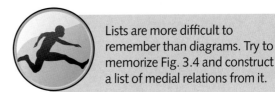

Lists are more difficult to remember than diagrams. Try to memorize Fig. 3.4 and construct a list of medial relations from it.

Hilum of the lung

The hilum or root of the lung (Fig. 3.6) consists of:

- Bronchi
- Vessels: pulmonary artery and vein
- Nerves
- Lymph nodes and lymphatic vessels
- Pulmonary ligament.

Bronchopulmonary segments

The trachea divides to form the left and right primary bronchi, which in turn divide to form lobar bronchi, supplying air to the lobes of each lung. The lobar bronchi divide again to give segmental bronchi, which supply air to regions of lung known as bronchopulmonary segments. The bronchopulmonary segment is both anatomically and functionally distinct. This is important because it means that a segment of diseased lung can be removed surgically (e.g., in tuberculosis).

Surface anatomy

The surface anatomy of the lungs is shown in Fig. 3.7.

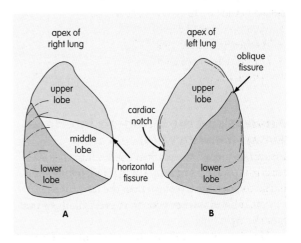

Fig. 3.4 Lateral aspect of the lungs. The outer surfaces show impression of the ribs. (A) Right lung; (B) left lung.

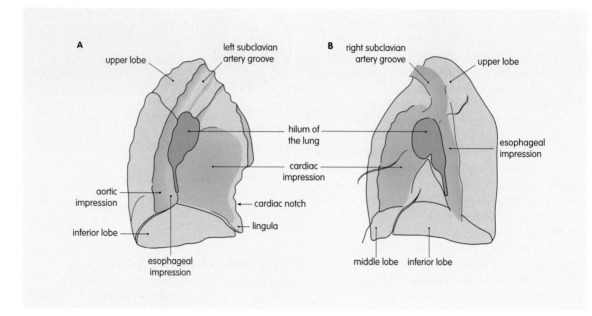

Fig. 3.5 Relations of the lung. (A) Left lung; (B) right lung.

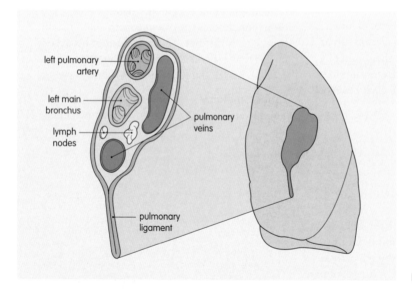

Fig. 3.6 Contents of the hilum.

Airways and the blood–air interface
Airways (respiratory tree)

Inside the thorax, the trachea divides into the left and right primary bronchi. The right main bronchus is shorter and more vertical than the left; for this reason, inhaled foreign bodies are more likely to pass into the right lung.

The primary bronchi within each lung divide into secondary or lobar bronchi. The lobar bronchi divide again into tertiary or segmental bronchi. The airways continue to divide, always splitting into two daughter airways of progressively smaller caliber until eventually forming bronchioles.

Figure 3.1 outlines the structure of the respiratory tree. Each branch of the tracheobronchial tree can be classified by its number of divisions (called the generation number); the trachea is generation number 0. The trachea and bronchi contain cartilage in their walls for support and to prevent collapse of the airway. At about generation 10 or 11, the airways

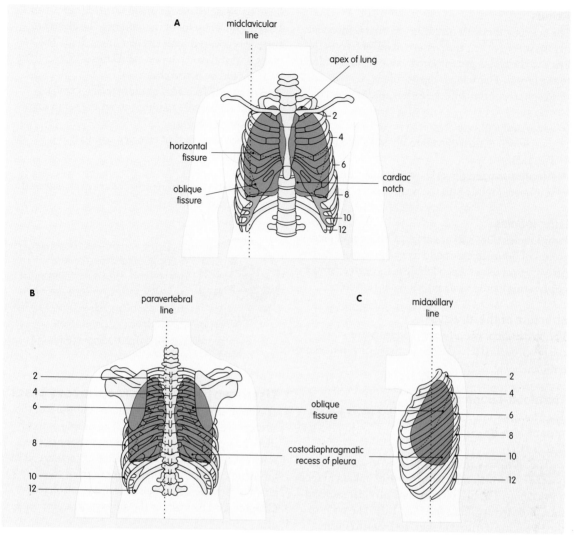

Fig. 3.7 Surface anatomy of the lungs and pleura (shaded area). (A) Anterior aspect; (B) posterior aspect; (C) lateral aspect. Rib numbers are labelled.

contain no cartilage in their walls and are known as bronchioles. Airways distal to the bronchi that contain no cartilage rely on lung parenchymal tissue for their support and are kept open by subatmospheric intrapleural pressure (radial traction).

Bronchioles continue dividing for up to 20 or more generations before reaching the terminal bronchiole. Terminal bronchioles are those bronchioles which supply the end respiratory unit (the acinus).

The tracheobronchial tree can be classified into two zones:

- The conducting zone (airways proximal to the respiratory bronchioles), involved in air movement by bulk flow to the end respiratory units
- The respiratory zone (airways distal to the terminal bronchiole), involved in gaseous exchange.

Because the conducting zone does not take part in gaseous exchange, it can be seen as an area of "wasted" ventilation and is described as anatomic dead space.

Acinus

The acinus is that part of the airway that is involved in gas exchange (i.e., the passage of oxygen from the lungs to the blood and carbon dioxide from the blood to the lungs). The acinus consists of:

- Respiratory bronchioles, leading to the alveolar ducts
- Alveolar ducts, opening into two or three alveolar sacs, which in turn open into several alveoli (see Fig. 1.2)
- Alveoli also open directly into alveolar ducts and a few open directly into the respiratory bronchiole.

Lung lobules

Lung lobules (Fig. 3.8) are areas of lung containing groups of between three and five acini surrounded by parenchymal tissue. Each lobule is separated from a neighboring lobule by an interlobular septum.

Structure of the airways

The structure of the airways changes as the tracheobronchial tree descends; these differences are outlined in Fig. 3.9.

The blood–air interface

The blood–air interface is a term that describes the site at which gas exchange takes place within the lung (Fig. 3.10).

The alveoli are microscopic blind-ending air pouches, of which there are 150–400 million in each normal lung. The alveoli open into alveolar sacs and then into alveolar ducts (see Fig. 1.2). The walls of the alveoli are extremely thin, and the alveoli are lined by a single layer of pneumocytes (types I and II) lying on a basement membrane. The alveolar surface is covered with alveolar lining fluid. The walls of the alveoli contain capillaries.

It should be noted that:

- Average surface area of the alveolar–capillary membrane = $50 - 100 \text{m}^2$ (about the same size as two tennis courts)
- Average thickness of alveolar–capillary membrane = $0.4\mu\text{m}$.

This allows an enormous area for gas exchange and a very short diffusion distance.

A common short-answer question in exams is: "Name the differences in structure between the bronchi and the bronchioles." It is a good idea to memorize the information in Fig. 3.9.

Tissues of the lower respiratory tract

The basic structural components of the walls of the airways are shown in Fig. 3.11. The proportions of these components vary in different regions of the tracheobronchial tree. The absence of cartilage in the bronchioles and distal airways means that these airways must be kept open by radial traction (see Chapter 4). The walls of the airways are composed of:

- Respiratory epithelium (ciliated columnar type)
- Basement membrane
- Lamina propria
- Elastic fibers
- Smooth muscle
- Cartilage.

Trachea

The respiratory epithelium of the trachea is tall and sits on a particularly thick basement membrane separating it from the lamina propria. The lamina propria of the trachea is loose and highly vascular, with a fibromuscular band of elastic tissue. Under the lamina propria lies a loose submucosa containing numerous glands that secrete mucinous and serous fluid. The C-shaped cartilage found within the trachea is hyaline in type and merges with the submucosa.

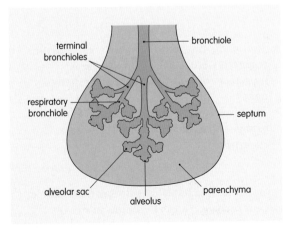

Fig. 3.8 The lung lobule.

Differences in structure of the airways						
Airway	Generation No.	Lining	Wall structure	Diameter	Function	Contractile
trachea	0	respiratory epithelium	membranous tube supported by C-shaped rings of cartilage; loose submucosa and glands	25 mm	Con	No
bronchus	1–11	respiratory epithelium	fibromuscular tubes containing smooth muscle; incomplete rings of cartilage	1–10 mm	Con	Yes
bronchiole	12–16	simple ciliated cuboidal epithelium and Clara cells	membranous and smooth muscle in the wall; no submucosal glands and no cartilage	1.0 mm	Con	Yes
respiratory bronchiole	18+	simple ciliated cuboidal epithelium and Clara cells	merging of cuboidal epithelium with flattened epithelial lining of alveolar ducts; membranous wall	0.5 mm	Con/Gas	Yes
alveolar duct	20–23	flat nonciliated epithelium; no glands	outer lining of spiral smooth muscle; walls of ducts contain many openings laterally into alveolar sacs	0.5 mm	Gas	Yes
alveolus	24	pneumocytes types I and II	types I and II pneumocytes lie on an alveolar basement membrane; capillaries lie on the outer surface of the wall and form the blood-air interface	75–300 μm	Gas	No

Fig. 3.9 Differences in structure of the airways. Function: Con = conduction of air; Gas = gas exchange.

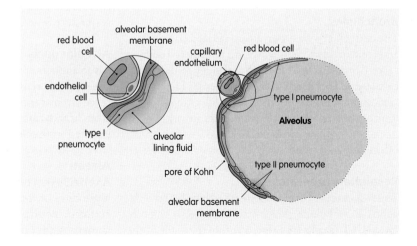

Fig. 3.10 Blood–air interface.

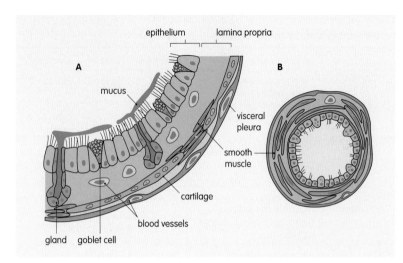

Fig. 3.11 Structure of the airways: (A) bronchial structure; (B) bronchiolar structure. Note there are no submucosal glands or cartilage in the bronchiole. (Redrawn with permission from *Respiratory Physiology*, 2nd ed., by J. G. Widdecombe and A. Davies. London, Edward Arnold, 1991.)

Bronchi

Respiratory epithelium of the bronchi is shorter than the epithelium of the trachea and contains fewer goblet cells. The lamina propria is denser with more elastic fibers and it is separated from the submucosa by a discontinuous layer of smooth muscle. The lamina propria also contains mast cells.

The cartilage of the bronchi forms discontinuous flat plates and there are no C-shaped rings.

Tertiary bronchi

The epithelium in the tertiary bronchi is similar to that in the bronchi. The lamina propria of the tertiary bronchi is thin and elastic, being completely encompassed by smooth muscle. Submucosal glands are sparse and the submucosa merges with surrounding adventitia. Mucosa-associated lymphoid tissue (MALT) is present.

Bronchioles

The epithelium of a bronchiole is ciliated cuboidal and contains clara cells, which are nonciliated and secrete proteinaceous fluid. Bronchioles contain no cartilage and no glands in the submucosa. The smooth muscle layer is prominent. Adjusting the tone of the smooth muscle layer alters airway diameter, enabling resistance to air flow to be effectively controlled.

Respiratory bronchioles

The respiratory bronchioles are lined by ciliated cuboidal epithelium, which is surrounded by smooth muscle. Clara cells are present within the walls of the

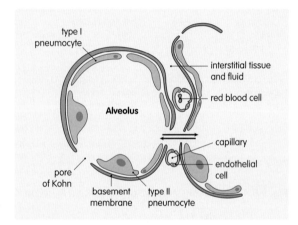

Fig. 3.12 The alveolus. Note communication between alveoli through pores of Kohn.

respiratory bronchioles. Goblet cells are absent, but there are a few alveoli in the walls; thus, the respiratory bronchiole is a site for gaseous exchange.

Alveolar ducts

Alveolar ducts consist of rings of smooth muscle, collagen, and elastic fibers. They open into two or three alveolar sacs, which in turn open into several alveoli. There are alveoli present in the walls and this is a site for gaseous exchange.

Alveoli

An alveolus is a blind-ending terminal sac of respiratory tract (Fig. 3.12). Most gaseous exchange occurs in the alveoli. Because alveoli are so numerous, they provide the majority of lung volume and surface area. The majority of alveoli open into the alveolar sacs. Communication between adjacent alveoli is possible through perforations in the alveolar wall called pores of Kohn. The alveoli are lined with type I and type II pneumocytes, which sit on a basement membrane. Type I pneumocytes are structural, whereas type II pneumocytes produce surfactant (see Chapter 4).

Layers through which gas exchange occurs are:
- Alveolar lining fluid
- Pneumocytes
- Alveolar basement membrane
- Capillary endothelium.

Type I pneumocytes
To aid gaseous diffusion, type I pneumocytes (also known as type I alveolar epithelial cells) are very thin; they contain flattened nuclei and few mitochondria. Type I pneumocytes make up 40% of the alveolar cell population and 90% of the surface lining of the alveolar wall. Cells are joined by tight junctions.

Type II pneumocytes
Type II pneumocytes (type II alveolar epithelial cells) are rounded cells containing rounded nuclei; their cytoplasm is rich in mitochondria and endoplasmic reticulum, and microvilli exist on their exposed surface. Type II pneumocytes make up 60% of the alveolar cell population and 5–10% of the surface lining of the alveolar wall. They produce surfactant.

Alveolar macrophages
Alveolar macrophages are derived from circulating blood monocytes. They lie on an alveolar surface lining or on alveolar septal tissue. The alveolar macrophages phagocytose foreign material and bacteria; they are transported up the respiratory tract by mucociliary clearance. They are discussed further under the lung defenses below.

Mucosa-associated lymphoid tissue (MALT)
The immune system has a major role in the defense of the respiratory tract against pathogens (see below). To aid this key role, lymphoid cells concentrate in the mucosal surfaces of the body to provide immunological protection. This specialized local system of lymphoid tissue is known as mucosa-associated lymphoid tissue (MALT).

MALT is noncapsulated lymphoid tissue located in the walls of the gastrointestinal, respiratory, and urogenital tracts, providing immunologic protection. These tissues are also a main site of lymphocyte activation, and activated lymphocytes will specifically return to respiratory mucosa.

Examples of MALT were mentioned among the tissues of the upper respiratory tract (e.g. the adenoids and the tonsils). MALT in the lung is termed BALT (bronchus-associated lymphoid tissue). BALT is located beneath the mucosa of the bronchi and is covered by M cells, specialized epithelial cells that sample and transport antigen to the lymphoid tissue.

The lymphoid tissue of the respiratory tract is similar to that in the gut; aggregates are a diffuse distribution of mostly B lymphocytes within the lamina propria, covered by similar antigen-targeting and antigen-transporting cells (M cells). The lymphatic vessels associated with MALT are all efferent lymphatics, which drain to regional (hilar) lymph nodes. Large aggregations function in a similar manner to lymph nodes, containing T-cell and B-cell zones.

Development of the lower respiratory tract

Development of the bronchi
The laryngotracheal diverticulum develops into the lung bud, which divides into two bronchial buds by the end of week 4 (Fig. 3.13). As the bronchial bud enlarges, it forms two primary bronchi: the right and left primary bronchi (occurring in week 5). The right main bronchus is slightly larger and more vertical than the left. By the end of week 5, the secondary bronchi start to form.

By week 8, the segmental bronchi develop and together with the splanchnic mesenchyme form the bronchopulmonary segment. The splanchnic mesenchyme forms:
- Visceral pleura (mesoderm)
- Pulmonary capillaries and vasculature
- Bronchial smooth muscle
- Pulmonary connective tissue.

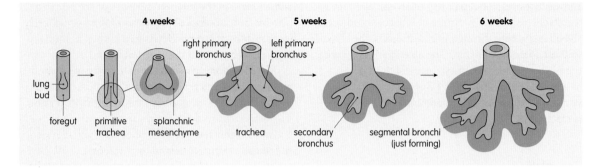

Fig. 3.13 Development of primary bronchi and the formation of the secondary and segmental bronchi.

Development of the lungs

Lung development is divided into four stages: pseudoglandular, canalicular, terminal sac, and alveolar periods.

Stage 1—pseudoglandular period

During the pseudoglandular period, the major parts of the lung are formed; however, because there are no areas for gaseous exchange, respiration is not possible, and babies born at this stage do not survive.

Stage 2—canalicular period

During the canalicular period, there are increases in the diameter of airways, bronchi, and terminal bronchioles. The lung vasculature develops, and primitive end respiratory units are formed: respiratory bronchiole, alveolar duct, and terminal sac (primitive alveolus). Some gaseous exchange is possible, and there is a very small chance of survival if born after week 22 (although intensive care is required).

Stage 3—terminal sac period

During the terminal sac period, numerous terminal sacs develop; there is thinning of the epithelial lining of terminal sacs. The squamous epithelium (type I pneumocytes) develops at about week 24, whereas secretory cells (type II pneumocytes) develop at around weeks 24–28. Type II pneumocytes produce surfactant, reducing surface tension within the liquid film within an alveolus and thus preventing alveolar collapse. After week 32, sufficient surfactant has been produced to allow the neonate to inflate its own lungs and allow the alveoli to continue to develop.

The formation of surfactant is an essential part of lung development. The first breath requires high pressures to inflate the lungs; less force is needed to generate subsequent breaths due to the action of surfactant in reducing surface tension. It is primarily lack of surfactant that causes ventilatory failure in premature babies.

Stage 4—alveolar period

During the alveolar period, clusters of primitive alveoli are formed. Breathing occurs in utero by aspiration of amniotic fluid. The lungs are half full of liquid at birth; fluid is emptied through the mouth and also absorbed into the blood and lymph. The alveoli mature after birth: for the first 3 years after birth, alveoli increase only in number, not size; between the ages of 3 and 8 years, alveoli increase in both size and number.

The pulmonary circulation

Blood vessels

The lungs have a dual blood supply from the pulmonary and bronchial circulations. The bronchial circulation is a small part of the systemic circulation.

Pulmonary circulation
Function
The primary function of the pulmonary circulation is to allow the exchange of oxygen and carbon dioxide between the blood in the pulmonary capillaries and air in the alveoli. Oxygen is taken up into the blood while carbon dioxide is released from the blood into alveolar air.

Anatomy
Mixed venous blood is pumped from the right ventricle through the pulmonary arteries and then through the pulmonary capillary network, which is in contact with the respiratory surface (Fig. 3.14). Gaseous exchange occurs (carbon dioxide given up by the blood, oxygen taken up by the blood) and the oxygenated blood returns through the pulmonary venules and veins to the left atrium. The pulmonary capillary network offers a huge gas exchange area of approximately 50–100 m².

Bronchial circulation
The bronchial circulation is part of the systemic circulation; bronchial arteries are branches of the descending aorta.

Function
The function of the bronchial circulation is to supply oxygen, water, and nutrients to:
- Lung parenchyma
- Airways—smooth muscle, mucosa, and gland
- Pulmonary arteries and veins
- Pleurae.

An additional function of the bronchial circulation is in the conditioning (warming) of inspired air. The airways distal to the terminal bronchiole are supplied only by alveolar wall capillaries. For this reason, a pulmonary embolus may result in infarction of the tissues supplied by the alveolar wall capillaries shown as a wedge-shaped opacity on the lung periphery of a chest x-ray.

Development of the pulmonary circulation
The primitive heart is divided into four chambers during weeks 4 and 5. This involves:
- Formation of endocardial cushions
- Division of the primitive atrium.

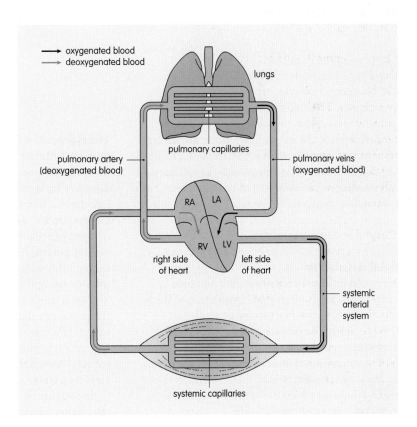

Fig. 3.14 Pulmonary circulation. The pulmonary capillaries lie within the lungs, situated in the alveolar walls. They are in contact with alveolar gas and this is the site where gaseous exchange takes place.

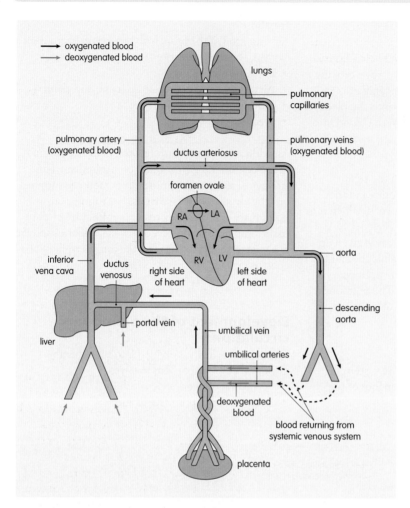

Fig. 3.15 Fetal circulation. A large proportion of blood entering the right atrium passes through the foramen ovale into the left atrium. A large proportion of blood entering the pulmonary artery passes along the ductus arteriosus directly to the aorta.

During week 6, the six primitive aortic arches are transformed into the adult arterial layout. However, the ductus arteriosus is still patent. For further information on development of the heart see *Crash Course: Cardiovascular System.*

Fetal circulation

The main difference between adult and fetal circulation (Fig. 3.15) is that oxygenation of the fetal blood is by the maternal placental circulation. Consequently, the pulmonary circulation is largely bypassed through:

- The foramen ovale—which connects the right atrium to the left atrium
- The ductus arteriosus—which connects the pulmonary artery to the aorta.

Deoxygenated fetal blood flows through the two umbilical arteries (branches of the common iliacs) to the placenta (see Fig. 3.15). Oxygen and nutrients are taken up from the maternal blood by the fetal circulation. Waste products of metabolism and carbon dioxide are passed from fetal blood to the maternal circulation.

Oxygenated blood returns back to the fetal heart through the umbilical vein, ductus venosus, and inferior vena cava. The oxygenated blood from the umbilical vein mixes with deoxygenated blood from the portal circulation and lower limbs and is returned to the right side of the heart. The majority of the fetal blood bypasses the pulmonary circulation, passing through the foramen ovale into the left atrium (see Fig. 3.15).

In fetal life, the pressure in the pulmonary circulation is greater than systemic circulation and less than one-third of the right ventricular output passes through the lungs; the remainder flows from the pulmonary artery through the ductus arteriosus into the aorta.

Changes of circulation after birth

At birth, blood flow through the umbilical vessels stops. When blood flow through the umbilical vein ceases, the ductus venosus, a thick-walled vessel with a muscular sphincter, closes. As the neonate takes its first breath, the lungs fill with air and pulmonary vascular resistance falls to 10% of its value before lung expansion. Left atrial pressure is raised above that in the inferior vena cava by three methods:

- Decreased pulmonary vascular resistance leading to a large increase in blood flow through the lungs to the left atrium
- Decreased blood flow to the right atrium caused by occlusion of the umbilical vein
- Increased resistance to the left ventricular output produced by occlusion of the umbilical arteries.

The reversal of pressure gradient between the atria closes the valve over the foramen ovale. Fusion of the septal leaflets occurs over a period of several days.

The fall in pulmonary arterial pressure reverses the flow through the ducus arteriosus, but within a few moments of birth the ductus arteriosus begins to constrict, producing a turbulent flow heard as a murmur in the newborn child. The constriction is progressive and usually complete within 1–2 days after birth.

The exact mechanism for closure of the ductus arteriosus is not entirely clear, although it is thought to involve bradykinin, prostaglandins (because indometacin can produce closure in premature infants when the ductus remains patent), and adenosine.

The following factors have been suggested as causes of closure of the ductus arteriosus:

- Cutting of the umbilical cord
- Exposure to cold air
- Increase in arterial partial pressure of oxygen
- Pressure difference between pulmonary and systemic circulations.

At birth, the walls of the left and right ventricles are the same thickness. After birth, the thickness of the right ventricular wall diminishes as the right heart pumps against lower resistance, whereas that of the

The following fetal vessels lose their function and become ligaments at birth:

- Ductus arteriosus—becomes the ligamentum arteriosum
- Ductus venosus—becomes the ligamentum venosum
- Umbilical arteries—become the medial umbilical ligaments
- Umbilical veins—become the ligamentum teres.

left ventricle increases as the left heart pumps against higher resistance.

Patent ductus arteriosus

Patent ductus arteriosus (PDA) is a common congenital heart defect, especially in girls. It is associated with maternal rubella (togavirus infection) in early pregnancy. As discussed above, the ductus arteriosus normally closes within 24 hours of birth. If closure fails to occur, blood flows from the aorta through the patent ductus and into the pulmonary artery (a left-to-right shunt). This increases pulmonary artery pressure (hydrodynamic pulmonary hypertension). The defect is classified as either small ductus or large ductus. The murmur heard has a machine-like quality and extends throughout the cardiac cycle. In newborns, patent ductus may be treated with indometacin. The treatment of choice at later stages or when indometacin fails is surgical ligation of the ductus. If the defect is large, the infant may require medical treatment to alleviate heart failure.

Atrial septal defect

Atrial septal defect (ASD) is a defect in the atrial septum around the area of the fossa ovalis, caused by a defect in the ostium secundum. Blood flows from the left atrium to the right atrium and then into the right ventricle (a left-to-right shunt), increasing the pulmonary blood flow, causing hydrodynamic pulmonary hypertension. Symptoms do not usually occur until about 30–40 years of age, when patients present with heart failure; at presentation, a soft heart murmur is usually heard, and a fixed splitting of the second heart sound.

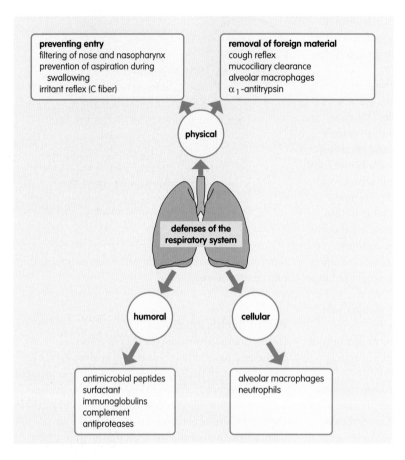

Fig. 3.16 Summary of defenses of the respiratory system.

Defense mechanisms of the lungs

Overview
The lungs have a very large surface area for gas exchange and present a small barrier to diffusion between air and the blood flowing through the lungs. In fact, they possess the largest surface area of the body in contact with the environment and, therefore, are extremely susceptible to damage by foreign material and provide an excellent gateway for infection. The lungs are exposed to many foreign materials:
- Dust particles
- Pollen
- Fungal spores
- Bacteria
- Viruses
- Airborne pollutants.

Therefore, it is necessary for defense mechanisms to prevent infection and reduce the risk of damage by inhalation of foreign material (Fig. 3.16). There are three main mechanisms of defense:
- Physical
- Humoral
- Cellular.

Physical defenses are particularly important in the upper respiratory tract, while at the level of the alveoli other defenses, such as alveolar macrophages, predominate.

Physical defenses
Preventing entry to distal lower respiratory tract
Entry is restricted by the following three mechanisms:
- Filtering at the nasopharynx—hairs within the nose act as a coarse filter for inhaled particles; sticky mucus lying on the surface of the respiratory epithelium traps particles, which are then transported by the wafting of cilia to the

nasopharynx; the particles are then swallowed into the gastrointestinal tract.

- Swallowing—during swallowing, the epiglottis folds back, the laryngeal muscles constrict the opening to the larynx, and the larynx itself is lifted; this prevents aspiration of food particles.
- Irritant C fibers—stimulation of receptors within the bronchi by inhalation of chemicals, particles, or infective material produces a reflex contraction of bronchial smooth muscle; this reduces the diameter of airways and increases mucus secretion, thus limiting the penetration of the offending material.

Airway clearance
Cough reflex
Inhaled material and material brought up the bronchopulmonary tree to the trachea and larynx by mucociliary clearance can trigger a cough reflex (see Chapter 8). This is achieved by a reflex deep inspiration, increasing intrathoracic pressure while the larynx is closed. The larynx is suddenly opened, producing a high-velocity jet of air, which ejects unwanted material at high speed through the mouth.

Mucociliary clearance
Mucociliary clearance deals with a lot of the large particles trapped in the bronchi and bronchioles and debris brought up by alveolar macrophages. Respiratory epithelium is covered by a layer of mucus secreted by goblet cells and submucosal glands. Approximately 10–100ml of mucus is secreted by the lung daily. The mucus film is divided into two layers:

- Periciliary fluid layer about 6µm deep, immediately adjacent to the surface of the epithelium. The mucus here is hydrated by epithelial cells. This reduces its viscosity and allows movement of the cilia.
- Superficial gel layer about 5–10µm deep. This is a relatively viscous layer forming a sticky blanket, which traps particles.

The cilia beat synchronously at 1000–1500 strokes per minute. Coordinated movement causes the superficial gel layer, together with trapped particles, to be continually transported towards the mouth at 1–3cm/min. The mucus and particles reach the trachea and larynx where they are swallowed or expectorated (coughed up and spat out).

Mucociliary clearance is inhibited by:
- Tobacco smoke
- Cold air
- Many drugs (e.g., general anesthetics)
- Sulfur oxides
- Nitrogen oxides.

It is possible to measure the efficiency of the cilia with a simple clinical test. The saccharin screening test establishes the amount of time it takes for saccharin placed in the anterior nares to taste sweet.

The importance of mucociliary clearance is illustrated by cystic fibrosis, in which a defect in chloride channels throughout the body leads to hyperviscous secretions. In the lung, inadequate hydration causes excessive stickiness of the mucus lining the airways, preventing the action of the cilia in effecting mucociliary clearance. Failure to remove bacteria leads to repeated severe respiratory infections, which progressively damage the lungs. Impaired mucociliary clearance is the major cause of morbidity and mortality in cystic fibrosis.

Smaller inhaled particles will travel further down the respiratory tract. The method that is used to deal with inhaled particles depends upon which area of the respiratory tract the particle finally reaches (e.g., large particles may be filtered out by the nasopharynx).

Humoral defenses
Lung secretions contain a wide range of proteins which defend the lungs by various different mechanisms.

Humoral and cellular aspects of the immune system are considered only briefly here; for more information see *Crash Course: Immunology and Microbiology*.

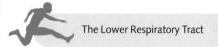

Antimicrobial peptides

A number of proteins in lung fluid have antibacterial properties. These are generally low molecular-weight proteins such as:

- Defensins
- Lysozyme
- Lactoferrin.

Surfactant

The alveoli are bathed in surfactant and this reduces surface tension and prevents the lungs from collapsing. Surfactant also contains proteins which play an important role in defending the host. Surfactant protein A (Sp-A) is the most abundant of these proteins; it has been shown to enhance phagocytosis of microorganisms by alveolar macrophages.

Immunoglobulins

Effector B lymphocytes (plasma cells) in the submucosa produce immunoglobulins. All classes of antibody are produced, but IgA production predominates. The immunoglobulins are contained within the mucous secretions in the respiratory tract and are directed against specific antigens.

Complement

Complement proteins are found in lung secretions in particularly high concentrations during inflammation and they play an important role in propagating the inflammatory response. Complement components can be secreted by alveolar macrophages (see below) and act as attractants for the migration of cells such as neutrophils to the site of injury.

Antiproteases

Lung secretions contain a number of enzymes (antiproteases) that break down the destructive proteases released from dead bacteria, macrophages, and neutrophils. One of the most important of these antiproteases is α_1-antitrypsin.

Cigarette smoke increases the number of pulmonary macrophages; these release a chemical that attracts leukocytes to the lung. The leukocytes in turn release proteases, including elastase, that attack elastic tissue in the lungs. This process is usually inhibited by α_1-antitrypsin, but this itself is inhibited by oxygen radicals released by leukocytes. The result is a protease–antiprotease imbalance that

leads to the destruction of lung tissue and the development of emphysema.

A deficiency in α_1-antitrypsin (inherited as an autosomal dominant condition) leads to a reduction in the breakdown of proteolytic enzymes, such as elastase, released from neutrophils during acute inflammation. This results in increased destruction of the alveolar wall and lung parenchymal tissue. Thus, any insult to the lungs (e.g., smoking) will lead to increased destruction of tissue and emphysema. It should be noted, however, that only 2% of individuals who have emphysema have α_1-antitrypsin deficiency; the vast majority of cases of emphysema are related to smoking alone.

Inherited defects in any of these humoral mechanisms can lead to lung disease. Patients with deficiencies in IgA or complement (C3) are prone to recurrent respiratory tract infections.

Cellular defenses

Alveolar macrophages

Alveolar macrophages are differentiated monocytes, and are both phagocytic and mobile. They normally reside in the lining of the alveoli where they ingest bacteria and debris, before transporting it to the bronchioles where it can be removed from the lungs by mucociliary clearance. Alveolar macrophages can also initiate and amplify the inflammatory response by secreting proteins that recruit other cells. These proteins include:

- Complement components
- Cytokines (e.g., IL-1, IL-6) and chemokines
- Growth factors.

Neutrophils

Neutrophils are the predominant cell recruited in the acute inflammatory response. Neutrophils emigrate from the intravascular space to the alveolar lumen where intracellular killing of bacteria takes place by two mechanisms:

- Oxidative—via reactive oxygen species
- Nonoxidative—via proteases.

In some cases, defense mechanisms can cause injury to lung tissue. Uncontrolled degranulation of neutrophils releases large amounts of elastase, damaging the lung parenchyma in diseases such as emphysema.

Metabolic functions of the lungs

Overview

The lungs, in addition to their role as gas exchange organs, have some important metabolic functions, notably:

- Conversion of angiotensin I to angiotensin II
- Deactivation of vasoactive substances
- Breakdown of arachidonic acid products
- Phospholipid synthesis
- Protein synthesis.

Angiotensin-converting enzyme

Renin released from the juxtaglomerular cells of the kidney enters the blood stream where it acts on a plasma protein, angiotensinogen, to produce angiotensin I (Fig. 3.17). Angiotensin I is further converted by angiotensin-converting enzyme (ACE) to angiotensin II, which stimulates aldosterone secretion and acts as a potent vasoconstrictor. ACE is produced by the vascular endothelial cells of the lungs.

Deactivation of vasoactive substances

Many different vasoactive substances are deactivated as they pass through the lungs. An example of this is the degradation of bradykinin (a potent vasodilator) to inactive peptides by ACE (Fig. 3.18).

The administration of an ACE inhibitor (such as captopril) inhibits both the production of angiotensin II and the breakdown of bradykinin.

Arachidonic acid product breakdown

The lungs are capable of both production and breakdown of arachidonic acid metabolites. The following metabolites are removed by the lung:

- Prostaglandin E_2
- Prostaglandin $F_{2\alpha}$
- Leukotrienes.

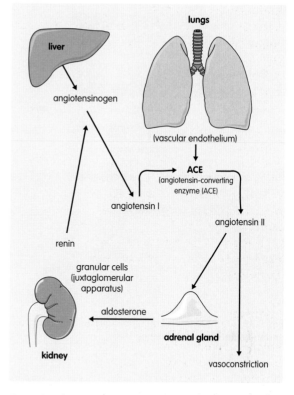

Fig. 3.17 The renin–angiotensin system. Conversion of angiotensin I to angiotensin II by angiotensin-converting enzyme (ACE) occurs mainly in the pulmonary vascular endothelium.

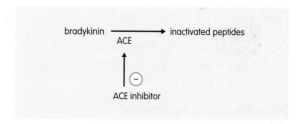

Fig. 3.18 Bradykinin degradation.

Arachidonic acid metabolism

Arachidonic acid is released from membrane phospholipids by the action of phospholipase A_2 (Fig. 3.19). Arachidonic acid is converted into endoperoxide intermediates by the action of cyclo-oxygenase (endoperoxides are subsequently converted into prostaglandins, prostacyclin, or thromboxane by additional enzymes) or into leukotrienes by the action of lipoxygenase. Cyclo-oxygenase is also known as COX. COX-1 is a

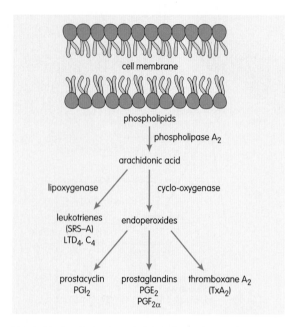

Fig. 3.19 Arachidonic acid metabolism. The production of endoperoxides and leukotrienes.

membrane. Synthesis occurs at the interface between cytosol and the endoplasmic reticular membrane. The synthesized phospholipids are transported to vesicles by "membrane budding" (endoplasmic reticular membrane fuses with the vesicle).

The surfactant mixture is extruded into the alveolus and lowers the surface tension. The synthesis is rapid and allows quick turnover of surfactant.

Protein synthesis

Structural proteins, collagen, and elastin form the parenchyma of the lung; their synthesis and breakdown are important to the normal functioning of the lung. An increase in their breakdown is associated with increased protease activity (as seen in α_1-antitrypsin deficiency) and leads to emphysema.

constitutive enzyme, while COX-2 is involved in inflammatory states.

Leukotrienes (LTB_4, LTC_4, LTD_4) are implicated as a cause of bronchoconstriction in asthma (see Chapters 6 and 7). Thromboxane A_2 increases platelet aggregation and vasoconstriction, whereas prostacyclin has opposite effects. The prostaglandins produced have vasodilatory and vasoconstrictory effects.

Phospholipid synthesis

Type II pneumocytes produce surfactant which contains an important phospholipid (dipalmitoyl phosphatidylcholine, DPC). As noted above, surfactant has the property of reducing surface tension in proportion to its surface concentration and plays an important role in defense.

Phospholipids are produced from fatty acids in association with smooth endoplasmic reticular

The effect of smoking on the lower respiratory tract

Smoking is associated with increased morbidity and mortality in many different diseases (e.g., ischemic heart disease, peripheral vascular disease, and carcinoma of the esophagus and bladder). Focusing on the respiratory system, smoking increases the number of deaths from laryngeal cancer and is strongly associated with the following lower respiratory tract diseases:

- Lung cancer
- Chronic obstructive pulmonary disease (COPD)
- Cor pulmonale.

The main mechanisms by which smoking causes harm include:

- The direct effect of toxic compounds in tobacco smoke (e.g., hydrocarbons and nitrosamines)
- The release of proteolytic enzymes from neutrophils and macrophages (see above)
- Reduction in endogenous nitric oxide production
- Increased permeability of blood vessel walls.

Smoking cessation is discussed in Chapter 6.

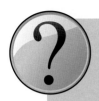

- Describe the anatomy and function of the pleurae.
- List the medial relations of the lungs and the contents of the hilum.
- Describe the structure of the tracheobronchial tree and define the differences between conducting and respiratory zones.
- Give an account of the blood–air interface.
- List the differences between bronchi and bronchioles.
- Describe the ultrastructure of the airways.
- Describe the differences in function between the pulmonary and bronchial circulations.
- Outline the fetal circulation.
- How does the circulation change at birth?
- Explain why the lungs are susceptible to damage.
- Describe the mechanisms available to the lung to prevent entry of particulate matter.
- Describe the key functions of the alveolar macrophage.
- List the metabolic functions of the lung.
- Describe with the use of a diagram the conversion of angiotensinogen to angiotensin II.
- Outline with the aid of a diagram arachidonic acid metabolism.

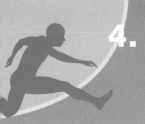

4. Ventilation and Gas Exchange

Overview

Ventilation is the flow of air in and out of the respiratory system (breathing); it is defined physiologically as the amount of air breathed in and out in a given time. The function of ventilation is to maintain blood gases at their optimum level, by delivering air to the alveoli where gas exchange can take place. The movement of air in and out of the lungs occurs due to pressure differences brought about by changes in lung volume. The respiratory muscles bring about these changes, but other factors are also involved, namely the physical properties of the lungs, including their elasticity and the resistance of the airways. Lung diseases that affect these physical properties therefore impair gas exchange by reducing the delivery of fresh gas to the lungs, ultimately leading to a mismatch in ventilation: perfusion.

Ventilation

Anatomic dead space

Not all of the air entering the respiratory system actually reaches the alveoli and takes part in gas exchange. Chapter 3 introduced the concept of anatomic dead space, or those areas of the airway not involved in gaseous exchange (i.e., the conducting zone). Included in this space are:

- Nose and mouth
- Pharynx
- Larynx
- Trachea
- Bronchi and bronchioles, down to and including the terminal bronchioles.

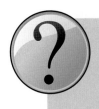 Respiratory physiology involves a number of equations, and you may find this aspect difficult. Memorizing these equations is less important than understanding the underlying concepts and being able to relate them to clinical practice. For this reason, in most cases we have separated the equations from the main body of the text; if you want more detail or need to memorize them for your exams, you will find the equations and brief explanations in the figures.

Inspired air held within these areas is referred to as dead air. The volume of the anatomic dead space (V_D) is usually about 150ml (or 2ml/kg of bodyweight). Anatomic dead space varies with the size of the subject and also increases with increased inspiration because greater expansion of the lungs lengthens and widens the conducting airways. Anatomic dead space can be measured using Fowler's method which is based on the single-breath nitrogen test. This test is described in Chapter 10.

Physiologic dead space

Anatomic dead space is not the only cause of "wasted" ventilation, even in the healthy lung. The total dead space is known as physiologic dead space and includes gas in the alveoli that does not participate in gas exchange.

Physiologic dead space
    = anatomic dead space + alveolar dead space

Fig. 4.1 The Bohr equation.

The Bohr equation is used in measuring physiological dead space

$V_D/V_T = (P_ACO_2 - P_ECO_2)/P_ACO_2$
V_D = Volume of dead space
V_T = Tidal volume
P_ACO_2 = Partial pressure of carbon dioxide in alveolar air
P_ECO_2 = Partial pressure of carbon dioxide in mixed expired air

Normally, the partial pressures of carbon dioxide in alveolar gas and arterial blood are the same.

The equation can therefore be shown as:
$V_D/V_T = (P_aCO_2 - P_ECO_2)/P_aCO_2$

Alveolar dead space comes about because gas exchange is less than optimal in some parts of the lung. If each acinus (or end respiratory unit) were perfect, the amount of air received by each alveolus would be matched by the flow of blood through the pulmonary capillaries. In reality:

- Some areas receive less ventilation than others
- Some areas receive less blood flow than others.

In a normal, healthy person, anatomic and physiologic dead space are almost equal, alveolar dead space being very small (<5 ml). However, when lung disease alters ventilation:perfusion relationships, the volume of alveolar dead space increases.

Measurement of physiologic dead space

Physiologic dead space is measured using the Bohr equation (Fig. 4.1).

The method requires a sample of arterial blood and involves the analysis of carbon dioxide in expired air. Knowing that carbon dioxide is not blown off from end respiratory units that are not perfused, and that carbon dioxide in air is almost zero, it is possible to carry out a component balance for carbon dioxide to establish the volume of physiologic dead space.

A component balance works on the basis of conservation of mass (i.e., what goes into a system must equal what comes out). Several tests in respiratory medicine (e.g., helium dilution, nitrogen washout) are based on this principle.

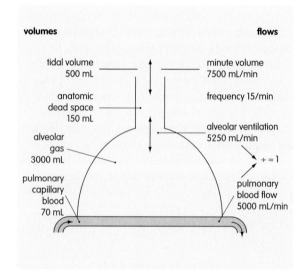

Fig. 4.2 Ventilation in the simplified lung. (From *Pulmonary Pathophysiology* by G. Criner and G. D'Alonzo. Madison, CT, Fence Creek Publishing, 1999, p. 38.)

Minute ventilation

Minute ventilation ($\dot{V}_E$) is the volume of gas moved in and out of the lungs in 1 minute (Fig. 4.2).

In order to calculate $\dot{V}_E$ you need to know:
- The number of breaths per minute
- The volume of air moved in and out with each breath (the tidal volume: V_T).

The normal frequency of breathing varies between 12 and 20 breaths per minute. Normal tidal volume is approximately 500 ml in quiet breathing. If a subject with a tidal volume of 500 ml took 12 breaths a minute, it would seem obvious that the volume exhaled per minute (minute ventilation) would be $500 \times 12 = 6000$ ml/min. Or, more generally:

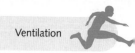

$$\dot{V}_E = V_T f$$

where V_E = minute ventilation, V_T = tidal volume, and f = the respiratory rate (breaths/minute).

Alveolar ventilation

We have already noted that not all the air inspired reaches the alveoli; some stays within the trachea or other conducting airways.

Therefore, two values of minute ventilation need to be considered:

- Minute ventilation ($\dot{V}_E$), as described above.
- Minute alveolar ventilation ($\dot{V}_A$), which is the amount of air that reaches the alveoli in 1 minute.

From our understanding of anatomic dead space, we can say that for one breath:

$$V_A = V_T - V_D$$

where V_A = the volume reaching the alveolus in one breath and V_D = the volume of dead space. Hence, in 1 minute:

$$\dot{V}_A = (V_T - V_D)f$$

Variation in ventilation within the lung

Not all regions of the lungs are ventilated equally. Ventilation per unit volume can be measured by inhalation of a radioactive isotope of xenon (^{133}Xe). If radiation counters are placed at different levels of the lungs, the volume of inhaled radioactive xenon in various areas of the lung can be measured.

It has been shown that the lower zones of the lungs are ventilated better than the upper zones. The causes of regional differences in ventilation will be discussed in the next section.

 Note that at this stage we are still considering the healthy lung. In clinical practice, disease has a much greater effect on variation of ventilation.

Lung volumes

The gas held by the lungs can be thought of in terms of subdivisions, or specific lung volumes. Some of these volumes can be measured using spirometry, a

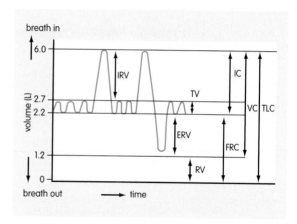

Fig. 4.3 Typical spirometer trace. Note that functional residual capacity (FRC) and residual volume (RV) cannot be measured using a spirometer; thus, neither can total lung capacity (TLC). ERV = expiratory reserve volume; IRV = inspiratory reserve volume; TV = tidal volume; IC = inspiratory capacity; VC = vital capacity.

technique which is described in Chapter 10. A trace from a spirometer, showing key lung volumes, is reproduced in Fig. 4.3. Note that one of the subdivisions shown here, tidal volume, has already been introduced above under the concept of minute ventilation. Definitions of all the lung volumes and capacities (combinations of two or more volumes) are given in Fig. 4.4.

Measuring lung volumes

There are four main methods of measuring lung volumes:

- Spirometry
- Nitrogen washout
- Helium dilution
- Plethysmography.

These techniques are considered in detail in Chapter 10.

Effect of disease on lung volumes

Understanding lung volumes is important because they can be affected by disease. Two particular volumes are important in common diseases such as asthma and COPD and are considered in more detail below. These are residual volume (RV) and functional residual capacity (FRC).

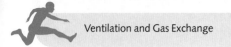

Descriptions of lung volumes and capacities	
Air in lungs is divided into 4 volumes	
tidal volume (TV)	volume of air breathed in and out in a single breath: 0.5 L
inspiratory reserve volume (IRV)	volume of air breathed in by a maximum inspiration at the end of a normal inspiration: 3.3 L
expiratory reserve volume (ERV)	volume of air that can be expelled by a maximum effort at the end of a normal expiration: 1.0L
residual volume (RV)	volume of air remaining in lungs at end of a maximum expiration: 1.2L
Pulmonary capacities are combinations of 2 or more volumes	
inspiratory capacity (IC) = TV + IRV	volume of air breathed in by a maximum inspiration at the end of a normal expiration: 3.8 L
functional residual capacity (FRC) = ERV + RV	volume of air remaining in lungs at the end of a normal expiration. Acts as buffer against extreme changes in alveolar gas levels with each breath: 2.2 L
vital capacity (VC) = IRV + TV + ERV	volume of air that can be breathed in by a maximum inspiration following a maximum expiration: 4.8 L
total lung capacity (TLC) = VC + RV	only a fraction of TLC is used in normal breathing: 6.0 L
Most of these volumes can be measured with a spirometer (see Fig. 4.3)	

Fig. 4.4 Descriptions of lung volumes and capacities.

Residual volume and functional residual capacity

After breathing out, the lungs are not completely emptied of air. A completely deflated lung would require a much greater amount of energy to inflate it than one in which the alveoli have not collapsed (see Fig. 4.17). Even a maximum respiratory effort (forced expiration) fails to expel all the air from the lungs. When the expiratory muscles contract, all the structures in the lungs (not only the alveoli but also the airways) are compressed by the positive intrapleural pressure. During forced expiration, the smaller airways collapse before the alveoli empty completely. Thus, some air remains within the lungs; this is known as the residual volume (see Fig. 4.3).

During normal breathing (quiet breathing), the lung volume oscillates between inhalation and exhalation. In quiet breathing, after the tidal volume has been expired:

- Pressure outside the chest is equal to pressure inside the alveoli (i.e. atmospheric pressure)
- Elastic forces tending to collapse the lung are balanced by the elastic recoil trying to expand the chest (Fig. 4.5)
- This creates a subatmospheric (negative) pressure in the intrapleural space.

The lung volume at this point is known as functional residual capacity. RV and FRC can be measured using nitrogen washout, helium dilution and plethysmography (see Chapter 10).

Patterns of lung function

Disease affects lung volumes in specific patterns, depending on the pathological processes. Diseases can be classified as obstructive, restrictive, or mixed, with each showing characteristic changes in lung volumes. Figures 4.6 and 4.7 summarize the common patterns seen.

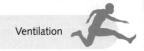

Fig. 4.5 Pressures within the thoracic cavity. The tendency for the lungs to collapse (elastic recoil) and for opposing forces to expand the chest wall creates a subatmospheric (negative) pressure in the intrapleural space at functional residual capacity.

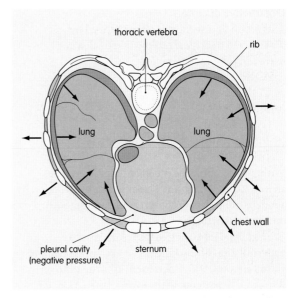

Fig. 4.6 Lung volumes in health, and in obstructive and restrictive disease. See Fig. 4.4 for abbreviations. Note that in obstructive diseases TLC and FRC are increased. VC may be entirely normal or reduced. In restrictive diseases all lung volumes are reduced. (From *Pulmonary Pathophysiology* by G. Criner and G. D'Alonzo. Madison, CT, Fence Creek Publishing, 1999, p. 128.)

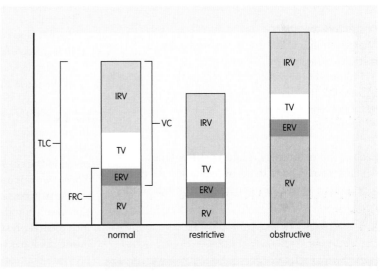

Patterns of lung function			
	Obstructive	Restrictive	Mixed
FEV$_1$	↓	↓	↓
FVC	N or ↓	↓	↓
FEV$_1$/FVC ratio	↓	N	↓
TLC	N or ↑	↓	↓
VC	N or ↓	↓	↓
RV	↑	N or ↓	N or ↑
RV/TLC ratio	↑	N or ↑	↑

Fig. 4.7 Patterns of lung function.

Obstructive disorders

This group of disorders is characterized by obstruction of normal airflow due to airway narrowing and includes:

- Asthma
- COPD
- Bronchiectasis
- Cystic fibrosis
- Tumors (inside or outside the airways).

Within this group, the mechanisms causing the airway narrowing differ. They include obstruction by a mucus plug, airway compression, and smooth muscle constriction.

In general, obstructive disorders lead to hyperinflation of the lungs as air is trapped behind closed airways. RV is increased, as is the ratio of RV:TLC. In patients with severe obstruction, air trapping is so extensive that vital capacity is decreased.

Restrictive disorders

A large number of disorders can be classifed as restrictive, including:

- Pulmonary fibrosis
- Sarcoidosis
- Silicosis
- Asbestosis.

Each of these disorders results in stiffer lungs which cannot expand to normal volumes. All the subdivisions of volume are decreased and the ratio of RV:TLC will be normal, or where VC decreases more quickly than RV, increased.

Mechanics of breathing

In order to understand ventilation we must also understand the mechanism by which it takes place: breathing. This section reviews the mechanics of breathing, including:

- The pressure differences which generate airflow
- The respiratory muscles that effect these pressure differences
- Tissue properties that influence how easily the lungs expand.

Flow of air into the lungs

To achieve air flow into the lungs, we require a driving pressure (remember air flows from high pressure to low pressure). Pressure at the entrance to the respiratory tract (i.e., at the nose and mouth) is atmospheric (P_{atm}). Pressure inside the lungs is alveolar pressure (P_A).

Therefore:

- If $P_A = P_{atm}$, no air flow occurs (e.g., at functional residual capacity)
- If $P_A < P_{atm}$, air flows into the lungs
- If $P_A > P_{atm}$, air flows out of the lungs.

Because we cannot change atmospheric pressure, alveolar pressure must be altered to achieve air flow. Thus, if the volume inside the lungs is changed, Boyle's law predicts that pressure inside the lungs will also change. How can this be achieved (Fig. 4.8)?

- The lungs contain no muscle that can actively expand or contract.
- Therefore, the chest must be expanded, which lowers intrapleural pressure, expanding the lungs.
- The majority of chest expansion in quiet breathing is caused by contraction of the diaphragm.
- Relaxation of the muscles of the chest wall allows the elastic recoil of the lungs to cause contraction of the lungs and expulsion of gas.

Intrapleural pressure

In the previous section, we saw that at FRC elastic recoil of the lungs is exactly balanced by the elastic recoil of the chest wall trying to expand the chest. These two opposing forces create a subatmospheric (negative) pressure within the intrapleural space; as the alveoli communicate with the atmosphere, the intrapleural pressure is also less than the pressure inside the lungs at FRC (Fig. 4.9). The intrapleural pressure fluctuates during breathing (Fig. 4.10) but is about $-5\,cmH_2O$ at the end of quiet expiration. In summary, there is a gradient between the pressure on the inside and the outside of the lungs, or across the lung walls; this is known as the transmural pressure. It is transmural pressure (caused by the negative pressure in the pleural space) that ensures that the lungs are held partially expanded in the thorax. It effectively links the lungs (which are like suspended balloons) with the chest wall.

On inspiration, intrathoracic volume is increased; this lowers intrapleural pressure making it more negative, causing the lungs to expand and air to enter. On expiration, the muscles of the chest wall relax and the lungs return to their original size by elastic recoil, with the expulsion of air.

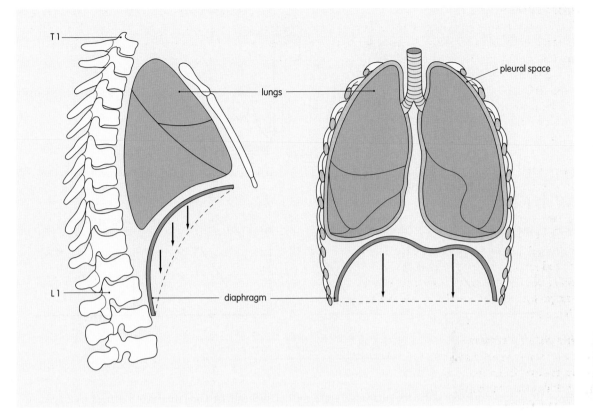

Fig. 4.8 Expanding the lungs to draw in air. Flattening the diaphragm increases the thoracic volume, lowering the intrapleural pressure and expanding the lungs.

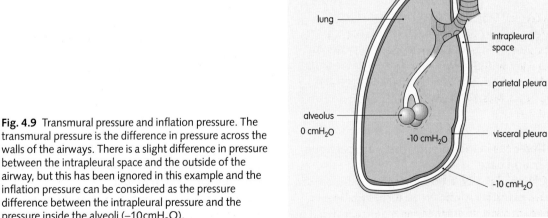

Fig. 4.9 Transmural pressure and inflation pressure. The transmural pressure is the difference in pressure across the walls of the airways. There is a slight difference in pressure between the intrapleural space and the outside of the airway, but this has been ignored in this example and the inflation pressure can be considered as the pressure difference between the intrapleural pressure and the pressure inside the alveoli (-10cmH$_2$O).

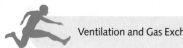

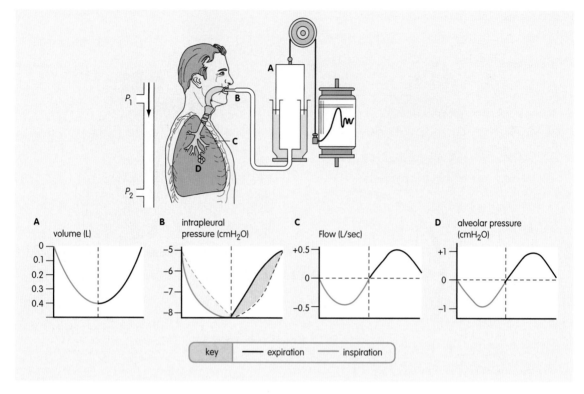

Fig. 4.10 Negative pressure within the intrapleural space and during breathing. Lung volume (A), change in intrapleural pressure (B), air flow (C), and alveolar pressure (D). All measurements are relative to inspiration and expiration. Note that intrapleural pressure becomes more negative during inspiration as intrathoracic volume increases.

It should be noted that during quiet breathing, intrapleural pressure is always negative. In forced expiration, however, the intrapleural pressure becomes positive, forcing a reduction in lung volume with the expulsion of air.

> Puncture wounds through the thorax can mean that the intrapleural space is open to the atmosphere—a pneumothorax. The pressures equilibrate and the lungs are no longer held expanded, leading to collapse.

Differences in intrapleural pressure between apex and base

The lungs are not rigid and therefore not self-supportive. As we pass vertically down the lung, each layer of lung hangs down from the layer of lung above and sits on the layer of lung below. Thus, at the apex, there is a larger weight of lung pulling away from the chest wall causing the intrapleural pressure to be more negative at the apex than at the base. For an upright subject at functional residual capacity (before inspiration) the intrapleural pressure at the apex is $-8\,cmH_2O$ and at the base about $-2\,cmH_2O$. The lung base is compressed compared with the apex.

It should be noted that:

- Alveolar volumes at the base and the apex of the lung are of different values before inspiration.
- However, intrapleural pressure changes at lung base and apex during breathing are of equal magnitude.

These two factors will be important later when we look at why ventilation varies from lung base to apex.

Muscles of respiration

We have seen that the chest must be expanded in order to reduce intrapleural pressure and drive air into the lungs. This section describes the muscles of respiration that bring about this change in volume.

Thoracic wall

The thoracic wall is made up of (from superficial to deep):
- Skin and subcutaneous tissue
- Ribs, thoracic vertebrae, sternum, and manubrium
- Intercostal muscles: external, internal, and thoracis transverses
- Parietal pleura.

Situated at the thoracic outlet is the diaphragm, which attaches to the costal margin, xyphoid process and lumbar vertebrae.

Intercostal muscles

The action of the intercostal muscles is to pull the ribs closer together. There are, therefore, two main actions:
- If the first rib is fixed by scalene muscle, the external intercostal muscles pull the ribs upward.
- If the last rib is fixed by quadratus lumborum, the internal intercostal muscles pull the ribs downward.

Their action during respiration is discussed in function of the respiratory muscles.

External intercostal muscles

External intercostal muscles span the space between each rib and originate from the inferior border of the upper rib, attaching to the superior border of the rib below. The muscle attaches along the length of the rib, from the tubercle to the costal chondral junction and its fibers run forward and downward (Fig. 4.11A).

Internal intercostal muscles

Internal intercostal muscles span the space between each rib and originate from the subcostal groove of the rib above and attach to the superior border of the rib below. The muscle attaches along the length of the rib from the angle of the rib to the sternum and its fibers run downward and backward (Fig. 4.11B).

Thoracis transverses

Thoracis transversus muscle is incomplete and has the parietal pleura and neurovascular bundle as its relations.

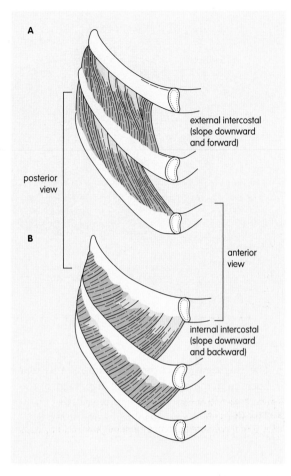

Fig. 4.11 Intercostal muscles. (A) External intercostal muscles; (B) internal intercostal muscles.

Diaphragm

The diaphragm is the main muscle of respiration (Fig. 4.12). The central region of the diaphragm is tendinous; the outer margin is muscular, originating from the borders of the thoracic outlet.

The diaphragm has right and left domes. The right dome is higher than the left to accommodate the liver below. There is a central tendon that sits below the two domes, attaching to the xiphisternum anteriorly and the lumbar vertebrae posteriorly.

Several important structures pass through the diaphragm:
- The inferior vena cava passes through the right dome at the level of the eighth thoracic vertebra (T8)

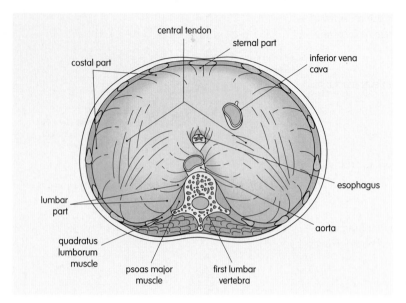

central tendon
sternal part
costal part
inferior vena cava
lumbar part
esophagus
quadratus lumborum muscle
aorta
psoas major muscle
first lumbar vertebra

Fig. 4.12 The diaphragm. Many structures pass through the diaphragm, notably the inferior vena cava, the aorta and the esophagus.

- The esophagus passes through a sling of muscular fibers from the right crus of the diaphragm at the level of the tenth thoracic vertebra (T10)
- The aorta pierces the diaphragm anterior to the twelfth thoracic vertebra (T12).

The diaphragm attaches to the costal margin anteriorly and laterally. Posteriorly, it attaches to the lumbar vertebrae by the crura (left crus at L1 and L2, right crus at L1, L2, and L3). In addition, the position of the diaphragm changes relative to posture: it is lower when standing than sitting.

The motor and sensory nerve supply of the diaphragm is from the phrenic nerve. Blood supply of the diaphragm is from pericardiophrenic and musculophrenic branches of the internal thoracic artery.

The phrenic nerve supplies the diaphragm (60% motor, 40% sensory). Remember, "nerve roots 3, 4, and 5 keep the diaphragm alive." Thus, if you break your neck at C3, you die.

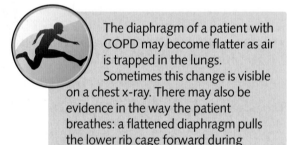

The diaphragm of a patient with COPD may become flatter as air is trapped in the lungs. Sometimes this change is visible on a chest x-ray. There may also be evidence in the way the patient breathes: a flattened diaphragm pulls the lower rib cage forward during inspiration (Hoover's sign).

Function of the muscles of respiration

Breathing can be classified into inspiration and expiration, quiet or forced.

Quiet inspiration

In quiet inspiration, contraction of the diaphragm flattens its domes. This action increases the length of the thorax and thus its volume. This lowers intrapleural pressure and draws air into the lungs. At the same time, the abdominal wall must relax to allow the abdominal contents to be displaced as the diaphragm moves down.

The main muscle in quiet breathing is the diaphragm, but the intercostal muscles are involved. With the first rib fixed, the intercostal muscles can expand the rib cage by two movements:

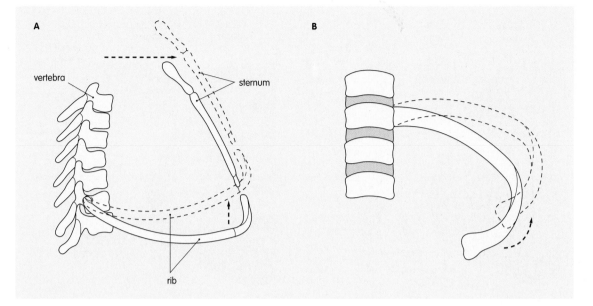

Fig. 4.13 Posterior (A) and lateral (B) expansion of the chest. (A) Note the expansion of the chest in a forward and upward movement (pump-handle action) and (B) an outward and upward movement (bucket-handle action).

- Forward movement of the lower end of the sternum—pump-handle action (Fig. 4.13A)
- Upward and outward—bucket-handle action (Fig. 4.13B).

During quiet inspiration, these actions are small and the intercostal muscles mainly prevent deformation of the tissue between the ribs, which would otherwise lower the volume of the thoracic cage (Fig. 4.14). The internal intercostal muscles carry out this role.

Quiet expiration

Quiet expiration is passive and there is no direct muscle action. During inspiration, the lungs are expanded against their elastic recoil. This recoil is sufficient to drive air out of the lungs in expiration. Thus, quiet expiration involves the controlled relaxation of the intercostal muscles and the diaphragm.

Forced inspiration

In addition to the action of the diaphragm:

- Scalene muscles and sternocleidomastoids raise the ribs anteroposteriorly, producing movement at the manubriosternal joint.
- Intercostal muscles are much more active and raise the ribs to a much greater extent than in quiet inspiration.
- The twelfth rib, which is attached to quadratus lumborum, allows forcible downward movement of the diaphragm.
- Arching the back using erector spinae also increases thoracic volume.

During respiratory distress, the scapulae are fixed by trapezius muscles, rhomboid muscles, and levator scapulae; pectoralis minor and serratus anterior raise the ribs; the arms can be fixed (e.g., by holding the back of a chair), allowing the use of pectoralis major.

The change in intrathoracic volume is mainly caused by the movement of the diaphragm downward. Contraction of the diaphragm comprises 75% of the energy expenditure during quiet breathing.

Use of the accessory muscles of inspiration and fixing of the torso are signs that you should look for when assessing a patient with dyspnea.

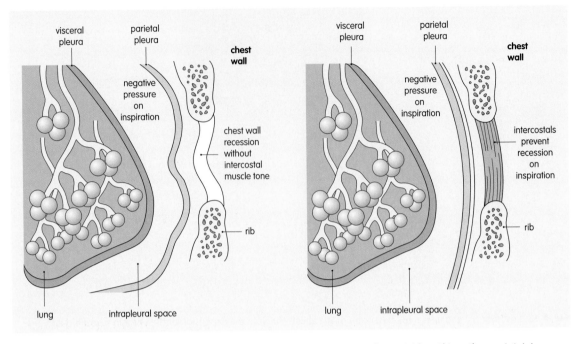

Fig. 4.14 The intercostal muscles: they prevent deformation of the thoracic wall in quiet breathing, thus maintaining thoracic volume.

Forced expiration

Elastic recoil of the lungs is reinforced by contraction of the muscles of the abdominal wall. These force the abdominal contents against the diaphragm, pushing it up (Fig. 4.15).

In addition, quadratus lumborum pulls the ribs down, thus adding to the force of the abdominal contents against the diaphragm. Intercostal muscles prevent outward deformation of the tissue between the ribs. Latissimus dorsi and serratus posterior inferior also may play some role.

Elastic properties of the lung

In order for ventilation to take place, the respiratory muscles described above must overcome the mechanical properties of the lungs and thorax, specifically their tendency to elastic recoil.

The elastic properties of the lung are caused by:
- Elastic fibers and collagen in the tissues in the lung
- Surface tension forces in the lung caused by the alveolar–liquid interface.

When we discuss the elastic properties of the lung, we often focus not on recoil but on stretch; the

capacity of the lung to stretch is known as compliance and is discussed below.

Compliance

Compliance describes the distensibility or ease of stretch of a material when an external force is applied to it. Elasticity (E) is the resistance to that stretch: Therefore,

$$C = 1/E$$

In respiratory physiology, we deal with:
- Compliance of the lung (C_L)
- Compliance of the chest wall (C_w)
- Total compliance (C_{TOT}) of the chest wall and lung together.

Lung compliance

Lung compliance is the ease with which the lungs expand under pressure. The pressure to inflate comes from the transmural pressure (i.e., the difference between the intrapleural pressure and the intrapulmonary pressure); this is plotted against the change in volume on a pressure–volume curve (Fig. 4.16). Compliance represents the slope of the curve ($\Delta V : \Delta P$).

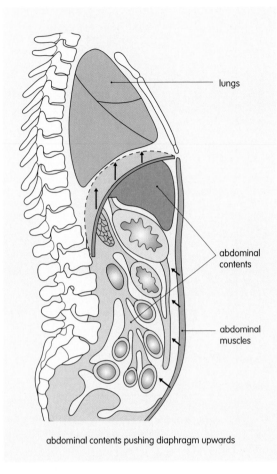

abdominal contents pushing diaphragm upwards

Fig. 4.15 Forced expiration. Note the abdominal contents pushing the diaphragm upward.

Lung mechanics are often categorized as static or dynamic. This can sometimes be confusing. As the name implies, static qualities do not change with time; lung statics help us to explore certain qualities of the lungs in isolation. Obviously, in real life, air in the respiratory tree flows (i.e., it changes with time). Therefore, lung dynamics give us a fuller picture of what actually happens during respiration.

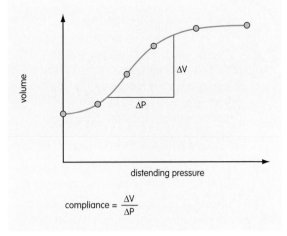

$$\text{compliance} = \frac{\Delta V}{\Delta P}$$

Fig. 4.16 The pressure–volume curve.

Lung compliance can be looked at in two ways:
- Static lung compliance
- Dynamic lung compliance.

Dynamic lung compliance is a measure of the change in volume of the lung during breathing and will thus include the work required to overcome airway resistance. This will be discussed later.

Static lung compliance involves the inflation of the lungs in steps of various inflating pressures and recording the volume at the new inflation pressure. The lungs are expanded from complete collapse to total lung capacity, and measurements are also taken in deflation (see dotted line in Fig. 4.17A). This is carried out *in vitro* because, in life, we cannot completely deflate the lungs. Why is there a difference between inflation and deflation curves? This difference is called hysteresis and will be explained later.

Figure 4.17B also shows the pressure–volume curve for inflation of the lungs from functional residual capacity to total lung capacity. The curve still shows hysteresis, but not to the extent of the pressure–volume curve from complete lung collapse to total lung capacity. The slope of the curve (i.e. compliance) varies with lung volume. It can be seen that compliance is greatest at the lower lung volumes and is smallest at higher lung volumes. For these reasons, lung compliance is sometimes quoted as specific lung compliance (sp.C_L):

$$\text{sp.}C_L = C_L/V_L$$

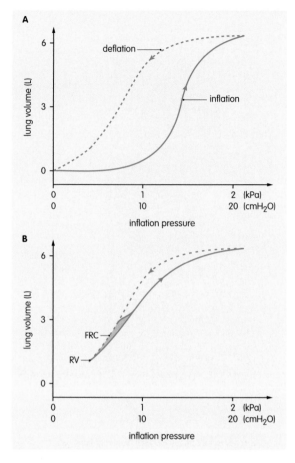

You can see from the pressure–volume curve that expanding the lung is like blowing up a balloon. At first high pressure is required for a small increase in volume. Then the slope becomes steeper before flattening again.

This change in lung compliance helps explain the difference in ventilation of the lung between apex and base.

The lung volume in the base is less (because it is compressed) relative to the apex. Thus, the base of the lung has greater initial compliance than that of the apex. Because both base and apex are subject to intrapleural pressure changes of the same magnitude during inspiration, the base of the lung will therefore expand to a greater extent than the apex. This explains in part the regional difference of ventilation.

Chest wall compliance

As we have discussed before, the chest wall has elastic properties; at functional residual capacity, these are equal and opposite to those in the lung (i.e., tending to expand the chest). If the sternum were cut (e.g., in surgery) or if air were introduced into the intrapleural space then this would cause the chest wall to spring open.

As we breathe in, elastic forces (tending to expand the chest wall) aid inflation; however, at about two-thirds of total lung capacity, the chest wall has reached its resting position and any expansion beyond this point requires a positive pressure to stretch the chest wall.

Below this resting position, the chest wall is being compressed by the pressure difference between atmospheric pressure and intrapleural pressure. Thus, if we plot inflation pressure against volume of the chest wall, the inflation pressure is negative below two-thirds of total lung capacity (the dashed line in Fig. 4.18). However, compliance (the slope of the pressure–volume curve for the chest wall) remains positive, because we are looking at the change in volume caused by a change in inflation pressure. Above the resting position the inflation pressure required to expand the chest is positive. Compliance of the lung is also plotted (dotted line in

Fig. 4.17 Pressure–volume curves for inflation of the lungs (A) *in vitro* and (B) in life, from residual volume to total lung capacity. Note the curve still shows hysteresis but to a lesser extent.

Fig. 4.18). Total compliance is plotted on the same graph and is derived from:

$$1/C_{TOT} = 1/C_L + 1/C_W$$

Effect of disease on compliance

Structural change in the thorax (e.g., kyphoscoliosis) may alter compliance of the chest wall; however, in practice, disease more often has an effect on compliance of the lung. Emphysema and pulmonary fibrosis (Fig. 4.19) represent two extremes of lung compliance in disease. In emphysema the compliance of the lung is increased, that is, it becomes more easily distended. This is due to the destruction of the normal lung architecture, including the elastic fibers and collagen. Impaired elastic recoil means that the lungs do not deflate as easily, contributing to air trapping.

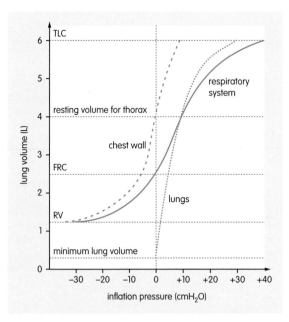

Fig. 4.18 Pressure–volume curve of the entire respiratory system. Only at functional residual capacity does the passively inflated lung–thorax system (respiratory system) have no pressure difference between the alveoli and the body surface.

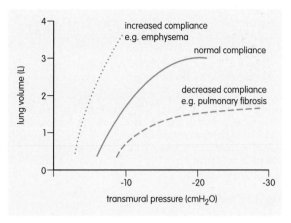

Fig. 4.19 Pressure–volume curves in disease.

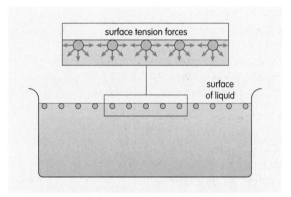

Fig. 4.20 Surface tension. (Adapted from *Physiology* 3rd ed, by R.M. Berne and M.N. Levy. St. Louis, Mosby Year Book, 1993.)

In diseases that cause fibrosis, scar tissue replaces normal interstitial tissue. As a result, the lungs become stiffer and compliance decreases.

Surface tension and surfactant

As noted above, the elasticity and therefore compliance of the lungs is dependent on two factors. The first is the elastic fibers in lung tissue. The second is the surface tension of the alveolar lining. This lining is a thin film of liquid, the main component of which is surfactant.

Surface tension

Surface tension is a physical property of liquids and arises because fluid molecules have a stronger attraction to each other than to air molecules (Fig. 4.20). Molecules on the surface of a liquid in contact with air are therefore pulled close together and act like a skin.

When molecules of a liquid lie on a curved surface (e.g., in a bubble), surface tension acts to pull that surface inwards. If the bubble is to be prevented from collapsing there must be an equal and opposite force tending to expand it. This is provided by a positive pressure within the bubble.

The alveoli are lined with liquid and are in contact with air. They can therefore be considered similar to tiny bubbles. Laplace's law (Fig. 4.21) tells us that the smaller a bubble, the greater the internal pressure needed to keep it inflated (Fig. 4.22). If a bubble of about the same size as an alveolus was made of interstitial fluid and filled with air it would require an internal pressure in the order of 25mmHg to prevent it from collapsing. The lungs would have a very low compliance and the forces involved in breathing would be extremely large. This would seem to argue against the lungs having a liquid lining.

This problem was investigated by von Neergaard, who measured the compliance of excised lungs, first using air to inflate them and then using saline (Fig. 4.23). He noticed that:

59

Laplace's law: states that "The pressure within a bubble is equal to twice the surface tension divided by the radius"

$$P = \frac{2T}{r}$$

P = pressure within bubble
T = surface tension
r = radius

The smaller a bubble (i.e. the more curved the surface) the greater the tendency to collapse.
Smaller bubbles must have a greater internal pressure to keep them inflated.

Fig. 4.21 Laplace's law.

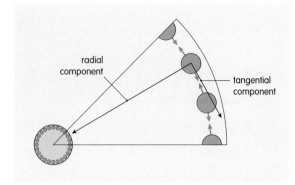

Fig. 4.22 Surface tension of a bubble. Radial forces tend to collapse the bubble and there must be a positive pressure inside the bubble to prevent it from collapsing. The smaller the bubble, the greater the internal pressure.

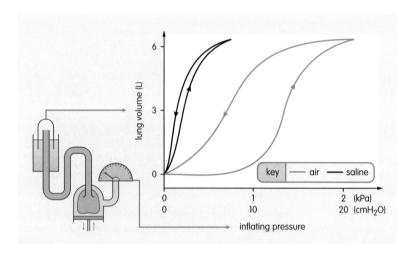

Fig. 4.23 Note the marked difference between the pressure–volume curves of air-filled and saline-filled lungs. It is much easier to inflate the lung without air. (Adapted with permission from *Physiology* 3rd ed, by R.M. Berne and M.N. Levy. St. Louis, Mosby Year Book, 1993.)

- Lungs were much easier to inflate (i.e. more compliant) with saline than air
- When he used air, the pressure required was greater during inflation than during deflation.

This phenomenon is called hysteresis.

Since there was no surface tension when saline was used, the alveoli did seem to have a liquid lining; surface tension was contributing to the elastic recoil of the lungs making them harder to inflate. However, the pressure needed to inflate the lungs was actually much lower than if the fluid were water or interstitial fluid. Something in the fluid lining the lungs reduces surface tension, making the lungs more compliant and therefore easier to expand.

This leads us to three questions:

- How is this low surface tension achieved?
- Laplace's law says that small bubbles have higher internal pressure than larger ones. If two bubbles of different sizes were connected, air would flow from the small bubble to the large, causing the small bubble to collapse (Fig. 4.24). Why does this not happen to alveoli?
- How does the phenomenon of hysteresis of the pressure–volume curve occur?

The answers to all these questions are linked to surfactant.

Surfactant

Surfactant is secreted by type II pneumocytes (type II alveolar epithelial cells) and contains a

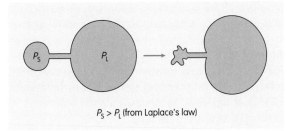

Fig. 4.24 The pressure in the smaller bubble (P_S) from Laplace's law. The smaller bubble collapses, emptying into the larger, lower-pressure bubble.

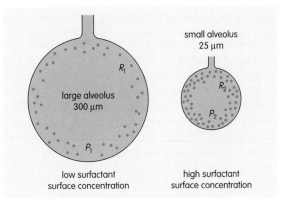

Fig. 4.25 The surface tension (T_1) within the larger alveolus (with radius R_1) is greater than the surface tension (T_2) within the smaller alveolus (with radius R_2). This is because the surfactant is more spread out in the larger alveolus. Thus, the T:R ratio remains constant and the same pressure is required to inflate alveoli of all sizes ($P_1 = P_2$).

phospholipid (dipalmitoyl phosphatidyl choline). Surfactant has three functions:

- Prevention of alveolar collapse (gives alveolar stability)
- Increase in lung compliance by reducing surface tension of alveolar lining fluid
- Prevention of transudation of fluid into alveoli.

Prevention of alveolar collapse Because of two factors, alveoli of different sizes do not collapse:

- Surface tension of the alveolar lining fluid varies with surface area. This is because surfactant reduces surface tension in proportion to its surface concentration. Surfactant is insoluble in water and floats on the surface of the alveolar lining fluid. In larger alveoli the surfactant is more spread out (dilute) and the surface tension is higher (Fig. 4.25).
- There is interaction between adjacent groups of alveoli. Therefore, collapsing alveoli pull on adjacent alveoli preventing further collapse. This is termed alveolar interdependence.

Prevention of transudation of fluid into alveoli
Surfactant reduces the surface tension in the alveolar lining fluid, which reduces the tendency for the alveolus to collapse. If the alveoli were lined with interstitial fluid, their collapse would cause a more negative pressure in the interstitial space. This would lead to an increase in hydrostatic pressure difference between the pulmonary capillary and the interstitial space, leading to transudation of fluid.

Hysteresis Hysteresis of the pressure–volume curve is explained by a property of surfactant. The surface tension of surfactant shows different values when being expanded (e.g., during inspiration) or compressed (e.g., during expiration). Because lung

compliance is dependent upon surface tension, this explains why hysteresis of the pressure–volume curve occurs.

Respiratory distress syndrome Respiratory distress syndrome (RDS) occurs in premature babies of less than 32 weeks' gestation; it is caused by a deficiency of surfactant production by type II pneumocytes. Difficulty in breathing occurs; breathing is rapid and labored, often with an expiratory grunt. There is diffuse damage to alveoli with hyaline membrane formation. Treatment is with high-concentration oxygen therapy, which reverses the hypoxemia.

Dynamics of ventilation

The previous section discussed the elastic properties of the lungs (i.e., those caused by surface tension and tissue elasticity). These were looked at under static conditions; however, if we inflate the lungs, dynamic conditions exist. So, in addition to overcoming the elastic properties of the lung during breathing, we must also overcome the dynamic resistance to inflation of the lungs.

The total pressure difference (P_{TOT}) required to inflate the lungs is the sum of the pressure to overcome lung compliance and the pressure to overcome dynamic resistance:

$$P_{TOT} = P_{COM} + P_{DYN}$$

where P_{COM} = pressure to overcome lung compliance and P_{DYN} = pressure to overcome the dynamic resistance.

Dynamic resistance itself comprises:

- Resistance presented by the airways to flow of air into the lungs—airway resistance
- Resistance to tissues as they slide over each other—viscous tissue resistance.

$$P_{DYN} = P_{AR} + P_{VTR}$$

where P_{AR} = pressure to overcome airways resistance and P_{VTR} = pressure to overcome viscous tissue resistance.

Viscous tissue resistance comprises approximately 20% of the total dynamic resistance, i.e. the vast majority of the total resistance is provided by the airways.

Dynamic lung compliance

Now that we have introduced dynamic conditions, in which airway resistance is a factor, we need to review our measurements of lung compliance. If a pressure–volume curve is plotted under dynamic conditions, the pressure–volume loop is widened when compared with the curve under static conditions (Fig. 4.26). Dynamic lung compliance is the slope of this curve at any one point. Dynamic lung compliance is less than static lung compliance.

Airway resistance

Airway resistance is an important concept because it is increased in common diseases such as asthma and COPD. It is defined as the resistance to flow of gas within the airways of the lung.

Before we discuss airway resistance, it is important to outline pattern of flow.

Pattern of flow

The pattern of fluid flowing through a tube (e.g., an airway or blood vessel) varies with the velocity and physical properties of the fluid. This was established by a French engineer, Reynolds, who injected a colored dye into the center of a clear pipe of water flowing at various velocities. He discovered two phenomena, which he described as laminar flow (which appeared at low flow rates; Fig. 4.27) and turbulent flow (which appeared at high flow rates; Fig. 4.28).

Figure 4.29 describes some of the differences between laminar and turbulent flow. Both types of flow are seen in the respiratory system.

Turbulent flow Turbulent flow is much more likely to occur with:

- High velocities (e.g., within the airways during exercise)
- Larger-diameter airways
- Low-viscosity, high-density fluids.

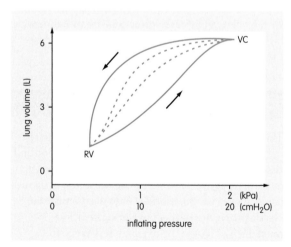

Fig. 4.26 Difference in pressure–volume relationships in lungs inflated and deflated (measurements made under static conditions with no air flowing: dotted lines; dynamic conditions with air flowing continuously into or out of the lung: solid lines).

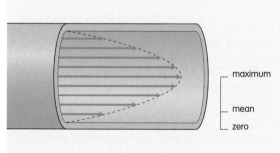

Fig. 4.27 Laminar flow in which the colored filament remained central. The flow occurs in streamlines, or laminae. The greatest velocity of flow is centrally and the velocity profile is parabolic. (Adapted with permission from *Physiology* 3rd ed., by R.M. Berne and M.N. Levy. St. Louis, Mosby Year Book, 1993.)

Branching or irregular surfaces can also initiate turbulence.

Laminar flow Laminar flow is described by Poiseuille's law (Fig. 4.30). In basic terms, Poiseuille's law means that the wider the tube, the lower the resistance to airflow. Importantly, the change in width is not directly proportional to the change in resistance: when the radius is cut in half, resistance is increased by a factor of 16. Narrower or longer pipes or a higher fluid viscosity have a higher resistance to flow and so flow rate is reduced.

Sites of airway resistance

Considering the whole respiratory system, approximately one-half of the resistance to airflow occurs in the upper respiratory tract when breathing through the nose. This is significantly reduced when mouth breathing. Thus, approximately one-half of the resistance lies within the lower respiratory tract.

Assuming laminar air flow, Poiseuille's law would predict that the major resistance to air flow would occur in the airways with a smaller radius. This is not the case because although the individual diameter of each airway is small, the total cross-sectional area for

Remembering Poiseuille's law isn't drastically important, but understanding it is! So, remember that in laminar flow:
A small change in radius greatly affects either flow rate or pressure drop required to achieve the same flow. An example of this is bronchoconstriction in asthma. In addition:
* Flow varies directly with pressure drop
* Flow varies inversely with viscosity (e.g., during scuba diving).

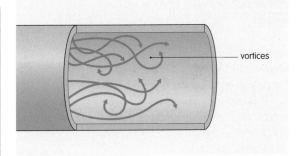

Fig. 4.28 Turbulent flow in which the colored filament broke up into eddies. (Adapted with permission from *Physiology* 3rd ed., by R.M. Berne and M.N. Levy. St. Louis, Mosby Year Book, 1993.)

Differences between laminar and turbulent flow	
Laminar	**Turbulent**
fluid moves parallel to walls only	flow has some movement at right angles
no mixing between fluid layers other than by diffusion	well-mixed flow eddies and diffusion
nonerosive flow	flow can be erosive
flow is quiet	may account for murmurs heard clinically
arterial thrombi unlikely but venous stasis may lead to thrombi	arterial thrombi more likely to form
resistance to flow is independent of surface roughness	resistance to flow is dependent on surface roughness
flow is proportional to the radius to the power 4	flow is proportional to radius to the power 4

Fig. 4.29 Differences between laminar and turbulent flow.

flow increases greatly (large number of small airways) as we go down the tracheobronchial tree. In fact, the greatest resistance is in the medium-sized bronchi.

Poiseuille's law: states that for a fluid under laminar flow conditions, the flow rate is directly related to the pressure drop between the two ends of a tube and the fourth power of the radius but inversely related to viscosity and length of pipe:

$$F = \frac{P\pi r^4}{8\eta L}$$

(F) = flow rate
(P) = pressure drop
(r) = radius
(η) = viscosity
(L) = length of pipe

Remember, Poiseuille's law applies to laminar, not turbulent, flow.

Fig. 4.30 Poiseuille's law.

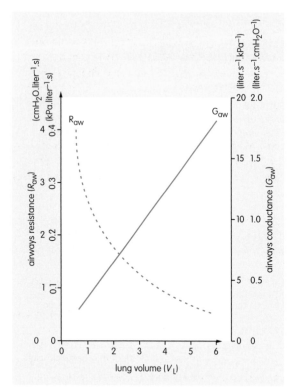

Fig. 4.31 The relationship between lung volume (V_L) and airway resistance (R_{aw}) and conductance (G_{aw}). Note that at low lung volumes, R_{aw} is high and G_{aw} is low. (Adapted with permission from *Respiratory Physiology* 2nd ed., by J. Widdicombe and A. Davies. London, Edward Arnold, 1991.)

In exercise, the airway resistance may increase significantly due to high air flows inducing turbulence. It is normal under these conditions to switch to mouth breathing to reduce airway resistance.

It is important to note that resistance of the smaller airways is difficult to measure. Thus, these small airways may be damaged by disease and it may be some time before this damage is detectable, thus representing a "silent" zone.

Factors determining airway resistance

Factors affecting airway resistance are:
- Lung volume
- Bronchial smooth muscle tone
- Altered airway caliber
- Change in density and viscosity of inspired gas.

Lung volume Airways are supported by radial traction of lung parenchyma and thus their diameter and resistance to flow are affected by lung volume (Fig. 4.31):
- Low lung volumes tend to collapse and compress the airways, reducing their diameter and thus increasing resistance to flow.
- High lung volumes tend to increase radial traction, increasing the length and diameter of airways.
- The increase in diameter reduces airway resistance. The increase in length has a much smaller effect of increasing resistance, which is explained by Poiseuille's law.

Things to remember:
- The major site of airway resistance is medium-sized bronchi
- 80% of the resistance of the upper respiratory tract is presented by the trachea and bronchi
- Less than 20% of airway resistance is caused by airways less than 2 mm in diameter.

Bronchial smooth muscle tone Motor innervation of the smooth muscle of the airways is via the vagus nerve. The muscle has resting tone determined by the autonomic nervous system. This tone can be affected by a number of factors (Fig. 4.32).

Factors acting to decrease the airway diameter include:

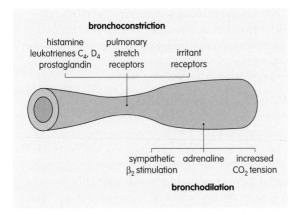

Fig. 4.32 Factors affecting bronchial motor tone. (Adapted from *Physiology* 3rd ed., by R.M. Berne and M.N. Levy. St. Louis, Mosby Year Book, 1993.)

- Irritant and cough receptors, C fiber reflex—reflex and bronchoconstriction act to close the airway
- Pulmonary stretch receptors
- Mediator release—inflammatory mediators (e.g., histamine, leukotrienes) cause bronchoconstriction.

Factors acting to increase the airway diameter include:
- Carbon dioxide
- Catecholamine release
- Other nerves—nonadrenergic, noncholinergic (NANC) nerves cause bronchodilation.

Reduced airway caliber can be caused either by disease or by an inhaled foreign body. A change in density and viscosity of gas occurs in scuba diving (Chapter 6).

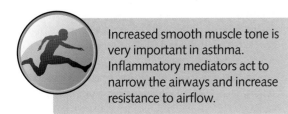

Increased smooth muscle tone is very important in asthma. Inflammatory mediators act to narrow the airways and increase resistance to airflow.

Effect of transmural pressure on airway resistance

Remember that the airways are not rigid tubes; they are affected by the pressures around them. The

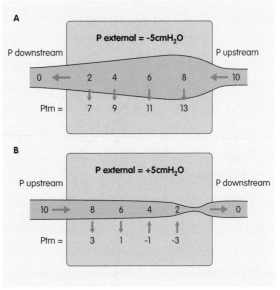

Fig. 4.33 Transmural pressure, (A) during inspiration; (B) during expiration. Ptm = transmural pressure.

pressure difference between the gas in the airway and the pressure outside the airway is known as the transmural pressure difference. The pressure outside the airway reflects the intrapleural pressure (Fig. 4.33).

During inspiration The pressure within the pleural cavity is always negative, and the alveolar pressure is greater than intrapleural pressure. The transmural pressure difference is always positive thus the airway is distended (radial traction).

During expiration The pressure within the alveolus is positive with respect to the intrapleural pressure; hence, the alveolus stays open. The transmural pressure difference, however, is dependent upon expiratory flow rate and intrapleural pressure.

During forced expiration, the positive intrapleural pressure is transmitted through the lungs to the external wall of the airways. In addition, there is a dynamic pressure drop from alveolus to the airway caused by airway resistance. This is greater at high expiratory flow rates. Thus, the pressure in the lumen of the airway may be lower than the external wall pressure (negative transmural pressure), leading to collapse of the airways.

Thus, the harder the subject tries to exhale forcibly, the more the airways are compressed, so the

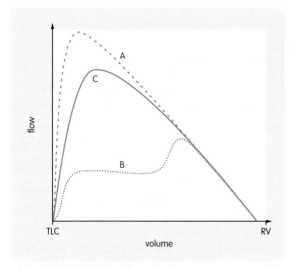

Fig. 4.34 Flow–volume curves made with a spirometer. (A) Maximum inspiration and forced expiration. (B) Slow expiration initially then forced. (C) Expiratory flow almost to maximum effort. Note that the three descending curves are almost superimposed.

rate of expiration does not rise as the increased pressure gradient (from alveoli to atmospheric pressure) is offset by the reduced caliber of the airways. This phenomenon is known as the dynamic compression of airways.

Dynamic compression of airways is greater at lower lung volumes because the effect of radial traction holding the airways open is less. Thus it can be seen that for a specific lung volume there is a maximum expiratory flow rate caused by dynamic compression of the airways (Fig. 4.34). Any rate of expiration below this flow rate is dependent on how much effort is made to expel the air from the lungs and the flow is said to be effort dependent. At maximum expiratory flow rate, any additional effort does not alter the expiratory flow rate (because of dynamic compression of airways) and the flow is said to be effort independent.

Dynamic compression in disease In patients with COPD, dynamic compression limits expiratory flow even in tidal breathing. The main reasons for this are:

- Loss of radial traction (due to destruction of the lung architecture) means the airways are more readily compressed
- Increased lung compliance, leading to lower alveolar pressure and less force driving air out of the lungs.

The clinical consequences are airway collapse on expiration and air trapping in the alveoli. Patients sometimes demonstrate pursed lip breathing as they attempt to increase pressure on expiration and reduce the amount of air trapped.

Measuring airway resistance

Airway resistance can be measured by plethysmography. In practice, estimates of airway resistance are made every day using simpler methods which rely on the relationship between resistance and airflow. Peak expiratory flow rate (PEFR) measures the maximum airflow achieved in a rapid, forced expiration. Spirometry measures the volume exhaled in a specified time (e.g., the forced expired volume in 1 second or FEV_1). These tests are described in Chapter 10.

The work of breathing

The work of breathing is the work done by the respiratory muscles to overcome the forces described above, i.e. resistance to airflow and the elastic recoil of the lungs.

The work done (W) to change a volume (ΔV) of gas at constant pressure (P) is shown by the relationship below:

$$W = P \cdot \Delta V$$

Work done is measured in joules; a volume change of 10 L at a pressure of $1\,cmH_2O = 1\,J$ of energy.

Respiration normally represents just a small fraction of the total cost of metabolism (approximately 2%). However, the work required to inflate the lungs, along with this percentage, will rise if:

- Lungs are inflated to a larger volume (e.g., COPD and chronic severe asthma)
- Lung compliance decreases (e.g., fibrotic lungs)
- Airway resistance increases (e.g., COPD and asthma)
- Turbulence is induced in the airways (e.g., in high flow rates experienced during strenuous exercise).

In contrast, the work of breathing is reduced by bronchodilators which act to decrease airway resistance.

The increased work requirement can be dramatic in patients with severe COPD; a great deal of energy is required just in order to breathe. This can also be understood in terms of the efficiency of ventilation (i.e., the amount of work done divided by energy

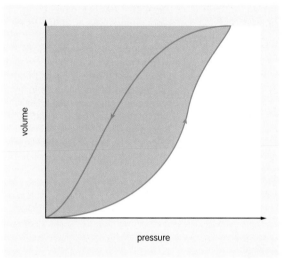

Fig. 4.35 Graph of normal lung volume against translung pressure. The shaded area is the inspiratory work of breathing. (Adapted with permission from *Respiratory Physiology* 2nd ed., J. Widdicombe and A. Davies. London, Edward Arnold, 1991.)

expenditure). Efficiency of normal quiet breathing is low (about 10%) even in good health. In COPD, efficiency decreases, and the work done increases, so much that all the oxygen supplied from increasing ventilation may be consumed by the respiratory muscles.

The work of breathing can be illustrated by volume–pressure curves (Fig. 4.35). Figure 4.36 shows the effect of disease on these curves. Figure 4.37 shows the effect of the pattern of breathing on work; there is an optimal balance between volume and rate of breathing at which the work of breathing is minimal.

Try to relate these concepts to respiratory failure. A patient with lung disease may be able to respond to impaired gas exchange by raising the ventilatory rate, leading to rapid, shallow breaths. This increases the work of breathing. If lung disease is severe, the work of breathing may become unsustainable. Respiratory muscles tire, ventilatory failure ensues, and the patient must be mechanically ventilated, to reduce the work of breathing.

Gas exchange in the lungs

This section discusses how gas is transferred from the alveoli to the bloodstream and from the bloodstream to the alveoli. A brief outline of how the laws of diffusion apply to the diffusion of gas from the airways to the circulation is given below. Time for diffusion and diffusion–perfusion limitations are also discussed.

Diffusion

Gas exchange between alveolar air and blood in the pulmonary capillaries takes place by diffusion.

Diffusion is the process in which molecules move due to their random motion (Brownian motion). The process of diffusion is seen to be a net movement of particles:

- Diffusion occurs from an area of high concentration to an area of low concentration. Thus, the driving force for diffusion is concentration difference (ΔC).
- Diffusion will occur until the concentration in the two areas is equalized (i.e., net movement has ceased). Random movement of particles continues to occur, and this is known as dynamic equilibrium.

Diffusion in the lungs occurs across a membrane and is therefore governed by Fick's law (Fig. 4.38). Fick's law tells us that the rate of diffusion of a gas increases:

- As the surface area of the membrane increases
- The thinner the membrane
- The greater the partial pressure gradient across the membrane
- The more soluble the gas.

It is clear that the blood–gas interface with its large surface area of 50–100m^2 and average thickness of 0.4µm permits the high rate of diffusion required by the body.

We can also see that the rate of diffusion across the alveoli is directly dependent upon the difference in partial pressures between a gas in the alveoli (P_A) and in arterial blood (P_a).

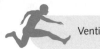

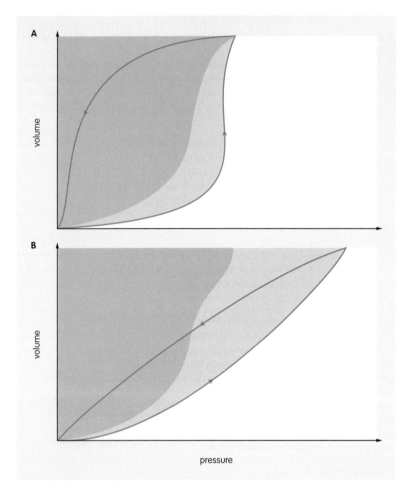

Fig. 4.36 Changes to breathing work during diseased states. Paler shading denotes disease state; dark shading shows the normal work prefills from Fig. 4.35. (A) Increased airway resistance (e.g., in asthma); (B) decreased compliance (e.g., in fibrotic lung disease). (Adapted with permission from *Respiratory Physiology* 2nd ed., by J. Widdicombe and A. Davies. London Edward Arnold, 1991.)

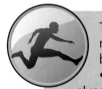
Henry's law states that at equilibrium, the amount of gas dissolved in a given volume of liquid at a given temperature is proportional to the partial pressure (*P*) of the gas in the gas phase and its solubility in the liquid (*S*).

$$C = S \cdot P$$

The following will increase the rate of oxygen diffusion into the blood:
- Increased surface area of the alveolus
- Decreased thickness of the alveolar wall
- Increased alveolar partial pressure of oxygen (oxygen therapy).

Partial pressures of respiratory gases

The partial pressure of a gas can be calculated by Dalton's law. Dalton's law states that "The pressure exerted by a mixture of nonreacting gases is equal to the sum of the partial pressures of the separate components." In other words, each gas in a mixture of gases exerts the same pressure as it would if it were present alone in the volume occupied by the mixture (Fig. 4.39).

From Dalton's law we see that:
- The total pressure of a gas is the sum of all the partial pressures of its constituents.

Fig. 4.37 The work done in breathing is altered by the pattern of breathing. (A) Optimal pattern; (B) increased frequency and decreased volume; (C) decreased frequency and increased volume. Note that the work of breathing is highest when frequency decreases and volume increases. (Adapted with permission from *Respiratory Physiology* 2nd ed., by J. Widdicombe and A. Davies. London, Edward Arnold, 1991.)

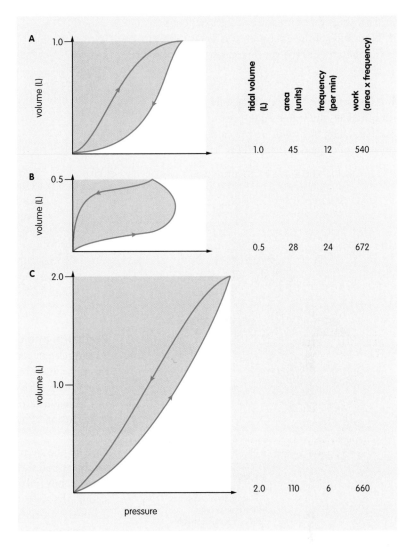

	tidal volume (L)	area (units)	frequency (per min)	work (area x frequency)
A	1.0	45	12	540
B	0.5	28	24	672
C	2.0	110	6	660

- The partial pressure of a gas can be calculated from its fractional concentration.

If we consider the total barometric pressure of air (P_{atm}, about 760mmHg at sea level), this is composed of the sum of all the partial pressures of its constituent gases:

$$P_{atm} = PO_2 + PN_2 + PCO_2 + PH_2O$$

Secondly, taking one of the constituent gases, we can multiply the fractional concentration of that gas by the total pressure to find the partial pressure that the gas exerts, or its tension:

$$PO_2 = FO_2 \times P_{atm}$$

where FO_2 is the fractional concentration of oxygen.

Dry air has a fractional concentration of oxygen of 21%; inserting this value into the equation above gives us an oxygen tension at sea level of 159mmHg.

We specified sea level because the partial pressure of a gas in a system will alter with total pressure. If atmospheric pressure is reduced (e.g., when climbing Mount Everest), so is the partial pressure of oxygen.

Water vapor pressure

Dry gas pressures are, however, of little relevance in respiratory medicine. On inspiration, air is warmed and humidified. Therefore water vapor also exerts a pressure, which reduces the pressure available to the partial pressures of the gases.

69

The water vapor pressure of a gas depends on:
- Saturation of the gas (quoted as % saturation)
- Temperature of the gas (increases as temperature rises).

It is important to know that for fully (100%) saturated air, the water vapor pressure at 37°C is 47 mmHg. Using this value we can calculate the partial pressure of oxygen in inspired (or "tracheal") air.

$$PO_2 = 0.21 \times (760 - 47) = 150\,mmHg$$

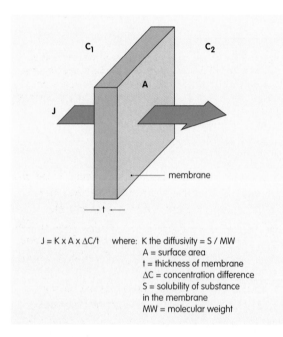

$J = K \times A \times \Delta C/t$ where: K the diffusivity = S / MW
A = surface area
t = thickness of membrane
ΔC = concentration difference
S = solubility of substance in the membrane
MW = molecular weight

Fig. 4.38 Diffusion—Fick's law. Fick stated that the rate of diffusion (J) of a gas through a membrane was: $J = K \times A \times \Delta C/t$, where $K = S/wt_{mol}$, A = surface area; t = thickness of membrane; ΔC = concentration difference; S = solubility of substance in the membrane; wt_{mol} = molecular weight.

The following will decrease the rate of oxygen diffusion into the blood:
- Reduction in the overall alveolar surface area (e.g., emphysema)
- Increased distance for diffusion within the alveoli (e.g., emphysema)
- Increased thickness of the alveolar wall (e.g., pulmonary fibrosis)
- Reduction in the alveolar partial pressure of oxygen (e.g., altitude)

Partial pressures are also expressed in kPa. 1 kPa is 7.5 mmHg.

Perfusion and diffusion limitation

At the gas exchange surface, gas transfer occurs through a membrane into a flowing liquid. There are two processes (Fig. 4.40) occurring:
- Diffusion across the alveolar capillary membrane
- Perfusion of blood through pulmonary capillaries.

Uptake of a gas into the blood is dependent on its solubility and the chemical combination (e.g., with hemoglobin (Hb)). If the chemical combination is strong, the gas is taken up by the blood with little rise in arterial partial pressure.

The solubility of nitrous oxide (N_2O) in the blood is low, and it does not undergo chemical combination with any component of the blood. Thus, rate of transfer of gas into the liquid phase is slow and partial pressure of the gas in the blood rises rapidly (Fig. 4.41). This reduces the partial pressure

Partial pressures of respiratory gases			
Gas	PO_2 (mmHg)	PCO_2 (mmHg)	PH_2O (mmHg)
atmosphere (dry air)	159	0	0
trachea (inspiration)	150	0	47*
alveolar gas	100	40	47

*note that inspired gas is fully saturated with water vapor before it enters the lungs

Fig. 4.39 Partial pressures of respiratory gases.

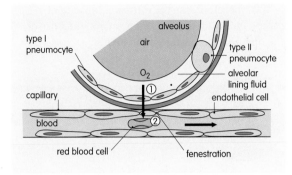

Fig. 4.40 Gas transfer across alveolar capillary membrane.
(1) Diffusion across membrane; (2) perfusion of blood
through pulmonary capillaries.

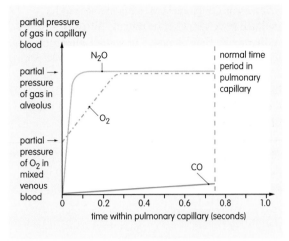

Fig. 4.41 Graph of partial pressure of respiratory gases
against time within the pulmonary capillary bed. Transfer
of N_2O is perfusion limited, transfer of CO is diffusion
limited. Transfer of O_2 is usually perfusion limited but may
change with diseased states.

difference between alveolar gas and the blood and
hence the driving force for diffusion. Nitrous oxide
is, therefore, an example of a gas that is said to be
perfusion limited. Thus, the amount of nitrous oxide
taken up by the blood is dependent almost solely
upon the rate of blood flow through the pulmonary
capillaries.

In the case of carbon monoxide (CO), the gas is
taken up rapidly and bound tightly by hemoglobin;
the arterial partial pressure rises slowly (Fig. 4.41).
Thus, there is always a driving force (partial pressure
difference) for diffusion (even at low perfusion
rates), and the overall rate of transfer will be
dependent on the rate of diffusion. This type of
transfer is said to be diffusion limited. Thus the
amount of carbon monoxide taken up by the blood is
dependent on the rate of diffusion of carbon
monoxide from the alveoli to the blood.

The transfer of oxygen is normally perfusion
limited because the arterial partial pressure of
oxygen (P_aO_2) reaches equilibrium with the alveolar
gas (P_AO_2) by about one-third of the way along the
pulmonary capillary (see Fig. 4.41); there is,
therefore, no driving force for diffusion after this
point. However, if the diffusion is slow because of
emphysematous changes to the lung, then P_aO_2 may
not reach equilibrium with the alveolar gas before the
blood reaches the end of the capillary. Under these
conditions, the transfer of oxygen is diffusion
limited.

Oxygen uptake in the capillary network
The time taken for the partial pressure of oxygen to
reach its plateau is approximately 0.25 seconds. The

pulmonary capillary volume under resting conditions
is about 75 ml, which is approximately the same
size as the stroke volume of the right ventricle.
Pulmonary capillary blood is therefore replaced with
every heart beat, approximately every 0.75 seconds.
This far exceeds the time for transfer of oxygen into
the bloodstream.

During exercise, however, the cardiac output
increases and the flow rate though the pulmonary
capillaries also increases. Because the lungs have the
ability to recruit new capillaries and distend already
open capillaries (see Chapter 5), the effect of
increased blood flow rate on the time allowed for
diffusion is not as great as one might expect. In
strenuous exercise, the pulmonary capillary
network volume may increase by up to 200 ml. This
helps maintain the time allowed for diffusion,
although it cannot keep it to the same value as at
rest.

Carbon dioxide transfer
Fick's is not the only law that describes the diffusion
of gases in the lung. Graham's law tells us that gases
with greater molecular weights diffuse more slowly
than those that are lighter.

However, we are also concerned with the
diffusion rates of gas in blood. Diffusion in liquids is
directly dependent upon the solubility of the gas, but

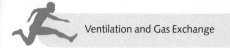

inversely proportional to the square root of its molecular weight. Carbon dioxide diffuses 20 times more rapidly than oxygen, but has a similar molecular weight. Thus, the difference in rates of diffusion is caused by the much higher solubility of carbon dioxide.

Under normal conditions, the transfer of carbon dioxide is not diffusion-limited.

Measuring diffusion

As we have already seen, gas transfer (J) can be calculated using Fick's law:

$$J = K \cdot A \cdot (P_A - P_a)/t$$

It is not possible to measure the area and thickness of a complex structure like the blood–gas barrier, so the equation is rewritten:

$$J = D_L(P_A - P_a)$$

where D_L is the diffusing capacity of the lung, defined as the ease of diffusion of gas into the blood (the rate of uptake of a gas divided by the partial pressure difference between alveoli and blood).

$$D_L = J/(P_A - P_a)$$

Carbon monoxide is the gas most commonly used to study diffusing capacity. Because carbon monoxide is taken up into the liquid phase very quickly, the rate of perfusion of pulmonary capillaries does not significantly affect the partial pressure difference between alveolar gas and the bloodstream. In addition, carbon monoxide binds irreversibly to hemoglobin and is not taken up by the tissues. Therefore, the rate of diminution of CO in alveolar gas after inspiration of air containing a small concentration of CO can be used to calculate diffusing capacity.

In contrast, oxygen is not a good candidate for calculating diffusing capacity because it binds reversibly to hemoglobin; thus, mixed venous partial pressure may not be the same as that of blood entering the pulmonary capillary bed. In addition, because oxygen is taken up less quickly than CO, perfusion has more of an effect.

We, therefore, use the diffusing capacity of carbon monoxide ($D_{L(CO)}$) as a general measure of the diffusion properties of the lung.

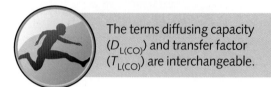
The terms diffusing capacity ($D_{L(CO)}$) and transfer factor ($T_{L(CO)}$) are interchangeable.

The partial pressure of carbon monoxide in the blood ($P_{a(CO)}$) is negligible, so the equation can be rewritten:

$$D_{L(CO)} = J_{(CO)}/P_{A(CO)}$$

One of the methods used to measure diffusion across the blood–gas interface is the single-breath method. A single breath of a mixture of carbon monoxide and air is taken. The breath is then held for approximately 10 seconds. The difference between inspiratory and expiratory concentrations of carbon monoxide is measured and therefore the amount of carbon monoxide taken up by the blood in 10s is known. If the lung volume is also measured by the helium dilution method, it is possible to determine the transfer coefficient (K_{CO}) or diffusion rate per unit of lung volume. This is a more useful measure of diffusion where lung volume has been lost, for example after surgery or in pleural effusion. Because there can be many causes of a reduction in diffusing capacity, it is not a specific test for lung disease. It is, however, a sensitive test; it is able to demonstrate minor impediments to gas diffusion.

Factors that decrease the rate of diffusion include:
- Thickening of the alveolar capillary membrane (e.g., in pulmonary fibrosis)
- Edema of the alveolar capillary walls
- Increased lining fluid within the alveoli
- Increased distance for gaseous diffusion (e.g., in emphysema)
- Reduced area of alveolar capillary membrane (e.g., in emphysema)
- Reduced flow of fresh air to the alveoli from terminal bronchioles
- Hypoventilation.

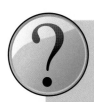

- **Define** minute ventilation and alveolar ventilation.
- Define anatomic dead space, quoting its normal value. Describe two methods of measuring anatomic dead space.
- Define all lung volumes and capacities, giving normal values. State the significance of each volume and capacity.
- Name four methods for measuring lung volume.
- Outline the regional variations in ventilation of the lung and how this might be measured.
- Explain why intrapleural pressure is negative. Describe its variation during breathing.
- Describe how breathing is brought about, naming the muscles involved and their actions.
- Define lung compliance and explain what is meant by static and dynamic lung compliance, including a description of the pressure–volume curve.
- Describe the role of surfactant.
- Define airway resistance and viscous tissue resistance.
- List the factors determining airway resistance.
- Describe how airway resistance is altered in asthma.
- Explain what is meant by dynamic compression of the airways.
- Summarize the mechanisms that impair ventilation in COPD.
- Which factors affect the rate of diffusion across the blood–air interface? What is the driving force for diffusion?
- Give the normal values of the partial pressures of carbon dioxide and oxygen within the respiratory system.
- Explain the terms "partial pressure of a gas" and "vapor pressure."
- Name three conditions that lower the transfer of oxygen to the blood. How do these conditions affect diffusion?
- Using examples, define perfusion limitation and diffusion limitation.
- Define diffusing capacity. How can diffusing capacity be measured?

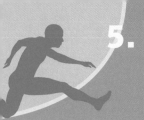

5. Perfusion and Gas Transport

Overview

The pulmonary circulation is a highly specialized system which is adapted to accommodate the entire cardiac output both at rest and during exercise. It is able to do this because it is:

- A low-pressure, low-resistance system
- Able to recruit more vessels with only a slight increase in arterial pulmonary pressure.

However, good perfusion is not enough to ensure that the blood is adequately oxygenated. The most important determinant in arterial blood gas composition is the way in which ventilation and perfusion are matched to each alveolus. Mismatching of ventilation:perfusion is the central mechanism in many common lung diseases.

The ability of the lungs to change minute ventilation, and therefore alter the rate of elimination of CO_2, gives the respiratory system a key role in maintaining the body's acid–base status. This chapter, therefore, also reviews the fundamentals of acid–base balance and discusses the common acid–base disturbances.

Pulmonary blood flow

Outline of pulmonary circulation

An outline of the pulmonary blood flow was given in Fig. 3.14. Venous blood returning from the body enters the right atrium and passively fills the right ventricle during diastole. During systole, the right ventricle contracts, ejecting its contents into the pulmonary artery (note the pulmonary artery contains deoxygenated blood).

Blood flows along the pulmonary arteries and arterioles, which closely follow the course of the airways. Blood enters the pulmonary capillaries (situated within the walls of the alveoli) and gaseous exchange takes place. Blood then returns to enter the left atrium through postcapillary venules and pulmonary veins (which contain oxygenated blood).

Mechanics of the circulation

The flow of blood through the pulmonary vasculature is slightly less than the systemic output of the left ventricle. This is because a small proportion of the coronary circulation from the aorta drains directly into the left ventricle. In addition, the bronchial circulation from the aorta drains into pulmonary veins, thus bypassing the lungs. However, we can consider the flow through the pulmonary artery to be equal to cardiac output.

Pressures within the pulmonary circulation are much lower than those equivalent regions within the systemic circulation (Fig. 5.1). Because the volume of blood flowing through both circulations is approximately the same, the pulmonary circulation must offer much lower resistance.

Pulmonary capillaries and arterioles cause the main resistance to flow in the pulmonary circulation. This low resistance is achieved in two ways:

- A large number of resistance vessels exist, which are usually dilated; thus, the total area for flow is very large.
- Small muscular arteries contain much less smooth muscle than equivalent arteries in the systemic circulation; they are more easily distended.

Many other factors affect pulmonary blood flow and pulmonary vascular resistance. These are discussed below.

Hydrostatic pressure

Hydrostatic pressure has three effects.

- It distends blood vessels: as hydrostatic pressure rises, distension of the vessel increases.
- It is capable of opening previously closed capillaries (recruitment).
- It causes flow to occur; in other words, a pressure difference (ΔP) between the arterial and venous

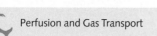
Normal pressures in the pulmonary circulation		
Site	Pressure (mmHg)	Pressure (cmH$_2$O)
Pulmonary artery Systolic/diastolic pressure	24/9	33/11
Mean pressure	14	19
Arteriole (mean pressure)	12	16
Capillary (mean pressure)	10.5	14
Venule (mean pressure)	9.0	12
Left atrium (mean pressure)	8.0	11

Fig. 5.1 Pressures within the pulmonary circulation. The pulmonary arterial and left atrial pressures are measured during cardiac catheterization, the former directly, the latter by wedging the arterial catheter into a branch of the pulmonary artery. The capillary pressure is computed by a standard equation. (Adapted from *Physiology* 3rd ed., by R.M. Berne and M.N. Levy. St. Louis, Mosby Year Book, 1993.)

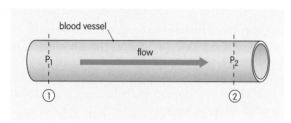

Fig. 5.2 Hydrostatic pressure in terms of driving force, $P_1 - P_2$, i.e., ΔP provides the driving force of the flow.

ends of a vessel provides the driving force for flow (Fig. 5.2).

Pulmonary ΔP is small compared with the systemic circulation, so R must be small to achieve the same flow rate.

Flow = driving force/resistance = $\Delta P/R$

Poiseuille's law tells us that the caliber of a vessel significantly affects resistance to flow and hence the flow rate through a vessel when a particular pressure difference is applied. The pulmonary circulation is, therefore, a low-pressure, low-resistance system.

In situations where increased pulmonary flow is required (e.g., during exercise), the cardiac output is increased, which raises pulmonary vascular pressure. This causes recruitment of previously closed capillaries and distension of already-open capillaries (Fig. 5.3). In turn, this reduces the pulmonary vascular resistance to flow; it is for this reason that resistance to flow through the pulmonary vasculature decreases with increasing pulmonary vascular pressure.

Remember, any resistance to flow causes a drop in downstream pressure; therefore, the hydrostatic pressure in postcapillary venules will be less than that within the capillaries.

Pressure outside pulmonary blood vessels

Pressure outside a vessel can tend either to compress or collapse the vessel if the pressure is positive, or to aid the distension of the vessel if the pressure is negative.

The tendency for a vessel to distend or collapse is also dependent on the pressure inside the lumen. Thus, it is the pressure difference across the wall (or the transmural pressure) which determines whether a vessel compresses or distends (Fig. 5.4).

Pulmonary vessels can be considered in two groups (Fig. 5.5): alveolar and extra-alveolar vessels.

Alveolar vessels

Remember that there is a dense network of capillaries in the alveolar wall; these are the alveolar vessels. External pressure is alveolar pressure (normally atmospheric pressure after inspiration). The diameter of these vessels (capillaries) is dependent on the transmural pressure (i.e., the difference between hydrostatic pressure within the capillary lumen and pressure within the alveolus). If the alveolar pressure is greater than capillary hydrostatic pressure, the capillary will tend to collapse.

Fig. 5.3 In order to minimize pulmonary vascular resistance when pulmonary arterial pressure increases, new vessels are recruited and vessels that are already open are distended.

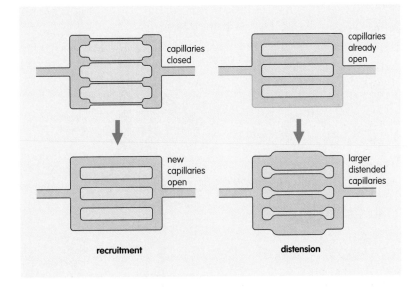

Fig. 5.4 Hydrostatic pressure. (A) Hydrostatic pressure $= \rho \cdot g \cdot h$ [ρ = density of liquid; g = gravity; h = height]. (B) $P_2 > P_1$ because of the height of the column of liquid. $P_3 = P_1$ because they are at the same height. (C) Hydrostatic pressure tends to distend pulmonary vessels, whereas the external pressure tends to collapse them.

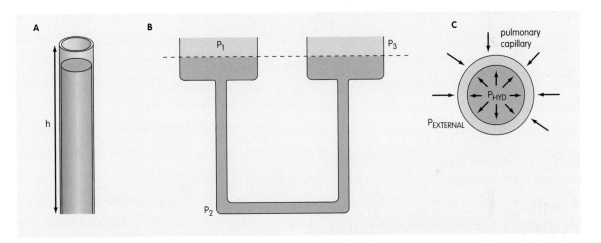

Vessels in the top of the lung, where capillary hydrostatic pressure is lowest, may collapse during inspiration (when vascular pressure is lower than pressure during expiration). This is much more likely during diastole when the venous (capillary) pressure falls below alveolar pressure (see Fig. 5.4).

Extra-alveolar vessels

Extra-alveolar vessels are arteries and veins contained within the lung tissue. As the lungs expand, these vessels are distended by radial traction. The external pressure is similar to intrapleural pressure (subatmospheric—negative).

Because extra-alveolar vessels have an external pressure that is almost always negative, transmural pressure tends to distend these vessels.

During inspiration, intrapleural pressure and thus the pressure outside the extra-alveolar vessels becomes even more negative, causing these vessels to distend even further, reducing vascular resistance and increasing pulmonary blood flow. At large lung

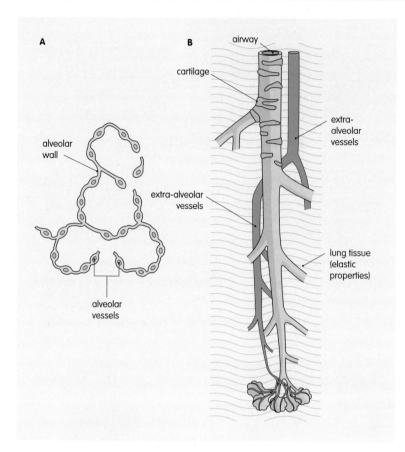

Fig. 5.5 Diagram of (A) alveolar vessels, which are subject to external pressures of alveolar gas, and (B) extra-alveolar vessels contained within lung tissue, subject to intrapleural pressure.

volumes, the effect of radial traction is greater, and the extra-alveolar vessels are distended more.

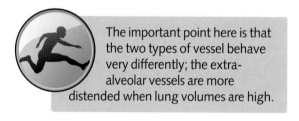

The important point here is that the two types of vessel behave very differently; the extra-alveolar vessels are more distended when lung volumes are high.

Lung volume

Extra-alveolar vessels are distended by increased radial traction associated with increased lung volumes. The capillary, however, is affected in several ways.

Hydrostatic pressure within the capillaries during deep inspiration is lowered. This is caused by a negative intrapleural pressure around the heart. This changes the transmural pressure and the capillaries tend to be compressed, increasing pulmonary vascular resistance (Fig. 5.6).

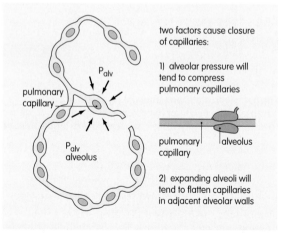

two factors cause closure of capillaries:

1) alveolar pressure will tend to compress pulmonary capillaries

2) expanding alveoli will tend to flatten capillaries in adjacent alveolar walls

Fig. 5.6 Alveolar pressure and capillary compression. The transmural pressure is the difference between hydrostatic pressure inside the capillary and alveolar pressure outside the capillary. P_{alv} = pressure in the alveolus.

At large lung volumes, the alveolar wall is stretched and becomes thinner, compressing the capillaries and increasing vascular resistance.

Smooth muscle within the vascular wall

Smooth muscle in the walls of extra-alveolar vessels tends to reduce their diameter. Thus, the forces caused by radial traction and hydrostatic pressure within the lumen tend to distend these vessels, whereas the tone of the vascular smooth muscle opposes this action. Drugs that lead to contraction of smooth muscle, therefore, increase pulmonary vascular resistance.

The factors affecting the capillary blood flow are:
- Hydrostatic pressure
- Alveolar air pressure
- Lung volume.

The factors affecting extra-alveolar vessels are:
- Hydrostatic pressure
- Intrapleural pressure
- Lung volume
- Smooth muscle tone.

Measurement of pulmonary blood flow

Pulmonary blood flow can be measured by three methods:
- Fick principle (Fig. 5.7)
- Indicator dilution method: a known amount of dye is injected into venous blood and its arterial concentration is measured
- Uptake of inhaled soluble gas (e.g., N_2O): the gas is inhaled and arterial blood values measured.

Both the first and second methods give average blood flow, whereas the third method measures instantaneous flow. The third method relies upon N_2O transfer across the gas exchange surface being perfusion limited.

Fick theorized that because of the laws of conservation of mass, the difference in oxygen concentration between mixed venous blood returning to the pulmonary capillary bed $(O_2)_{pv}$ and arterial blood leaving the heart $(O_2)_{pa}$ must be caused

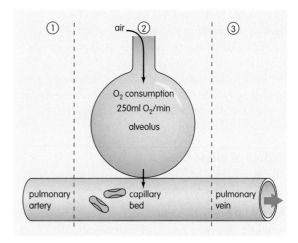

Fig. 5.7 Fick principle for measuring pulmonary blood flow. Fick theorized that the difference in oxygen content between pulmonary venous blood and pulmonary arterial blood must be due to uptake of oxygen in the pulmonary capillaries, therefore the pulmonary blood flow can be calculated.

by uptake of oxygen within the lungs. This uptake must be equal to the body's consumption of oxygen (see Fig. 5.7).

Distribution of blood within the lung

Blood flow within the normal, healthy upright lung is not uniform. Blood flow at the base of the lung is greater than at the apex. Why is this the case?

Because the lungs are vertical in an upright human, they are under the influence of gravity and the pulmonary vessels at the lung base will therefore have a greater hydrostatic pressure than vessels at the apex.

The hydrostatic pressure exerted by a vertical column of fluid is given by the relationship:

$$P = \rho \cdot g \cdot h$$

where ρ = density of the fluid, h = height of the column, and g = acceleration due to gravity.

From the equation above, it can be seen that:
- Vessels at the lung base are subjected to a higher hydrostatic pressure
- The increase in hydrostatic pressure will distend these vessels, lowering the resistance to blood flow. Thus, pulmonary blood flow in the base will be greater than in the apex.

Ventilation also increases from apex to base but is less affected than blood flow because the density of air is much less than blood. In diastole, the hydrostatic pressure in the pulmonary artery is $11\,cmH_2O$. The apex of each lung is approximately 15 cm above the right ventricle, and the hydrostatic pressure within these vessels is lowered or even zero. Vessels at the apex of the lung are therefore narrower or even collapse because of the lower hydrostatic pressure within them.

Pattern of blood flow
The distribution of blood flow within the lung can be described in three zones (Fig. 5.8).

Zone 1 (at the apex of the lung)
In zone 1, arterial pressure is less than alveolar pressure: capillaries collapse and no flow occurs. Note that under normal conditions, there is no zone 1 because there is sufficient pressure to perfuse the apices.

Zone 2
In zone 2, arterial pressure is greater than alveolar pressure, which is greater than venous pressure. Postcapillary venules open and close depending on hydrostatic pressure (i.e., hydrostatic pressure difference in systole and diastole). Flow is determined by the arterial–alveolar pressure difference (transmural pressure).

Zone 3 (at the base of the lung)
In zone 3, arterial pressure is greater than venous pressure, which is greater than alveolar pressure. Blood flow is determined by arteriovenous pressure difference as in the systemic circulation.

Control of pulmonary blood flow
We have already mentioned how the pulmonary circulation adapts to changes of hydrostatic pressure and how it can recruit capillaries during exercise. These effects are passive and caused by changes in hydrostatic pressure. The pulmonary blood flow can also be controlled by other local mechanisms to improve efficiency of gaseous exchange. Like the systemic circulation, other mediators such as thromboxane, histamine, and prostacylin also alter pulmonary vascular tone.

Contraction and relaxation of smooth muscle contained within the walls of arteries, arterioles, and veins is the mechanism for active control of pulmonary blood flow. An important mechanism of control, particularly in disease, is hypoxic vasoconstriction.

Hypoxic vasoconstriction
The aim of breathing is to oxygenate the blood sufficiently. This is achieved by efficient gaseous

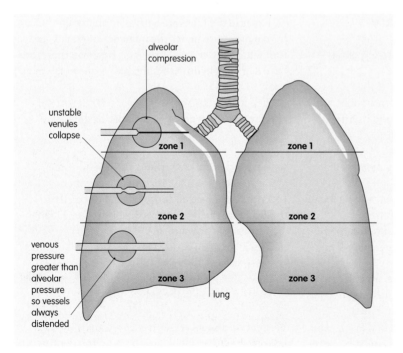

Fig. 5.8 Zones of pulmonary blood flow.

exchange between alveolar gas and the bloodstream. If an area of lung is poorly ventilated and the alveolar partial pressure of oxygen (alveolar oxygen tension) is low, perfusion of this area with blood will lead to inefficient gaseous exchange. It would be more beneficial to perfuse an area that is well ventilated. This is the basis behind hypoxic vasoconstriction. Small pulmonary arteries and arterioles are in close proximity to the gas exchange surface, and vessels in and around the alveolar wall are surrounded by alveolar gas. Oxygen passes through the alveolar walls into the smooth muscle of the blood vessel by diffusion. The extremely high oxygen tension to which these smooth muscles are normally exposed acts to dilate the pulmonary vessels. In contrast, if the alveolar oxygen tension is low, pulmonary blood vessels are constricted, which leads to reduced blood flow in the area of lung which is poorly ventilated and diversion to other regions where alveolar oxygen tension is high.

It should be noted that it is the partial pressure of oxygen in the alveolus (P_AO_2) and not in the pulmonary artery (P_aO_2) that causes this response.

The actual mechanism and the chemical mediators involved in hypoxic vasoconstriction are not known. Many mediators have been investigated, and nitric oxide has been shown to reverse the vasoconstriction. Factors that regulate pulmonary vascular tone are shown in Fig. 5.9.

In summary:
- The aim of ventilation is to oxygenate blood sufficiently and blow off carbon dioxide.
- High levels of alveolar oxygen dilate pulmonary vessels.
- Low levels of alveolar oxygen constrict pulmonary blood vessels.
- This aims to produce efficient gaseous exchange.

Higher than normal alveolar carbon dioxide partial pressures also cause pulmonary blood vessels to constrict, thus reducing blood flow to an area that is not well ventilated.

Pulmonary water balance

Figure 5.10 shows the structure of the alveolar–capillary membrane. Note that on one side there is the interstitial space while on the other the epithelial and endothelial membranes are fused and there is only a tiny membrane between pulmonary capillary blood and the alveolus. It is essential for gas exchange that this surface is kept dry; the mechanisms by which liquid is prevented from entering are discussed below.

Fluids in the pulmonary capillary and interstitial spaces obey Starling's forces (Fig. 5.11). In addition, surfactant lowers the surface tension of the alveolar lining fluid, thus reducing the transudation of liquid into the alveolus by increasing the interstitial pressure to −4mmHg. Without surfactant, the higher surface tension would produce a greater negative interstitial hydrostatic pressure. Hydrostatic

Factors that regulate vascular tone	
Vasodilation	**Vasoconstriction**
Nitric oxide	Histamine
Prostacyclin	Serotonin
Prostaglandin	Thromboxane
Bradykinin	Leukotrienes
Acetylcholine	Platelet activating factor
	Angiotensin II
	Endothelin

Fig. 5.9 Factors that regulate vascular tone.

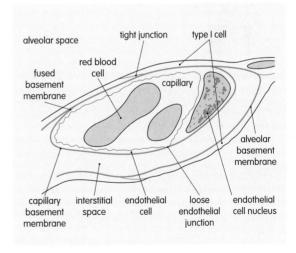

Fig. 5.10 The alveolar–capillary membrane. Note that the basement membranes of the alveolus and capillary are fused on one side; on the other is the interstitial space. (Adapted with permission from *Crofton and Douglas's Respiratory Diseases*, Vol 1, 5th ed. London, Blackwell Science, 2000.)

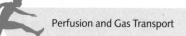

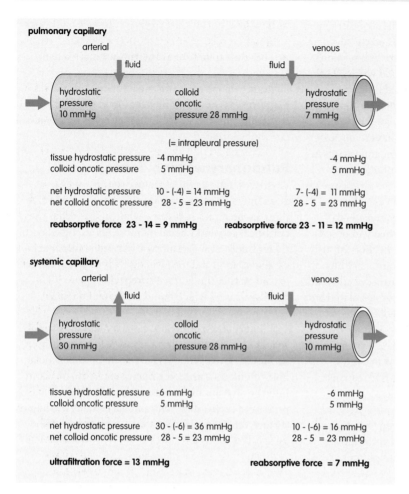

Fig. 5.11 Comparison of Starling's forces between pulmonary and systemic capillary beds. The resorptive force is positive and hence fluid is reabsorbed into the pulmonary capillary. Without surfactant in the alveoli the tissue hydrostatic pressure could be −23 mmHg and the reabsorptive force would be −10 mmHg, causing transudation of fluid into the alveolus.

pressure within the capillary tends to force fluid out into the interstitial space. The colloid osmotic pressure difference between interstitial space and capillary tends to force fluid into the capillary.

The resultant fluid flow from capillary to interstitial space is small and normally fluid drains to lymphatics and the perivascular space. Under pathologic conditions, fluid can reside either in the interstitial space (interstitial edema) or in the alveoli (alveolar edema). This may be due to an increase in:

• Hydrostatic pressure in the pulmonary capillaries
• Permeability of the capillaries.

Adult respiratory distress syndrome (ARDS) is noncardiogenic pulmonary edema caused by capillaries which have become acutely inflamed and "leaky."

The ventilation:perfusion relationship

Basic concepts

To achieve efficient gaseous exchange, it is essential that the flow of gas (ventilation: $\dot{V}$) and the flow of blood (perfusion: $\dot{Q}$) are closely matched.

The ideal situation would be where:

• All alveoli are ventilated equally with gas of identical composition and pressure
• All pulmonary capillaries in the alveolar wall are perfused equally with mixed venous blood.

Unfortunately, this is not the case. Ventilation is not uniform throughout the lung; neither is perfusion.

The partial pressure of oxygen in the alveoli

determines the amount of oxygen transferred to the blood. Two factors affect the partial pressure of oxygen in the alveoli: the amount of ventilation (i.e., the addition of oxygen to the alveolar compartment) and the perfusion of blood through pulmonary capillaries (i.e., the removal of oxygen from the alveolar compartment).

It is the ratio of ventilation to perfusion that determines the concentration of oxygen in the alveolar compartment.

Ventilation : perfusion ratio

By looking at the ventilation : perfusion ratio, we can see how well ventilation and perfusion are matched.

By definition, ventilation : perfusion ratio = $\dot{V}_A/\dot{Q}$, where $\dot{V}_A$ = alveolar minute ventilation (usually about 4.2 L/min); $\dot{Q}$ = pulmonary blood flow (usually about 5.0 L/min).

Thus, normal $\dot{V}_A/\dot{Q} = 0.84$ (i.e., approximately 1).

This is an average value across the lung. Different ventilation : perfusion ratios are present throughout the lung from apex to base (Fig. 5.12).

Extremes of ventilation : perfusion ratio

Looking at the ventilation : perfusion ratio, it can be seen that there are two extremes to this relationship. These extremes were introduced in Chapter 1. Either there is:

- No ventilation (a shunt): $\dot{V}_A/\dot{Q} = 0$
- No perfusion (dead space): $\dot{V}_A/\dot{Q} = \infty$.

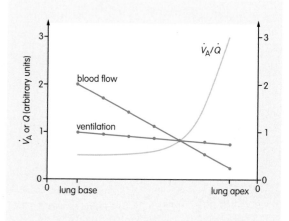

Fig. 5.12 Distribution of ventilation ($\dot{V}_A$) and perfusion ($\dot{Q}$). Blood flow and ventilation are both higher at the lung base but the difference in blood flow is more striking. (Adapted from *Respiratory Physiology*, 2nd ed., by J. Widdicombe and A. Davies. London, Edward Arnold, 1991.)

Right-to-left shunt

A right-to-left shunt is described when the pulmonary circulation bypasses the ventilation process (Fig. 5.13), either by:

- Bypassing the lungs completely (e.g. transposition of great vessels, see Chapter 3)
- Perfusion of an area of lung that is not ventilated.

The shunted blood will not have been oxygenated or been able to given up its carbon dioxide. Therefore, its levels of PO_2 and PCO_2 are those of venous blood. When added to the systemic circulation, this blood will proportionally decrease arterial PO_2; it is called the venous admixture.

A right-to-left shunt may cause a low arterial PO_2 but a normal PCO_2—how can this be explained? The venous admixture has a low arterial PO_2 and high PCO_2. This initially causes the arterial PO_2 to be lowered and the arterial PCO_2 to be increased. This high PCO_2 causes an increase in ventilation, which reduces PCO_2 in those areas of lung that are well ventilated, giving them a lower than normal PCO_2. This reduction in PCO_2 lowers the arterial PCO_2 to its normal value. This additional ventilation in well-ventilated areas, however, has very little effect on the arterial oxygen content because of the shape of the oxyhemoglobin dissociation curve (i.e., hemoglobin is already saturated in the well-ventilated areas). Only a small increase in oxygen content is seen because of increased dissolved oxygen from the overventilated areas. This small increase in PO_2 from

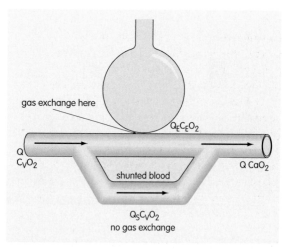

Fig. 5.13 Shunted blood. The shunted blood has a low oxygen concentration (i.e., of venous blood) and is known as the venous admixture.

overventilated areas is unable to increase the arterial PO_2 to its normal value. Thus, the mixed blood has a lower PO_2 and normal PCO_2.

In normal subjects, there is only a very small amount of shunt (about 1%). However, right-to-left shunt makes a significant contribution to abnormal gas exchange in some disease states, notably:

- Cyanotic congenital heart disease
- Pulmonary edema
- Severe pneumonia.

Giving oxygen to patients with shunt does not increase arterial oxygen tension. This makes sense because:

- Shunted blood is not actually exposed to the oxygen
- Hemoglobin is already saturated in well-ventilated areas.

Effect of V̇/Q̇ mismatch on blood gases

The easiest way to imagine how the ventilation:perfusion ratio affects the arterial oxygen concentration is to look at the extremes of ventilation:perfusion.

Ventilation but no perfusion

If a unit of lung is ventilated but not perfused, that unit will have a PO_2 and PCO_2 of inspired gas, because no gas exchange with the blood has taken place (Fig. 5.14C). If the perfusion of the unit increases (lowering the ventilation:perfusion ratio), alveolar PCO_2 will rise and the PO_2 will fall (an example of lung normally perfused is shown in Fig. 5.14A).

Perfusion but no ventilation

If the perfusion is increased further and the ventilation reduced until the unit of lung is perfused but not ventilated, the gas within that unit will be in equilibrium with the blood perfusing the alveolar capillaries (venous blood), because no gas exchange has taken place (Fig. 5.14B). This relationship is also described in Fig. 5.15; read the caption to work through the figure.

It should be noted that:

- Alveolar (and thus end capillary) PO_2 varies to a much greater extent than PCO_2 with small changes from normal in ventilation:perfusion ratio.
- Overall, variation in PO_2 is much greater than that of PCO_2.
- PCO_2 cannot rise above that of mixed venous blood.

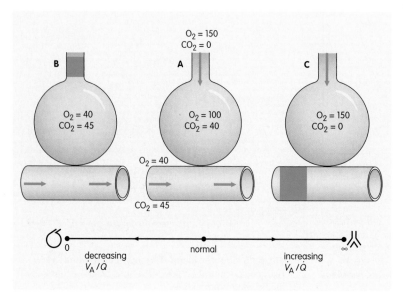

Fig. 5.14 The effect of altering the ventilation:perfusion ratio on the P_AO_2 and P_ACO_2 in a lung unit. (A) Normal lung; (B) lung unit is not ventilated; O_2 falls and CO_2 rises within lung unit; (C) lung unit is not perfused; O_2 is not taken up and CO_2 does not diffuse into the alveolus.

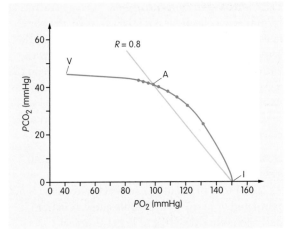

Fig. 5.15 The effect of altering the ventilation:perfusion ratio on both PO_2 and PCO_2. Point A represents normal arterial values of PO_2 and PCO_2 at a value of ventilation:perfusion ratio of 0.84 when the respiratory exchange ratio (R) = 0.8. (R is the ratio of CO_2 produced to oxygen consumed; 0.8 is the normal value.) Increasing ventilation:perfusion ratios reduces PCO_2 but causes a corresponding rise in PO_2. Eventually point I is reached, where PCO_2 is zero and PO_2 is equal to that of inspired gas; this relates to a point of infinite ventilation:perfusion (i.e., there is no perfusion). Point V represents the opposite end of the ventilation:perfusion spectrum where the lung is not ventilated at all. The alveolar end capillary blood partial pressures of oxygen and carbon dioxide are the same as mixed venous values. Thus values of ventilation:perfusion ratio greater than normal are to the right of point A and those that are less are to the left. (Adapted from *Physiology*, 3rd ed., by R.M. Berne and M.N. Levy. St. Louis, Mosby Year Book, 1993.)

Regional variation of ventilation and perfusion

Both ventilation and perfusion increase towards the lung base because of the effects of gravity.

Because the blood has a greater density than air, the gravitational effects on perfusion are much greater than on ventilation. This leads to a regional variation (see Fig. 5.12) in ventilation:perfusion ratio from lung apex (high $\dot{V}/\dot{Q}$) to lung base (low $\dot{V}/\dot{Q}$).

These regional variations in ventilation:perfusion ratio are caused by the lung being upright; thus, changes in posture will alter the ventilation:perfusion ratio throughout the lung. For example, when lying down, the posterior area of the lung has a low ventilation:perfusion ratio and the anterior area has a high ventilation:perfusion ratio. The effect of high and low ventilation:perfusion ratios on carbon dioxide and oxygen in the alveolus and blood is highlighted in Fig. 5.16 and described below.

At low ventilation:perfusion ratios (e.g., at the lung base)

Effect on carbon dioxide concentrations Carbon dioxide diffuses from the blood to alveoli; however, because ventilation is low relative to perfusion, carbon dioxide is not taken away as rapidly. Thus, carbon dioxide tends to accumulate in the alveolus until a new, higher steady-state P_ACO_2 is reached.

Diffusion occurs only until equilibrium is achieved, when P_aCO_2 is equal to P_ACO_2. If there were no ventilation, the P_ACO_2 of this lung unit would rise quickly to meet mixed venous P_vCO_2, and no diffusion could take place.

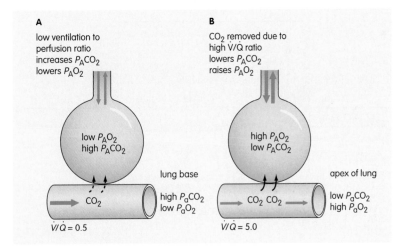

Fig. 5.16 Ventilation and perfusion at lung base (A) and apex (B). At the lung base perfusion is high and the $\dot{V}/\dot{Q}$ ratio is low. This reduces alveolar O_2 and raises CO_2. At the apex the $\dot{V}/\dot{Q}$ ratio is higher, leading to a high alveolar O_2 and more CO_2 blown off.

A low ventilation to perfusion ratio increases P_ACO_2 lowers P_AO_2

low P_AO_2 high P_ACO_2

lung base

CO_2

high P_aCO_2 low P_aO_2

$\dot{V}/\dot{Q} = 0.5$

B CO_2 removed due to high $\dot{V}/Q$ ratio lowers P_ACO_2 raises P_AO_2

high P_AO_2 low P_ACO_2

apex of lung

CO_2 CO_2

low P_aCO_2 high P_aO_2

$\dot{V}/\dot{Q} = 5.0$

85

Assuming that the overall lung function is normal, this regional variation in P_aCO_2 will not affect overall P_vCO_2. Thus, reducing the ventilation:perfusion ratio will not increase P_aCO_2 above the mixed venous value.

Effect on oxygen concentrations Oxygen diffuses from the alveolus into the blood; however, because ventilation is low, oxygen taken up by the blood and metabolized is not replenished fully by new air entering the lungs. Oxygen in the alveolus is depleted until a new, lower steady-state P_AO_2 is reached. Because diffusion continues until equilibrium is achieved, the P_aO_2 of this unit will also be low (Fig. 5.16A).

At high ventilation:perfusion ratios (e.g. at the lung apex)

Effect on carbon dioxide concentrations The carbon dioxide diffusing from the blood is nearly all removed; carbon dioxide in the alveolus is depleted until a new, lower steady-state P_ACO_2 is reached. Diffusion continues until equilibrium is achieved: P_aCO_2 will also be low.

If we take this to the extreme, then as ventilation:perfusion ratios tend to infinity, P_ACO_2 tends to zero.

Effect on oxygen concentrations Oxygen diffusing from the alveolar gas is not taken away by the blood in such large amounts because the relative blood flow is reduced; in addition, oxygen is replenished with each breath. Thus, oxygen tends to accumulate in the alveolus until a new steady-state concentration is reached (Fig. 5.16B).

Diffusion occurs until a new higher equilibrium is achieved; thus, P_aO_2 is also higher.

How do regional variations in $\dot{V}/\dot{Q}$ affect overall gas exchange?

As mentioned previously, a normal healthy lung is not ventilated or perfused uniformly and ventilation:perfusion ratios vary (Fig. 5.17). The actual difference between gaseous exchange in a healthy lung and in an ideal lung is perhaps smaller than one might expect. The ideal lung is capable of only 2–3% more gaseous exchange.

However, if the ventilation:perfusion inequality from lung apex to base becomes more severe, the transfer of oxygen and carbon dioxide will be significantly affected. The majority of the blood will come from poorly ventilated areas at the lung base, where P_AO_2 is low; thus P_aO_2 will be low. P_aCO_2 will similarly be raised at the base of the lung.

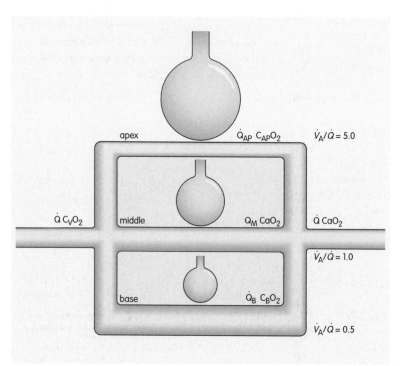

Fig. 5.17 Ventilation and perfusion at the lung apex, middle, and base.

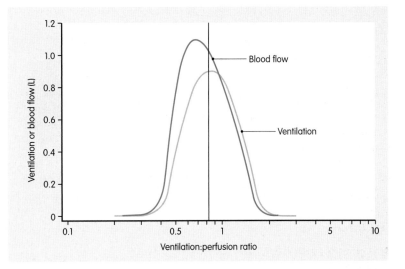

Fig. 5.18 Normal human ventilation:perfusion curves. Note that ventilation and perfusion are matched in health. At the average $\dot{V}/\dot{Q}$ ratio of 0.8, blood flows to the areas that are well ventilated.

The nonlinear shape of the oxyhemoglobin dissociation curve does not allow areas with high ventilation:perfusion ratios to compensate for areas of low ratio.

Ventilation:perfusion distributions If we look at the variation in ventilation and blood flow in relation to $\dot{V}/\dot{Q}$ in the normal lung (Fig. 5.18), it should be noted that:

• Where the ventilation:perfusion ratio is high, absolute values of ventilation are low
• Where the ventilation:perfusion ratio is low, absolute values of blood flow are also low.

Thus, the majority of blood flow and ventilation go to areas of lung that have a ventilation:perfusion ratio that is close to the average value. In the diseased lung, this might not be the case and blood may flow to areas where ventilation:perfusion ratios are extremely low; this is effectively a shunt.

Areas with extremely high ventilation:perfusion ratios may be ventilated to high absolute values and receive very poor blood flow. This is effectively wasted ventilation.

Measurement of ventilation and perfusion
Ventilation:perfusion scans
In clinical practice, ventilation:perfusion ratios are assessed primarily by means of radioisotope scans. Ventilation is detected by inhalation of a gas or aerosol labeled with the radioisotope, Xe^{133}. The distribution of pulmonary blood flow is tested with an intravenous injection of Tc^{99m}-labeled macroaggregated albumin (MAA). These radioactive particles are larger than the diameter of the pulmonary capillaries, and they remain lodged for several hours. A gamma camera is then used to detect the position of the MAAs.

The two scans are then assessed together for "filling defects," or areas where ventilation and perfusion are not matched. The technique is primarily used to detect pulmonary emboli. Spiral CT scans are now superseding this technique. Figure 5.19 shows a lung scan following pulmonary embolism.

Multiple inert gas procedure
As noted above, radioisotope scans can allow only a broad comparison to be made between areas of ventilation and perfusion in the lungs. The multiple inert gas procedure measures the actual ratio of ventilation:perfusion, but is a much more complicated technique. In the multiple inert gas procedure, six inert gases are infused into the venous bloodstream. Each gas has a different partition coefficient in gas and blood (i.e., different solubility in gas and blood).

Steady state is reached by a constant rate of infusion and expiration. From component balances for each gas of amount infused and amount expired the ventilation:perfusion distribution is calculated.

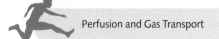
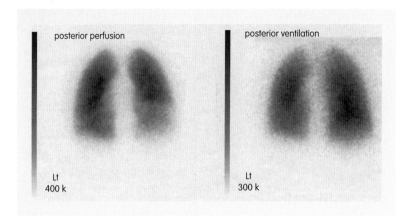

Fig. 5.19 Ventilation:perfusion scan following pulmonary embolus. (Courtesy of Ivor Jones and the Nuclear Medicine staff, Derriford Hospital, Plymouth.)

$$\text{Amount infused} = P\text{in} \cdot S \cdot \dot{Q}$$
$$\text{Amount expired} = P\text{ex} \cdot \dot{V}$$

where S = solubility of the gas.

Thus, ventilation and perfusion can be calculated giving a ventilation:perfusion distribution.

Gas transport in the blood

Oxygen transport
Oxygen is carried in the blood in two forms:
- Dissolved in plasma
- Bound to hemoglobin.

Dissolved oxygen
To meet the metabolic demands of the body, large amounts of oxygen must be carried in the blood. We have seen that the amount of gas dissolved in solution is proportional to the partial pressure of the gas (Henry's law). The solubility of oxygen in the blood is low: 0.000225ml of oxygen per kilopascal per milliliter of blood. With normal arterial P_aO_2 (100mmHg; 13.3kPa), for each milliliter of blood there is only 0.003ml of dissolved oxygen.

Normal cardiac output is 5.0L/min; it is therefore capable of supplying:

$$5 \times 1000 \times 0.003 = 15\text{ml of oxygen per minute}$$

At rest, the body requires approximately 250ml of oxygen per minute. Thus, if all the oxygen in the blood was carried in the dissolved form, cardiac output would meet only 6% of the demand at rest.

In fact, in contrast to the tiny amounts calculated above, the oxygen content of blood is approximately 200ml of oxygen per liter of arterial blood.

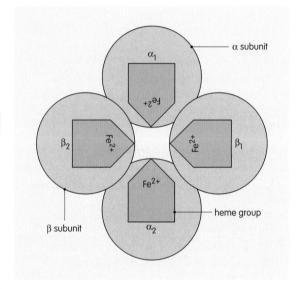

Fig. 5.20 Schematic diagram of hemoglobin: α subunit consists of a polypeptide chain of 141 amino acids and one heme group; β subunit consists of a polypeptide chain of 146 amino acids and one heme group.

Therefore, most of the oxygen must be carried in chemical combination, not in simple solution. Oxygen is combined with hemoglobin.

Hemoglobin
Hemoglobin (Hb) is found in red blood cells and is a conjugate protein molecule, containing iron within its structure. The molecule consists of four polypeptide subunits, two α and two β. Associated with each polypeptide chain is a heme group that acts as a binding site for oxygen (Fig. 5.20).

The heme group consists of a porphyrin ring containing iron and is responsible for binding of oxygen:

- Hemoglobin contains iron in a ferrous (Fe^{2+}) or ferric (Fe^{3+}) state.
- Only hemoglobin in the ferrous form can bind oxygen.
- Methemoglobin (containing iron in a ferric state) cannot bind oxygen.

The quaternary structure of hemoglobin determines its ability to bind oxygen.

In its deoxygenated state, hemoglobin (known as reduced hemoglobin) has a low affinity for oxygen. The binding of one oxygen molecule to hemoglobin causes a conformational change in its protein structure; this positive cooperativity allows easier access to the other oxygen-binding sites, thus increasing hemoglobin's affinity for further binding of oxygen. Hemoglobin is capable of binding up to four molecules of oxygen.

$$Hb + 4O_2 \rightarrow Hb(O_2)_4$$

It should be noted that during this reaction the iron atom of the heme group remains in the ferrous Fe^{2+} form. It is not oxidized to the ferric Fe^{3+} form. The interaction of oxygen with hemoglobin is oxygenation, not oxidation.

The main function of hemoglobin is to take up oxygen in the blood at the alveolar capillary membrane and to transport oxygen within the blood and release it into the tissues. However, hemoglobin also has other functions:

- Buffering of H^+ ions
- Transport of CO_2 as carbamino compounds.

Hemoglobin binding

Hemoglobin has four binding sites; the amount of oxygen carried by hemoglobin in the blood depends on how many of these binding sites are occupied. Therefore, the hemoglobin molecule can be said to be saturated or partially saturated:

- Saturated—all four binding sites are occupied by O_2
- Partially saturated—some oxygen has bound to hemoglobin, but not all four sites are occupied.

If completely saturated, each gram of hemoglobin can carry 1.34ml of oxygen. There are 15g of

hemoglobin per deciliter of blood; therefore, the maximum binding of oxygen to hemoglobin we could expect is:

$$15 \times 1.34 = 20.1ml \text{ of oxygen per deciliter of blood}$$

In addition, there is approximately 0.3ml/dl of O_2 in solution. The total (20.4ml) is called the oxygen-carrying capacity; the hemoglobin is said to be 100% saturated ($SO_2 = 100\%$). The actual amount of oxygen bound to hemoglobin and dissolved in the blood at any one time is called the oxygen content.

The oxygen saturation (SO_2) of the blood is defined as the amount of oxygen carried in the blood, expressed as a percentage of oxygen-carrying capacity:

$$SO_2 = O_2 \text{ content} \div O_2 \text{ capacity} \times 100$$

Cyanosis

Hemoglobin absorbs light of different wavelengths, depending on whether it is in the reduced or oxygenated form. Oxyhemoglobin appears bright red, whereas reduced hemoglobin appears purplish, giving a bluish pallor to skin. This is called cyanosis, which can be described as either central or peripheral. Cyanosis depends on the absolute amount of deoxygenated hemoglobin in the vessels, not the proportion of deoxygenated:oxygenated hemoglobin. In central cyanosis, there is more than 5g/dl deoxygenated hemoglobin in the blood and this can be seen in the peripheral tissues (e.g., lips, tongue). Peripheral cyanosis is due to a local cause (e.g., vascular obstruction of a limb).

It follows that an anemic patient with low hemoglobin may become dangerously desaturated without appearing cyanotic!

Oxygen dissociation curve

How much oxygen binds to hemoglobin is dependent upon the partial pressure of oxygen in the blood. This relationship is represented by the oxygen dissociation curve (Fig. 5.21A); this is an equilibrium curve at specific conditions:

- 15g of hemoglobin per deciliter of blood
- pH 7.4
- Temperature 37°C.

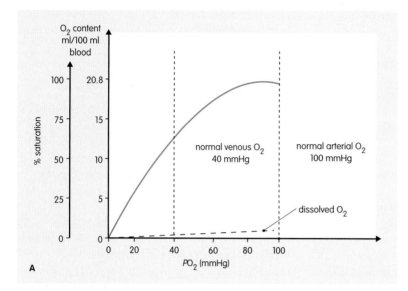

Fig. 5.21 (A) Oxyhemoglobin dissociation curve. (B) The effect of temperature, PCO_2, pH, and 2,3-DPG on the oxyhemoglobin dissociation curve. In both graphs, O_2 content is based on the assumption of hemoglobin concentration of 15g/100ml of blood.

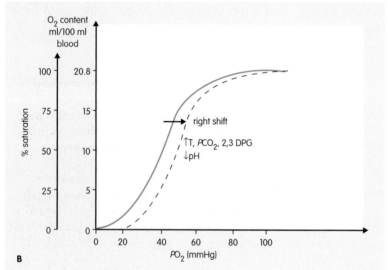

You will need to be able to visualize the oxygen dissociation curve in your exams. The easiest way to remember it is by using four points. Values at 25%, 50%, 75%, and 100% saturation are useful markers, and the curve is easily drawn from the origin through these points. You will also need to remember arterial and mixed venous blood partial pressures of oxygen.

Factors affecting the oxygen dissociation curve

The shape of the curve, and therefore oxygen delivery to the tissues, is affected by a number of factors, including:
- pH
- CO_2
- Temperature
- Other forms of hemoglobin.

These factors shift the oxygen dissociation curve to the right or to the left:
- A shift to the right allows easier dissociation of oxygen (i.e., lower oxygen saturation at any

particular PO_2) and increases the oxygen release from oxyhemoglobin.

- A shift to the left makes oxygen binding easier (i.e., higher oxygen saturation at any particular PO_2) and increases the oxygen uptake by hemoglobin.

The following factors shift the curve to the right (Fig. 5.21B):

- Increased PCO_2 and decreased pH (increased hydrogen ion concentration), known as the Bohr shift
- Increased temperature
- Increase in 2,3-diphosphoglycerate (2,3-DPG), which binds to the β chains.

2,3-Diphosphoglycerate is a product of anaerobic metabolism. Red blood cells possess no mitochondria and therefore carry out anaerobic metabolism to produce energy. 2,3-DPG binds more strongly to reduced hemoglobin than to oxyhemoglobin. Concentrations of 2,3-diphosphoglycerate increase in chronic hypoxia (e.g., in patients with chronic lung disease) or at high altitude.

If you cannot remember how the above factors affect the oxygen dissociation curve, it is helpful to think of exercising muscle. It would be useful if its blood supply gave up oxygen more easily (right shift of the curve). An exercising muscle produces carbon dioxide (increased carbon dioxide), which forms carbonic acid in the blood, which in turn dissociates to form hydrogen ions (lowers the pH). Exercising muscle is hot (increased temperature) and uses up oxygen forming more reduced hemoglobin in red blood cells (increased 2,3-DPG concentration).

Other forms of hemoglobin
Myoglobin
Myoglobin is an iron-containing molecule found within skeletal muscle and cardiac muscle. It consists of a single polypeptide chain with a heme group:

- Myoglobin is capable of binding oxygen.

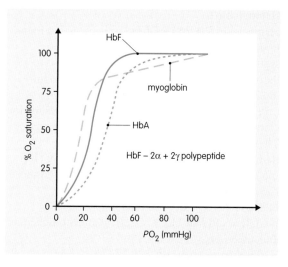

Fig. 5.22 Comparison of oxygen dissociation curves for myoglobin, fetal hemoglobin (HbF), and adult hemoglobin (HbA). (Adapted from *Physiology*, 3rd ed., by R.M. Berne and M.N. Levy. St. Louis, Mosby Year Book, 1993.)

- It acts as a temporary storage of oxygen within skeletal muscle.
- Myoglobin has a higher affinity for oxygen than does normal adult hemoglobin (HbA), seen as a shift to the left of the dissociation curve (Fig. 5.22).
- Myoglobin is unsuitable for oxygen transport, because it binds oxygen at partial pressures below those of mixed venous blood (<40mmHg) and so could not readily release O_2 to the tissues.

Fetal hemoglobin (HbF)
Fetal hemoglobin differs from adult hemoglobin by having two γ chains instead of two β chains (see Fig. 5.22).

Fetal hemoglobin has a higher affinity for oxygen because its γ chains bind 2,3-DPG less avidly than the β chains of adult hemoglobin and are therefore able to bind oxygen at lower partial pressures (maternal venous P_vO_2 is low: <40mmHg).

Release of carbon dioxide from fetal hemoglobin causes a shift to the left of the fetal oxyhemoglobin dissociation curve, thus increasing its affinity for oxygen. This released carbon dioxide binds to maternal hemoglobin, causing a shift to the right of maternal hemoglobin, thus reducing the affinity of the latter for oxygen. Oxygen is therefore released by maternal hemoglobin and bound by fetal hemoglobin. This is known as the double Bohr shift.

Hemoglobin S

Hemoglobin S (HbS) is a form of hemoglobin found in sickle cell anemia. Sickle cell anemia is an autosomal recessive disorder in which there is a defect in the β-globulin chain of the hemoglobin molecule.

There is a substitution of the amino acid valine for glutamine at position 6 of the β chain, forming HbS. The heterozygote has sickle cell trait and the homozygote sickle cell anemia. The abnormal HbS molecules polymerize when deoxygenated and cause the red blood cells containing the abnormal hemoglobin to sickle. The fragile sickle cells hemolyze and may block vessels, leading to ischemia and infarction.

The heterozygous patient may have painful crises with bone and abdominal pain; there may also be intrapulmonary shunting.

Thalassemia

The thalassemias are autosomal recessive disorders due to decreased production of either the α or the β chain of hemoglobin.

There are two genes for the β chain and, depending on the number of normal genes, the β thalassemia is quoted as major or minor. There are four genes which code for the α chain, leading to various clinical disorders depending on the genetic defect.

HbA_2 is present in a small amount in the normal population and consists of two α and two δ chains. It is markedly raised in β thalassemia minor.

Carboxyhemoglobin (carbon monoxide poisoning)

Carbon monoxide (CO) displaces oxygen from oxyhemoglobin because the affinity of hemoglobin for carbon monoxide is more than 200 times that for oxygen. This changes the shape of the oxyhemoglobin dissociation curve. Note that in Fig. 5.23, showing the effects of carbon monoxide poisoning:

- In this instance, oxygen capacity is 50% of normal (i.e., 50% HbO_2 and 50% HbCO). The actual value will depend on the partial pressure of CO (e.g., with a PCO of 16mmHg, 75% of Hb will be in the form of HbCO).
- Saturation is achieved at a PO_2 of <40mmHg (below venous PO_2).
- HbCO causes a shift to the left for the oxygen dissociation curve (i.e., HbCO has a higher affinity for oxygen than normal HbO_2).

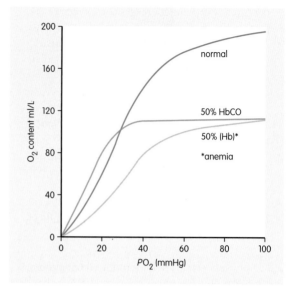

Fig. 5.23 Oxyhemoglobin curve showing effects of anemia and carbon monoxide poisoning (50% HbCO and anemia compared with normal hemoglobin). (Adapted from *Physiology*, 3rd ed., by R.M. Berne and M.N. Levy. St. Louis, Mosby Year Book, 1993.)

- Carbon monoxide binds to two of the four available heme groups.
- Carbon monoxide takes a long time to be cleared, but this can be speeded up by ventilation with 100% oxygen.
- The patient is not cyanosed, because HbCO is cherry-red.

Carbon dioxide transport

There are three ways in which carbon dioxide can be transported in the blood:
- Dissolved in plasma
- As bicarbonate ions
- As carbamino compounds.

Dissolved carbon dioxide

The solubility of carbon dioxide in the blood is much greater than that of oxygen (20 times greater); so, unlike oxygen, a significant amount (approximately 10%) of carbon dioxide is carried in solution.

The solubility of carbon dioxide = 0.07ml of carbon dioxide per mmHg per deciliter of blood.

Normal P_aCO_2 = 40mmHg

So the normal dissolved carbon dioxide = 27.4ml of carbon dioxide per liter of blood.

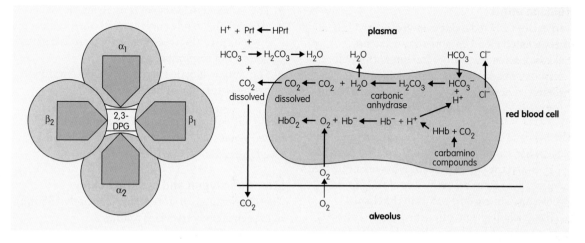

Fig. 5.24 Exchange of CO_2 from the blood to the alveolus in pulmonary capillaries. The reactions illustrated are reversed in the tissues of the systemic circulation, where O_2 is taken up by the tissues and CO_2 is taken up by the blood and erythrocytes. (Adapted from *Physiology*, 3rd ed., by R.M. Berne and M.N. Levy. St. Louis, Mosby Year Book, 1993.)

Bicarbonate ions

Approximately 60% of carbon dioxide added to blood in systemic capillaries is transported as bicarbonate ions. Dissolved carbon dioxide interacts with water to form carbonic acid as follows:

$$CO_2 + H_2O \leftrightarrow H_2CO_3 \qquad (1)$$

Carbonic acid rapidly dissociates into ions:

$$H_2CO_3 \leftrightarrow H^+ + HCO_3^- \qquad (2)$$

The total reaction being:

$$CO_2 + H_2O \leftrightarrow H_2CO_3 \leftrightarrow H^+ + HCO_3^-$$

The first reaction is very slow in plasma, but within the red blood cell it is dramatically speeded up by the enzyme, carbonic anhydrase. Reaction (2) is very fast, but if allowed to proceed alone, a large amount of H$^+$ ions would be formed, slowing down or halting the reaction. Hemoglobin has the property that it can bind H$^+$ ions and act as a buffer, thus allowing the reaction to proceed rapidly.

$$H^+ + HbO_2^- \leftrightarrow HHb + O_2$$
$$H^+ + Hb^- \leftrightarrow HHb$$

Reduced Hb can bind H$^+$ more actively; this is because reduced Hb is less acidic. The buffering capacities of hemoglobin and oxyhemoglobin are conferred by the imidazole groups of the 36 histidine residues in the hemoglobin molecule. The imidazole groups dissociate less readily in the deoxygenated form of hemoglobin, which is therefore a weaker acid and so a better buffer. This action reduces H$^+$ ions in the plasma and also pulls the second reaction to the right.

The bicarbonate produced in the red blood cells diffuses down its concentration gradient into the plasma in exchange for chloride ions (Cl$^-$). This process is known as the chloride shift. In the lung, these reactions are reversed. Bicarbonate is taken up by red blood cells in exchange for Cl$^-$, H_2CO_3 is converted to $CO_2 + H_2O$ by carbonic anhydrase, and the CO_2 diffuses down its concentration gradient to the plasma and alveolus (Fig. 5.24).

Carbamino compounds

Carbon dioxide is capable of combining with proteins, interacting with their terminal amine groups to form carbamino compounds. In the lung, the reverse reaction occurs (see Fig. 5.24). The most important protein involved is hemoglobin, as it is the most abundant in the blood. It is also important to note that:

- The interaction of carbon dioxide and hemoglobin is rapid.
- No enzyme is involved.
- Hemoglobin binds carbon dioxide in its deoxygenated state (reduced hemoglobin).
- Approximately 30% of carbon dioxide added to blood in systemic capillaries is transported as carbamino compounds.

Haldane effect

Carriage of carbon dioxide is increased in deoxygenated blood because of two factors:
- Reduced hemoglobin has a greater affinity for carbon dioxide than oxyhemoglobin.
- Reduced hemoglobin is less acidic (i.e., a better proton acceptor: H buffer) than oxyhemoglobin.

The Haldane effect minimizes changes in pH of the blood when gaseous exchange occurs. The decrease in pH due to the oxygenation of Hb is offset by the increase that results from the loss of CO_2 to the alveolar air. The reverse occurs in the tissues.

This is an important effect because:
- In peripheral capillaries, the unloading of oxygen from hemoglobin aids the binding of carbon dioxide to hemoglobin.
- In pulmonary capillaries, the loading of oxygen on hemoglobin reduces the binding of carbon dioxide to hemoglobin.

This allows efficient gaseous exchange of carbon dioxide in the tissues and the lungs.

Carbon dioxide dissociation curve

The carriage of carbon dioxide is dependent upon the partial pressure of carbon dioxide in the blood. This relationship is described by the carbon dioxide dissociation curve (Fig. 5.25). Compared with the oxygen dissociation curve:

- The carbon dioxide curve is more linear.
- The carbon dioxide curve is much steeper than the oxygen curve (between venous and arterial partial pressure of respiratory gases).
- The carbon dioxide curve varies according to oxygen saturation of hemoglobin.

Two main carbon dioxide dissociation curves, for mixed venous and arterial blood, can be drawn (see Fig. 5.25).

Stores of oxygen and carbon dioxide

There are only small stores (approximately 1550ml) of oxygen in body tissues as follows:
- Lungs—450ml
- Blood—850ml
- Myoglobin—200ml
- Tissue fluids—50ml

On the other hand, carbon dioxide has vast stores (approximately 120L):
- Blood carbonates
- Bone carbonates
- Tissue carbonates (including fat tissue).

A change in ventilation will affect both P_aO_2 and P_aCO_2. Because oxygen stores are small in comparison with those of carbon dioxide, a short-term variation in ventilation will affect P_aO_2. A persistent change in ventilation will be shown by a change in P_aCO_2. Clinically, ventilation is assessed by measurement of P_aCO_2.

Hypoventilation and hyperventilation

If P_aCO_2 is a measure of ventilation, it is appropriate in a review of carbon dioxide transport to consider two key concepts in respiratory medicine: hypoventilation and hyperventilation.

For the body to function normally, ventilation must meet the metabolic demand of the tissues (Fig. 5.26).

Thus, metabolic tissue consumption of oxygen must be equal to the oxygen taken up in the blood from alveolar gas. Or, metabolic tissue production of carbon dioxide must be equal to the amount of carbon dioxide blown off at the alveoli.

Hypoventilation

The term hypoventilation refers to a situation when ventilation is insufficient to meet metabolic demand.

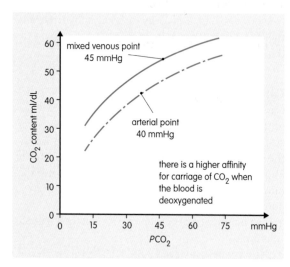

Fig. 5.25 Ventilation effects on oxygen and carbon dioxide levels in the blood. The top line (solid) is the carbon dioxide dissociation curve in mixed venous blood; the bottom (dashed curve) is the carbon dioxide dissociation curve for arterial blood.

Fig. 5.26 Differences between hyperventilation and hypoventilation.

Comparison of hyperventilation and hypoventilation	
Hyperventilation	**Hypoventilation**
Causes	**Causes**

anxiety
brainstem lesion
drugs
	obstruction:
	  asthma
	  chronic obstructive airways disease
	  foreign body (e.g. peanut)
	brainstem lesion
	pneumothorax or lung collapse
	trauma (e.g. fractured rib)
	drugs, notably opioids

Consequences	**Consequences**
ventilation too great for metabolic demand too much CO_2 blown off from lungs $P_aCO_2 < 40\,mmHg$ respiratory alkalosis	ventilation is too low for metabolic demand not enough CO_2 is blown off at the lungs $P_aCO_2 > 40\,mmHg$ respiratory acidosis

The alveolar ventilation equation: states that the alveolar PCO_2 is inversely proportional to the alveolar ventilation (as long as CO_2 production is constant).
$$P_ACO_2 = K \cdot \dot{V}CO_2 / \dot{V}_A$$

$\dot{V}CO_2$ = the volume of CO_2 exhaled per unit time
$\dot{V}_A$ is alveolar ventilation
K is a constant.

CO_2 exhaled ($\dot{V}CO_2$) = minute ventilation ($\dot{V}_E$) × the fractional concentration of CO_2 in the expired air (F_ECO_2).
CO_2 produced in the tissues = exhaled CO_2

$$\dot{V}CO_2 = \dot{V}_E \cdot F_ECO_2$$

CO_2 expired = the amount of CO_2 released at the alveoli, so:

$$\dot{V}CO_2 = \dot{V}_A \cdot F_ACO_2$$

where $\dot{V}_A$ = alveolar ventilation; F_ACO_2 = fractional concentration of CO_2 at the alveoli.

$$F_ACO_2 = \dot{V}CO_2 / \dot{V}_A$$

Using Dalton's law, relating the partial pressure to fractional concentration:

$$P_ACO_2 \propto \dot{V}CO_2 / \dot{V}_A$$

Or:

$$P_ACO_2 = K \cdot \dot{V}CO_2 / \dot{V}_A$$

Fig. 5.27 The alveolar ventilation equation.

Hyperventilation

The term hyperventilation refers to a situation where ventilation exceeds metabolic demand.

The alveolar ventilation equation (see Fig. 5.27 for derivation) states that if carbon dioxide produced in the tissues equals carbon dioxide exhaled (as is usual at rest), then alveolar PCO_2 (i.e., P_ACO_2) is inversely proportional to the alveolar ventilation:

$$P_ACO_2 = K \times \dot{V}CO_2 / \dot{V}_A$$

where $\dot{V}CO_2$ is the volume of CO_2 exhaled per unit time, V_A is the alveolar ventilation, and K is a constant.

We can see that this makes sense: increasing alveolar ventilation reduces the concentration of CO_2 in alveolar air at steady state.

Because alveolar gas is in equilibrium with the blood, P_ACO_2 can be estimated as P_aCO_2. Thus, it can be seen how ventilation will affect partial pressures of carbon dioxide and that hypoventilation and hyperventilation can be shown clinically by the partial pressure of carbon dioxide in the blood.

In order to relate P_ACO_2 to P_AO_2, so that we can see how hyperventilation and hypoventilation affect alveolar oxygen, we use the alveolar gas equation:

$$P_ACO_2 = P_IO_2 - (P_ACO_2/R) + K$$

where P_IO_2 = partial pressure of oxygen in inspired air and R = respiratory exchange ratio (or the ratio of CO_2 production to O_2 consumption: normally about 0.8).

Mild or moderate exercise in a normal subject does not cause hyperventilation: the depth of breathing is increased to balance the increased metabolic demand in exercise.

Hypercapnia and hypocapnia
Hypercapnia
A high partial pressure (concentration) of carbon dioxide in the blood ($P_aCO_2 > 45\,mmHg$) is termed hypercapnia (Fig. 5.28).

Hypocapnia
A low partial pressure of carbon dioxide in the blood ($P_aCO_2 < 40\,mmHg$) is termed hypocapnia.

Respiratory failure
Hypercapnia and hypocapnia are important concepts in the assessment of respiratory failure (see Chapter 8). Respiratory failure is defined as a $P_aO_2 < 60\,mmHg$ and is divided into type I and type II, depending on the P_aCO_2.

In type I respiratory failure (hypoxemic respiratory failure), $P_aCO_2 < 50\,mmHg$. P_aO_2 is low (hypoxemic), but P_aCO_2 may be normal or low; this represents a ventilation:perfusion mismatch, as occurs in pneumonia and adult respiratory distress syndrome (ARDS) or at high altitude.

In type II respiratory failure (hypercapnic/hypoxemic respiratory failure), $P_aCO_2 > 50\,mmHg$. Both P_aO_2 and P_aCO_2 indicate that the lungs are not well ventilated. Type II respiratory failure is more common than type I and has diverse etiologies.

The significance of this classification is that in type II respiratory failure the patient may have developed tolerance to increased levels of P_aCO_2; in other words, the drive for respiration no longer relies on hypercapnic drive (high P_aCO_2) but on hypoxic drive (low P_aO_2). Thus, if the patient is given high-concentration oxygen therapy, the hypoxic drive for ventilation may decrease and the patient may stop breathing and die!

Acid–base balance

Normal pH
The pH of the intracellular and extracellular compartments must be tightly controlled for the body to function efficiently, or at all. The normal arterial pH lies within a relatively narrow range: 7.35–7.45 ([H⁺] range, 45–35 mmol/L). An acid–base disturbance arises when arterial pH lies outside this range. If the blood pH is less than 7.35, an acidosis is present; if pH is greater than 7.45, the term alkalosis is used. Although a larger variation in pH can be tolerated (pH 6.8–7.8) for a short time, recovery is often impossible if blood remains at pH 6.8 for long.

Such a tight control on blood pH is achieved by a combination of blood buffers and the respiratory and renal systems which make adjustments to return pH toward its normal levels.

Before we review the mechanism of compensation, and discuss the acid–base disturbances, it is useful to review some key concepts.

Key concepts in acid–base balance
Metabolic production of acids
Products of metabolism (e.g., carbon dioxide, lactic acid, phosphate, sulfate) form acidic solutions, thus increasing the hydrogen ion concentration and reducing pH. We also have an intake of acids in our diet (approximately 50–100 mmol H⁺ per day).

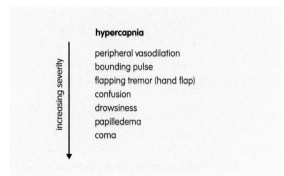

hypercapnia

peripheral vasodilation
bounding pulse
flapping tremor (hand flap)
confusion
drowsiness
papilledema
coma

increasing severity

Fig. 5.28 Clinical signs of hypercapnia.

We rely on three methods to control our internal hydrogen ion concentration:
- Dilution of body fluids
- The physiologic buffer system
- Excretion of volatile and nonvolatile acids.

Buffers

A buffer is a substance that can either bind or release hydrogen ions, therefore keeping the pH relatively constant even when considerable quantities of acid or base are added. There are four buffers of the blood:
- Hemoglobin
- Plasma proteins
- Phosphate
- Bicarbonate.

It is the bicarbonate system that acts as the principal buffer and which is of most interest in respiratory medicine.

We have already seen that CO_2 dissolves in water and reacts to form carbonic acid and that this dissociates to form bicarbonate and protons:

$$CO_2 + H_2O \leftrightarrow H_2CO_3 \leftrightarrow H^+ + HCO_3^-$$

This equilibrium tells us that changes in either CO_2 or HCO_3^- will have an effect on pH. For example, increasing CO_2 will drive the reaction to the right, increasing hydrogen ion concentration.

Remember that increasing the hydrogen ion concentration makes a solution more acid, i.e., it *reduces* pH.

As changes in CO_2 and bicarbonate can alter pH, controlling these elements allows the system to control acid–base equilibrium. This is why the bicarbonate buffer system is so useful; the body has control over both elements:
- Carbon dioxide is regulated through changes in ventilation
- Bicarbonate concentrations are determined by the kidneys.

The Henderson–Hasselbalch equation

We can calculate the pH resulting from the dissociation of carbonic acid by using the Henderson–Hasselbalch equation:

$$pH = pK_A + \log \frac{[HCO_3^-]}{\alpha PCO_2}$$

or

$$pH = 6.1 + \log \frac{[HCO_3^-]}{0.03 PCO_2}$$

where α is solubility of CO_2 (0.03 for plasma at 37°C).

In its simplest form this states:

$$[H^+] \propto PCO_2/[HCO_3^-]$$

The effect on pH of changing carbon dioxide or bicarbonate is now even clearer: if carbon dioxide rises, and there is no change in bicarbonate, then the hydrogen ion concentration will rise.

Acid–base disturbances

As noted above, blood pH can either be higher than normal (alkalosis) or lower (acidosis). From the Henderson–Hasselbalch equation we can see that an acidosis could be caused by either:
- A rise in PCO_2
- A fall in HCO_3^-.

Similarly alkalosis could occur through:
- A fall in PCO_2
- A rise in HCO_3^-.

When the primary change is in CO_2, we term the disturbance respiratory, and when it is in bicarbonate, we term the disturbance metabolic. This allows us to classify four types of disturbance:
- Respiratory alkalosis
- Respiratory acidosis
- Metabolic alkalosis
- Metabolic acidosis.

The disturbance was described as primary because the kidneys and lungs may try to return the acid–base disturbance towards normal values. This is called compensation and means that even in respiratory disturbances it may not be just CO_2 that is abnormal, bicarbonate may have altered too. Similarly CO_2 may be abnormal in a metabolic disturbance. The ways in which the two systems compensate are:
- The respiratory system alters ventilation; this happens quickly
- The kidney alters excretion of bicarbonate; this takes 2–3 days.

It is now clear that lung disease that affects gas exchange and therefore PCO_2 will have major effect on the body's acid–base status. It is also clear that while the respiratory system can act quickly to compensate for metabolic disturbances, it will take time for compensation to take place in respiratory disease; the renal system cannot act as quickly. We see this in clinical practice: a change in bicarbonate is characteristic of chronic lung disease rather than acute.

Assessing acid–base disturbances

Assessing acid–base disorders is relatively simple if you appoach the problem in stages (Fig. 5.29).
1. Start with the pH—is it outside the normal range?
2. If there is an acidosis or alkalosis, can it be explained by a change in CO_2?

3. If it can, then the primary disturbance is respiratory.
4. Now look at bicarbonate—has this moved to return the ratio to normal?
5. If it has, it is a respiratory disorder with metabolic compensation.

Davenport diagram

The Davenport diagram (Fig. 5.30) demonstrates the relationship between plasma $[HCO_3^-]$, pH, and PCO_2 in a graphical form.

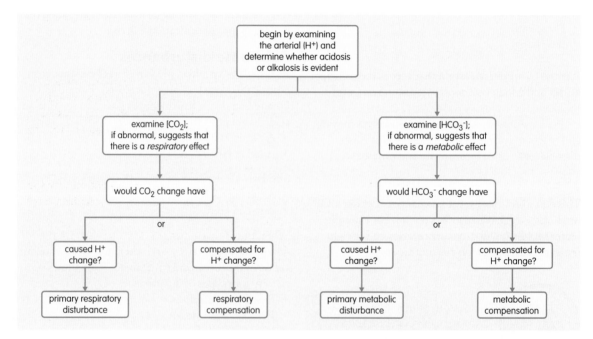

Fig. 5.29 Assessing acid–base disorders.

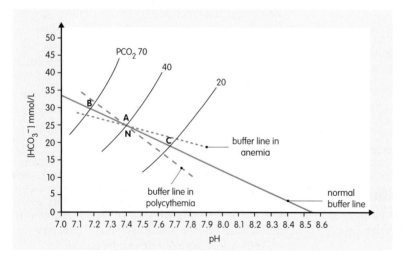

Fig. 5.30 The relationship between plasma $[HCO_3^-]$, pH, and PCO_2. A buffer line runs from points A to B. Any change in PCO_2 will have an associated change in $[HCO_3^-]$ because of bicarbonate buffering of hydrogen ions; this can be shown by moving up and down the buffer line. Point N shows the normal plasma pH and $[HCO_3^-]$. Lines running perpendicular to the buffer line are of constant PCO_2.

Respiratory acidosis

Respiratory acidosis results from an increase in PCO_2 caused by:

- Hypoventilation (less CO_2 is blown off)
- Ventilation:perfusion mismatch.

From the Henderson–Hasselbalch equation, we see that an increase in PCO_2 causes an increase in hydrogen ion concentration (i.e., a reduction in pH). Thus, plasma bicarbonate concentration increases to compensate for the increased hydrogen ion concentration (Fig. 5.31).

It is easiest to follow the principles of acid–base balance by using the Davenport diagram.

Renal compensation

The increase in hydrogen ion concentration in the blood results in increased filtration of hydrogen ions at the glomeruli, thus:

- Increasing HCO_3^- reabsorption
- Increasing HCO_3^- production.

Thus, plasma HCO_3^- rises, compensating for the increased [H^+], i.e., renal compensation raises pH toward normal in chronic respiratory acidosis.

Causes of respiratory acidosis

Mechanisms reducing ventilation or causing $V:Q$ mismatch include:

- COPD
- Asthma
- Blocked airway (by tumor or foreign body)
- Spontaneous lung collapse, brainstem lesion
- Injury to the chest wall
- Drugs that reduce respiratory drive (ventilation), including morphine, barbiturates, and general anesthetics.

Respiratory alkalosis

Respiratory alkalosis results from a decrease in PCO_2, generally caused by alveolar hyperventilation (more carbon dioxide is blown off). This causes a decrease in hydrogen ion concentration and thus an increase in pH (Fig. 5.32).

Renal compensation

The reduction in hydrogen ion concentration in the blood results in decreased hydrogen ion filtration at the glomeruli, thus:

- Reducing HCO_3^- reabsorption
- Reducing HCO_3^- production.

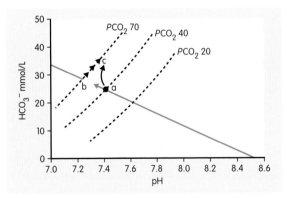

Fig. 5.31 Respiratory acidosis causes increases in PCO_2 and, to some extent, HCO_3^- and reduction in pH shown as a move from a to b. The kidneys compensate by increasing HCO_3^- reabsorption and production shown from point b to point c, with a return of pH toward the normal level. Arrow a–c shows a real-life situation.

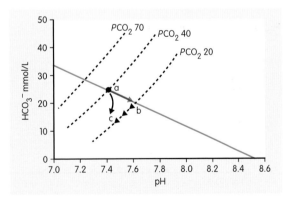

Fig. 5.32 Respiratory alkalosis causes reduced PCO_2 and somewhat reduced HCO_3^- and increases the pH. Shown as a move from point a to point b. The kidneys compensate by reducing the rate of renal excretion of H^+ so that less HCO_3^- is reabsorbed or produced by the kidney. This is shown as a move from point b to point c. The real-life situation is shown from point a to point c.

Thus, plasma HCO_3^- falls, compensating for the reduced $[H^+]$, i.e. renal compensation reduces pH toward normal.

Causes of respiratory alkalosis

The causes of respiratory alkalosis include:
- Increased ventilation—caused by hypoxic drive in pneumonia, diffuse interstitial lung diseases, high altitude, etc.
- Hyperventilation—brainstem damage, infection causing fever, drugs (e.g., aspirin), hysterical overbreathing.

Metabolic acidosis

Metabolic acidosis results from an excess of hydrogen ions in the body, which reduces bicarbonate concentration (shifting the equation below to the left). Respiration is unaffected; therefore, PCO_2 is initially normal (Fig. 5.33).

Respiratory compensation

$$CO_2 + H_2O \leftrightarrow H_2CO_3 \leftrightarrow H^+ + HCO_3^-$$

The reduction in pH is detected by the peripheral chemoreceptors. This causes an increase in ventilation, which lowers PCO_2. Also:
- The above equation is driven further to the left, reducing hydrogen ion concentration and bicarbonate.
- The decrease in hydrogen ion concentration raises pH toward normal.

Respiratory compensation cannot fully correct the values of PCO_2, $[HCO_3^-]$, and $[H^+]$, as there is a limit to how far PCO_2 can fall with hyperventilation. Correction can be carried out only by removing the excess hydrogen ions from the body or restoring the lost bicarbonate (i.e., correcting the metabolic fault).

Causes of metabolic acidosis

Causes of metabolic acidosis are:
- Ingestion of acid
- Loss of HCO_3^- from the kidneys
- Metabolic production of hydrogen ions. The kidneys may not be able to excrete the excess hydrogen ions immediately, or at all (as in renal failure).

Metabolic alkalosis

Metabolic alkalosis results from an increase in bicarbonate concentration or a fall in hydrogen ion concentration. Removing hydrogen ions from the right of the equation (below) drives the reaction to the right, increasing bicarbonate concentration. Decrease in hydrogen ion concentration raises pH; initially, PCO_2 is normal (Fig. 5.34).

Respiratory compensation

$$CO_2 + H_2O \leftrightarrow H_2CO_3 \leftrightarrow H^+ + HCO_3^-$$

The increase in pH is detected by the peripheral chemoreceptors. This causes a decrease in ventilation which raises PCO_2. Also:

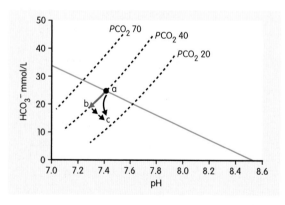

Fig. 5.33 Metabolic acidosis causes a rise in H^+, reduced HCO_3^-, and reduced pH. Shown as a move from point a to point b. The lungs compensate by blowing off CO_2 and therefore increasing the pH, shown as a move from point b to point c. The arrow from point a to point c shows the real-life situation.

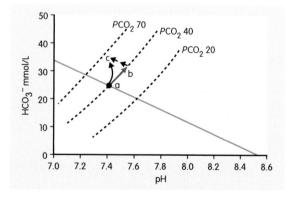

Fig. 5.34 Metabolic alkalosis due to loss of H^+ ions and increase in HCO_3^- with increase in pH shown as a move from point a to point b. The lungs compensate by reducing ventilation and increasing PCO_2, shown as a move from point b to point c. The arrow from point a to point c shows the real situation.

- The above equation is driven further to the right, increasing hydrogen ion and bicarbonate concentrations.
- The decrease in hydrogen ion concentration raises pH toward normal.

Respiratory compensation is through alveolar hypoventilation, but ventilation cannot reduce enough to correct the disturbance. This can only be carried out by removing the problem either of reduced hydrogen ion concentration or increased bicarbonate concentration. This is done by reducing renal hydrogen ion secretion.

More bicarbonate is excreted because more is filtered at the glomerulus and less is reabsorbed in combination with hydrogen ions.

Causes of metabolic alkalosis
The causes of metabolic alkalosis include:
- Vomiting (hydrochloric acid loss from the stomach)
- Ingestion of alkaline substances
- Increased plasma bicarbonate.

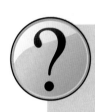

- What are the normal diastolic and systolic pressures in the pulmonary circulation?
- Describe recruitment and distension. How do these affect pulmonary vascular resistance?
- Outline what factors affect pulmonary blood flow and resistance of the pulmonary vasculature.
- Describe the pattern of blood flow through the lungs in terms of three zones.
- Explain the term hypoxic vasoconstriction and its importance.
- Describe what is meant by the ventilation:perfusion ratio.
- State the two extremes of ventilation:perfusion ratio.
- Define venous admixture.
- Describe with the aid of a diagram how disease might affect the ventilation:perfusion ratio distribution.
- Describe the structure of hemoglobin and its ability to bind oxygen.
- Draw and explain the oxygen dissociation curve for hemoglobin. What factors affect the curve?
- Describe how fetal hemoglobin differs from adult hemoglobin and explain the double Bohr shift.
- Explain the terms hypoventilation and hyperventilation.
- State the normal blood pH range.
- What is a buffer? Give four examples of buffers in the blood and their relative importance.
- Draw a Davenport diagram.
- Explain what is meant by an acid–base disturbance. Explain the four deviations.
- List the causes for respiratory acidosis and alkalosis.
- List the causes for metabolic acidosis and alkalosis.

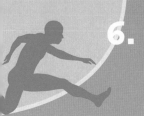

6. Control of Respiratory Function

Basics of control

Every control system needs certain key elements for it to function correctly. These are:

- A control variable—a variable to be kept within certain limits (e.g., P_aCO_2 or P_aO_2)
- A desired value for that control variable, often quoted as normal physiological range (e.g., P_aCO_2 of around 40 mmHg)
- A measured value for the control variable (e.g., actual $P_aCO_2 = 46$ mmHg, 35 mmHg, etc.)
- Sensors to detect the measured value or a difference from the desired value (e.g., muscle spindle stretch receptors or chemoreceptors)
- Effectors (e.g., respiratory muscles, which alter ventilation and thus change P_aCO_2)
- A controller that relates the measured value to the desired value and changes output to the effectors (respiratory muscles), altering ventilation.

There are two types of control system: feedback and feed-forward:

- Feedback control—the system detailed below (Fig. 6.1), in which the controller looks at the measured value of the control variable (e.g., P_aCO_2) and relates this to the desired value. Adjustments to the system are then made
- Feed-forward control—the system detailed below (Fig. 6.2), which anticipates the effects of external factors to the system and makes adjustments to the system in an attempt to control their effect. An example of this is behavioral control of breathing when we sing.

Control within the respiratory system

When considering control of breathing, the main control variable is P_aCO_2 (we try to control this value near to 40 mmHg). This can be carried out by adjusting the respiratory rate, the tidal volume, or both.

By controlling P_aCO_2 we are effectively controlling alveolar ventilation (see Chapter 3) and thus P_ACO_2.

> Note that we move between P_aO_2 and P_AO_2 here and throughout the chapter. Remember that these are different—if you are unclear, the abbreviations are explained in Chapter 4.

Although P_aCO_2 is the main control variable, P_aO_2 is also controlled, but normally to a much lesser extent than P_aCO_2. However, the P_aO_2 control system can take over and become the main controlling system when the P_aO_2 drops below 50 mmHg.

Control can seem to be brought about by:

- Metabolic demands of the body (metabolic control)—tissue oxygen demand and acid–base balance
- Behavioral demands of the body (behavioral control)—singing, coughing, laughing (i.e., control is voluntary).

These are essentially feedback and feed-forward control systems, respectively. The behavioral control of breathing overlays the metabolic control. Its control is derived from higher centers of the brain. The axons of neurons whose cell bodies are situated in the cerebral cortex bypass the respiratory centers in the brainstem and synapse directly with lower motor neurons that control respiratory muscles. This system will not be dealt with within this text; we will deal only with the metabolic control of respiration.

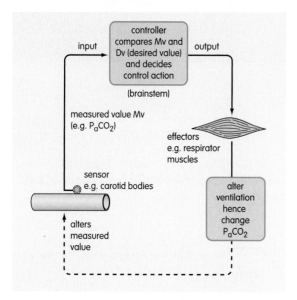

Fig. 6.1 Example of feedback control in the respiratory system. P_aCO_2 is used as the control variable.

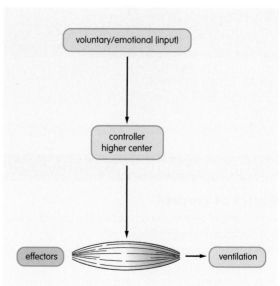

Fig. 6.2 Example of feed-forward control in the respiratory system. Higher centers predict the effect of external changes (e.g., emotion or singing) and alter the output to the effectors (respiratory muscles) to achieve the required ventilation.

Metabolic control of breathing

Metabolic control of breathing is a function of the brainstem (pons and medulla). The controller can be considered as specific groups of neurons (previously called respiratory centers).

Pontine neurons

Those located in the pons are the pontine respiratory group and consist of two groups of neurons:
- Expiratory neurons in the nucleus parabrachialis medialis
- Inspiratory neurons in the lateral parabrachial nucleus and Kölliker's fuse nucleus.

The role of the pontine respiratory group (PRG) is to regulate (i.e., affect the activity of) the dorsal respiratory group (DRG) and possibly the ventral respiratory group (VRG, neuron groups in the medulla).

Medullary neurons

It is believed that the medulla is responsible for respiratory rhythm.

Three groups of neurons associated with respiratory control have been identified in the medulla:
- The dorsal respiratory group, situated in the nucleus of tractus solitarius

- The ventral respiratory group, situated in the nucleus ambiguus and the nucleus retroambigualis
- The Bötzinger complex, situated rostral to the nucleus ambiguus.

These groups receive sensory information, which is compared with the desired value of control; adjustments are made to respiratory muscles to rectify any deviation from ideal. The dorsal respiratory group (Fig. 6.3) contains neuron bodies of inspiratory upper motor neurons. These inhibit the activity of expiratory neurons in the ventral respiratory group and have an excitatory effect on lower motor neurons to the respiratory muscles, increasing ventilation.

Ventral respiratory group neurons in the nucleus ambiguus (Fig. 6.4) are again inspiratory upper motor neurons.

Ventral respiratory group neurons in the rostral part of the nucleus retroambigualis (Fig. 6.5) contain inspiratory upper motor neurons which go on to supply through their lower motor neurons external intercostal muscles and accessory muscles.

Ventral respiratory group neurons in the caudal part of the nucleus retroambigualis (Fig. 6.6) are expiratory upper motor neurons.

Fig. 6.3 Dorsal respiratory group. Note the output to respiratory muscle and inhibition of expiratory neurons in the ventral respiratory group. UMN = upper motor neuron; LMN = lower motor neuron; VRG = ventral respiratory group; DRG = dorsal respiratory group.

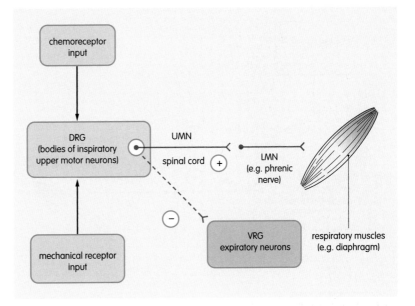

Fig. 6.4 Ventral respiratory group in the nucleus ambiguus. LMN = lower motor neuron; UMN = upper motor neuron; VRG = ventral respiratory group.

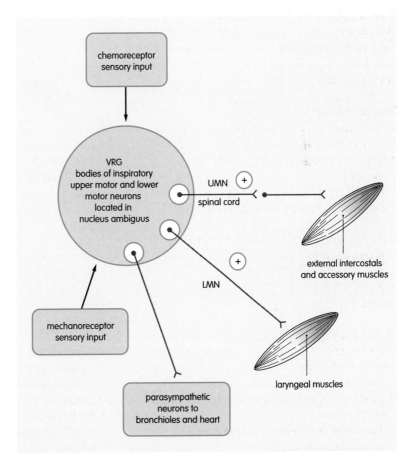

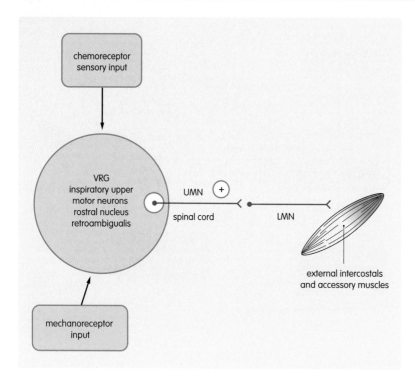

Fig. 6.5 Ventral respiratory group located in rostral nucleus retroambigualis. UMN = upper motor neuron; LMN = lower motor neuron; VRG = ventral respiratory group.

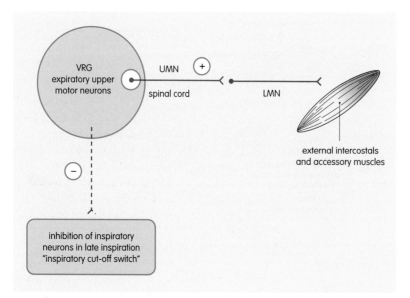

Fig. 6.6 Ventral respiratory group located in caudal nucleus retroambigualis (expiratory neurons).

The Bötzinger complex (Fig. 6.7) contains only expiratory neurons. Its sensory input is through the nucleus tractus solitarius. It has two functions:
- Inhibition of inspiratory neurons of the dorsal and ventral respiratory groups
- Excitation of expiratory neurons in the ventral respiratory group.

Two main theories exist as to how the medulla influences respiratory rhythm:
- Dorsal respiratory group inspiratory pacemaker—neurons discharge in a phasic manner, inhibiting expiratory neurons
- Neural networks—local re-excitation causes phasic firing in both inspiratory and expiratory neurons with reciprocal inhibition.

Fig. 6.7 Bötzinger complex (BC); located first rostral to nucleus ambiguus and comprised entirely of expiratory neurons. PRG = pontine respiratory group; DRG = dorsal respiratory group. (Adapted from *Decision Making in Medicine*, by H.L. Green and W.P. Johnson. St. Louis, Mosby Year Book, 1993.)

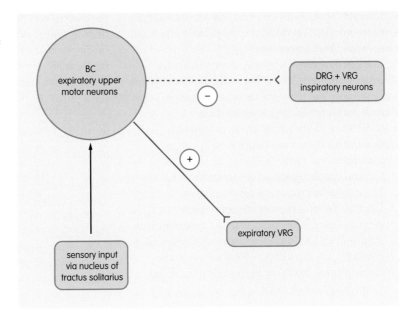

Effectors (muscles of respiration)

The muscles involved in respiration have been described in Chapter 4. The major muscle groups involved are the diaphragm, internal and external intercostals, and abdominal muscles.

Effectors carry out the control action for the central controller. Thus, the strength of contraction and coordination of these muscles is set by the central controller. If the muscles are not coordinated, this will result in abnormal breathing patterns.

Sensors (receptors)

Sensors report current values or discrepancies from ideal values for the various variables being controlled (e.g., P_aCO_2, P_aO_2, and pH) to the central controller.

There are many types of sensors and receptors involved with respiratory control:
- Chemoreceptors—central and peripheral
- Lung receptors—irritant, pulmonary stretch, and juxtapulmonary
- Receptors in the chest wall—muscle spindles and Golgi tendon organs
- Other receptors—nasal, tracheal, and laryngeal receptors, arterial baroreceptors, pain receptors.

Chemoreceptors

Chemoreceptors monitor blood gas tensions, P_aCO_2, P_aO_2, and pH, and help keep minute volume appropriate to metabolic demands of the body. Therefore, chemoreceptors respond to:

- Hypercapnia
- Hypoxia
- Acidosis.

There are both central and peripheral chemoreceptors.

Central chemoreceptors

Central chemoreceptors are tonically active and vital for maintenance of respiration; 80% of the drive for ventilation is a result of stimulation of the central chemoreceptors. When they are inactivated, respiration ceases. These receptors are readily depressed by drugs (e.g., opiates and barbiturates).

The receptors are located in the brainstem on the ventrolateral surface of the medulla, close to the exit of cranial nerves IX and X. They are anatomically separate from the medullary respiratory control center.

Central chemoreceptors respond to hydrogen ion concentration within the surrounding brain tissue and cerebrospinal fluid.
- Raised hydrogen ion concentration increases ventilation.
- Lowered hydrogen ion concentration decreases ventilation.

Diffusion of ions across the blood–brain barrier is poor. Blood levels of hydrogen ions and bicarbonate have little effect in the short term on the concentrations of hydrogen ions and bicarbonate in the cerebrospinal fluid and thus have little effect on the central chemoreceptors.

Carbon dioxide, however, can pass freely by diffusion across the blood–brain barrier. On entering the cerebrospinal fluid, the increase in carbon dioxide increases the free hydrogen ion concentration. This increase in hydrogen ion concentration stimulates the central chemoreceptors. Thus:

- Central chemoreceptors are sensitive to P_aCO_2 not arterial hydrogen ion concentration
- Central chemoreceptors are not sensitive to P_aO_2
- Because there is less protein in the cerebrospinal fluid (<0.4g/L) than in the plasma (60–80g/L), a rise in P_aCO_2 has a larger effect on pH in the cerebrospinal fluid than in the blood (CSF has lower buffering capacity).

Longstanding raised P_aCO_2 causes the pH of the cerebrospinal fluid to return towards normal. This is because prolonged hypercapnia alters production of bicarbonate by the glial cells and allows bicarbonate to cross the blood–brain barrier. It can therefore diffuse freely into the CSF and alter the CSF pH.

Peripheral chemoreceptors

Figure 6.8 shows the location of chemoreceptors around the carotid sinus and aortic arch. These are

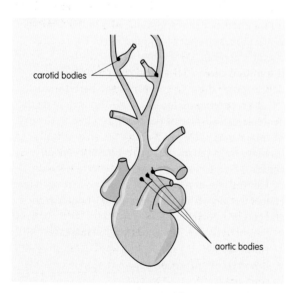

the carotid bodies and aortic bodies, respectively. Stimulation of peripheral chemoreceptors has both cardiovascular and respiratory effects. Of the two receptor groups, the carotid bodies have the greatest effect on respiration.

Carotid bodies   The carotid bodies contain two different types of cells: type I (glomus) cells and type II (sustentacular) cells. Type I cells are stimulated by hypoxia; they connect with afferent nerves to the brainstem. Type II cells are supportive (structural and metabolic), similar to glial cells of the central nervous system.

There is a rich blood supply to the carotid bodies (blood flow per mass of tissue far exceeds that to the brain); venous blood flow, therefore, remains saturated with oxygen. The exact mechanism of action of the carotid bodies is not known. It is believed that type I (glomus) cells are activated by hypoxia and release transmitter substances that stimulate afferents to the brainstem.

Peripheral chemoreceptors are sensitive to:
- P_aO_2
- P_aCO_2
- pH
- Blood flow
- Temperature.

The carotid bodies are supplied by the autonomic nervous system, which appears to alter their sensitivity to hypoxia by regulating blood flow to the chemoreceptor:
- Sympathetic action vasoconstricts, increasing sensitivity to hypoxia
- Parasympathetic action vasodilates, reducing sensitivity to hypoxia.

The relationship between P_aO_2 and the response from the carotid bodies is not a linear one. At a low P_aO_2 (< 50mmHg), a further decrease in arterial oxygen tension significantly increases ventilation (Fig. 6.9). However, at levels of oxygen tension close to 100mmHg, changes have little effect on ventilation. If P_aO_2 increases above 100mmHg (achieved when breathing high-concentration oxygen), ventilation is only slightly reduced.

Unlike central chemoreceptors, peripheral chemoreceptors are directly stimulated by blood pH. Although peripheral chemoreceptors are stimulated by P_aCO_2, their response is much less than that of central chemoreceptors (less than 10% of the effect).

Fig. 6.8 Peripheral chemoreceptors. Carotid bodies are situated around the carotid sinus and are sensitive both to P_aCO_2 and P_aO_2. Aortic bodies are situated around the aortic arch and are sensitive only to P_aCO_2.

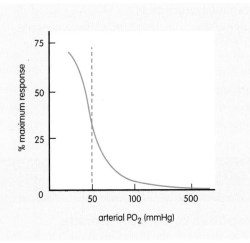

Fig. 6.9 Response of ventilation to P_aO_2. The response to a lowered P_aO_2 is small until the P_aO_2 falls below a value of 50mmHg, after which point the response increases dramatically.

In summary:
- Lowered P_aO_2 (especially below 50mmHg) increases ventilation.
- Increased P_aCO_2 increases ventilation (but this is < 10% of the effect of central receptors).
- Raised hydrogen ion concentration increases ventilation (however, aortic bodies do not respond).
- The response of these receptors is very fast and can oscillate within a respiratory cycle.

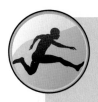 It is the peripheral chemoreceptors that are responsible for the ventilatory response to hypoxemia that occurs at high altitude.

Receptors in the lung

The receptors in the lung monitor mechanical activity. There are three types of receptors in the lung:
- Pulmonary stretch receptors—slowly adapting
- Pulmonary and bronchial C fiber receptors—formerly juxtapulmonary, J receptors
- Irritant receptors—rapidly adapting.

Stretch receptors

These receptors are situated in the smooth muscle of the bronchial walls and respond to changes in transmural pressure. They are slowly adapting, producing a maintained response to a maintained stimulus.

Primarily, these receptors are concerned with physiological control and regulatory reflexes. They are stimulated by inflation (which stretches the lungs):
- Inflation leads to decreased respiration (inflation reflex or Hering–Breuer reflex).
- Deflation leads to increased respiration (deflation reflex).

These reflexes are active in the first year of life, but are weak in adults. Therefore, they are not thought to determine the rate and depth of breathing in adults. However, these reflexes are seen to be more active if the tidal volume increases above 1.0L and therefore might have a role in exercise.

Afferent fibers travel to the respiratory centers through the vagus nerve. The functions of these receptors are:
- The termination of inspiration
- Regulation of the work of breathing
- Reinforcement of respiratory rhythm in the first year of life.

However, if the nerve is blocked by anesthesia, there is no change seen in the rate and depth of breathing of adults.

Pulmonary and bronchial C fiber receptors

These receptors are stimulated by:
- Large inflation
- Forced deflation
- Pulmonary vascular congestion
- Edema—interstitial fluid in the alveolar wall
- Chemical mediators—histamine and capsacin.

The receptors are thought to be situated in the alveolar wall close to pulmonary capillaries and in the bronchial mucosa. Afferent fibers travel to respiratory centers through the vagus nerve (nonmyelinated C fibers).

When stimulated, they cause:
- Closure of the larynx
- Rapid, shallow breathing
- Bradycardia
- Hypotension.

They also contribute to the breathlessness of heart failure.

Irritant receptors

These receptors are scattered through the airways and lie between epithelial cells. In contrast to the slowly adapting stretch receptors, they are rapidly adapting receptors. They are stimulated by inhaled particles, noxious gases, increased airflow, pulmonary congestion, and mechanical deformation. Chemical mediators of allergic reactions also stimulate these receptors, which in part account for an increase in ventilation in asthma.

Stimulation of these receptors in the trachea causes a cough reflex, thereby eliminating the particles from the airways. Receptors in lower areas cause bronchoconstriction, laryngeal constriction, and rapid, shallow breathing. This is an attempt to limit how far a particle is inhaled.

In the nose and upper airways, there are irritant receptors (Chapter 2), which act to protect the lower airway.

Receptors in the chest wall

Receptors in the chest wall consist of:

- Joint receptors—measure the velocity of rib movement
- Golgi tendon organs—found within the muscles of respiration (e.g., diaphragm and intercostals) and detect the strength of muscle contraction
- Muscle spindles—monitor the length of muscle fibers both statically and dynamically (i.e., detect muscle length and velocity).

These receptors help to minimize changes to ventilation imposed by an external load (e.g., lateral flexion of the trunk). They achieve this by modifying motor neuron output to the respiratory muscles. The aim is to achieve the most efficient respiration in terms of tidal volume and frequency. Thus, reflexes from muscles and joints stabilize ventilation in the face of changing mechanical conditions.

It is thought that stimulation of mechanoreceptors in the chest wall, along with hypercapnia and hypoxemia, leads to increased respiratory effort in a patient with sleep apnea. It is this sudden respiratory effort that then wakes the patient up.

Arterial baroreceptors

Hypertension stimulates arterial baroreceptors, which inhibit ventilation. Hypotension has the opposite effect.

Pain receptors

Stimulation of pain receptors causes a brief apnea, followed by a period of hyperventilation.

Coordinated responses of the respiratory system

Response to carbon dioxide

Carbon dioxide is the most important factor in the control of ventilation. Under normal conditions P_aCO_2 is held within very tight limits and ventilatory response is very sensitive to small changes in P_aCO_2.

The response of ventilation to carbon dioxide has been measured by inhalation of mixtures of carbon dioxide, raising the P_aCO_2 and observing the increase in ventilation (Fig. 6.10).

Note that a small increase in P_aCO_2 causes a significant increase in ventilation. The response to P_aCO_2 is also dependent upon the arterial oxygen tension. At lower values of P_aO_2 the ventilatory response is more sensitive to changes in P_aCO_2 (steeper slope) and ventilation is greater for a given P_aCO_2. If the P_aCO_2 is reduced, this causes a significant reduction in ventilation.

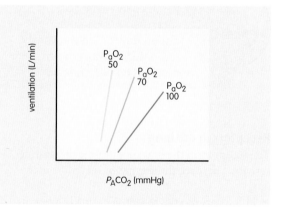

Fig. 6.10 The response of ventilation to CO_2. Note that at higher levels of P_aO_2 an increase in P_aCO_2 has less effect on ventilation (the curve is less steep).

Factors that affect ventilatory response to P_aCO_2 are:

- P_aO_2
- Blood pH
- Genetics
- Age
- Psychiatric state
- Fitness
- Drugs (e.g., opiates, such as morphine and diamorphine, reduce respiratory and cardiovascular drive).

Response to oxygen

As mentioned above, the response to reduced P_aO_2 is by stimulation of the peripheral chemoreceptors. This response, however, is not significant until the P_aO_2 drops to around 50mmHg. The relationship between P_aO_2 and ventilation has been studied by measuring changes in ventilation while a subject breathes hypoxic mixtures (Fig. 6.11). It is assumed that end expiratory P_AO_2 and P_ACO_2 are equivalent to arterial gas tensions.

The response to P_aO_2 is also seen to change with different levels of P_ACO_2.

- The greater the carbon dioxide tension, the earlier the response to low oxygen tension.

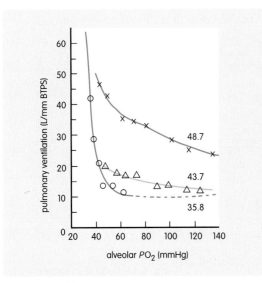

Fig. 6.11 The response of ventilation to P_AO_2 at three values of P_ACO_2. Lowered P_AO_2 has a much greater effect on ventilation when increased values of P_ACO_2 are present.

- Therefore, at high P_ACO_2, a decrease in oxygen tension below 100mmHg causes an increase in ventilation.

Under normal conditions, P_aO_2 does not fall to values of around 50mmHg and, therefore, daily control of ventilation does not rely on hypoxic drive. However, under conditions of severe lung disease or at high altitude, hypoxic drive becomes increasingly important. A patient with COPD may rely almost entirely on hypoxic drive alone, having lost ventilatory response to carbon dioxide (described above). Central chemoreceptors have become unresponsive to carbon dioxide; in addition, ventilatory drive from the effects of reduced pH on peripheral chemoreceptors is also lessened by renal compensation for the acid–base abnormality. Administration of high-concentration oxygen therapy (e.g., 100% O_2) may abolish any hypoxic drive the patient was previously relying upon, depressing ventilation and worsening the patient's condition.

Response to pH

From earlier in the chapter you should remember that hydrogen ions do not cross the blood–brain barrier and therefore affect only peripheral chemoreceptors. It is difficult to separate the response from increased P_aCO_2 and decreased pH. Any change in pH may be compensated in the long term by the kidneys and therefore has less effect on ventilation than might be expected.

An example of how pH may drive ventilation is seen in the case of metabolic acidosis. The patient will try to achieve a reduction in hydrogen ion concentration by blowing off more carbon dioxide from the lungs. This is achieved by increasing ventilation.

Response to exercise

As human beings, we are capable of a huge increase in ventilation in response to exercise: approximately 15 times the resting level. In moderate exercise, the carbon dioxide output and oxygen uptake are well matched. The increase in respiratory rate and tidal volume do not cause hyperventilation, and the subject is said to be hyperpneic:

- P_aCO_2 does not increase, but may fall slightly
- P_aO_2 does not decrease
- In moderate exercise, arterial pH varies very little.

111

Hyperpnea is an increased depth of breathing and occurs in exercise. Tachypnea is an abnormally high respiratory rate (over 20 breaths per minute), often seen in patients with pneumonia. Both are responses to increased metabolic demand and are therefore different from hyperventilation (defined as ventilation that is too great for metabolic needs).

So where does the drive for ventilation come from? There have been many possible causes of the increase in ventilation seen during exercise, but none is completely satisfactory:

- Carbon dioxide load within venous blood returning to the lungs affects ventilation
- Change in pattern of oscillations of P_aCO_2 (Fig. 6.12)
- Central control of P_aCO_2 is reset to a lower value and held constant during exercise
- Movement of limbs activates joint receptors, which contribute to increased ventilation
- Increase in body temperature during exercise may also stimulate ventilation
- The motor cortex stimulates respiratory centers
- Adrenaline (epinephrine) released in exercise also stimulates respiration.

The possible role of oscillations of P_aCO_2

It is suggested that there are cyclical changes of P_aCO_2, with inspiration and expiration. Although mean P_aCO_2 does not change during moderate exercise, the amplitude of these oscillations may increase, providing the stimulus for ventilation.

In heavy exercise, there can be measurable changes in P_aO_2 and P_aCO_2, which stimulate respiration. In addition, the pH falls because anaerobic metabolism leads to production of lactic acid (blood lactate levels increase 10-fold). This lactic acid is not oxidized because the oxygen supply cannot keep up with the demands of the exercising muscles (i.e., an "oxygen debt" is incurred). Rises in potassium ion concentration and temperature may also contribute to the increase in ventilation.

When exercise stops, respiration does not immediately return to basal levels. It remains elevated to provide an increased supply of oxygen to the tissues to oxidize the products of anaerobic metabolism ("repaying the oxygen debt").

Abnormalities of ventilatory control
Cheyne–Stokes respiration

In Cheyne–Stokes respiration, a breathing disorder occurring mainly during sleep, ventilation alternates between progressively deeper breaths and then progressively shallower breaths in a cyclical manner, alternating with brief periods of apnea. Ventilatory control is not achieved and the respiratory system appears to become unstable:

- Arterial carbon dioxide and oxygen tensions vary significantly
- Tidal volumes wax and wane (Fig. 6.13)

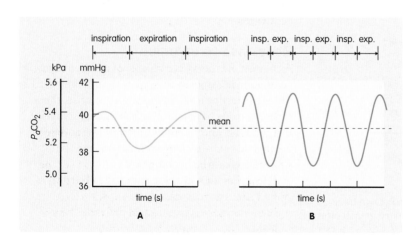

Fig. 6.12 Cyclical changes of P_aCO_2 with inspiration and expiration, (A) at rest, (B) during exercise. Larger oscillations are thought to alter ventilation.

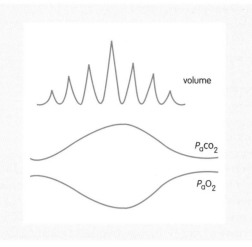

Fig. 6.13 Cheyne–Stokes respiration. (Adapted from *Physiology*, 3rd ed., by R.M. Berne and M.N. Levy. St. Louis, Mosby Year Book, 1993.)

- There are short periods of apnea separated by periods of hyperventilation.

Cheyne–Stokes breathing is observed at various times:
- At altitude—often when asleep
- During sleep
- During periods of hypoxia
- After voluntary hyperventilation
- During disease, particularly with combined right and left heart failure and uremia
- Secondary to brainstem lesions or compression.

Respiratory response to extreme environments

Response to high altitude

At high altitude, the barometric pressure is much lower than at sea level; for example, at the top of Mount Everest (8848 m), the barometric pressure is only 250 mmHg compared with 760 mmHg at sea level. Hence, the partial pressure of oxygen is lower. Dalton's law of partial pressures states that "The pressure exerted by a mixture of nonreacting gases is equal to the sum of the partial pressures of the separate components." Thus:

$$P_{atm} = PO_2 + PN_2 + PCO_2 + PH_2O$$

In addition, the partial pressure of water vapor is constant, because inspired air is saturated at body temperature. Therefore, the partial pressure of oxygen in the alveoli (and in the blood) is significantly lower than at sea level.

The content of oxygen in the blood is dependent on:
- Partial pressure of oxygen in the blood
- Hemoglobin concentration
- The oxyhemoglobin dissociation curve.

At altitude the partial pressure of oxygen in the blood is lowered. This would tend to limit the oxygen content. To combat this problem, the body can:
- Hyperventilate in an attempt to decrease the partial pressure of carbon dioxide in the alveoli and therefore increase the partial pressure of oxygen
- Increase the amount of hemoglobin in the blood, thereby increasing oxygen-carrying capacity
- Shift the oxygen dissociation curve
- Alter the circulation
- Increase anerobic metabolism in tissues, increase cytochrome oxidase activity, and increase myoglobin in muscle tissue.

Hyperventilation

It can be seen by looking at the alveolar gas equation that if we hyperventilate, thereby reducing P_ACO_2, it is possible to bring the partial pressure of oxygen in the alveolar gas much closer to the partial pressure of inspired gas.

$$P_AO_2 = P_IO_2 - (P_ACO_2/R) + K$$

This is very advantageous at altitude—at 8000 ft, the barometric pressure is 564 mmHg. Thus, for saturated air entering the lungs:

$$P_IO_2 = (564 - 47):21 = 108.5 \, mmHg$$

If a subject's P_ACO_2 was 40 mmHg and $R = 0.8$, then from the alveolar gas equation:

$$P_AO_2 = 108.5 - (40/0.8) = 58.5 \, mmHg$$

If the P_ACO_2 were reduced to 30 mmHg, then the P_AO_2 would be 71 mmHg.

At higher altitudes, because of the shape of the oxyhemoglobin dissociation curve, the effect on oxygen content in the blood is more dramatic.

Hyperventilation is stimulated by the effect of hypoxia on peripheral chemoreceptors.

Polycythemia

The function of the polycythemia that is experienced by those living at altitude is not to give a rosy-cheeked complexion, but to increase the hemoglobin concentration and therefore the oxygen-carrying capacity of the blood. The P_aO_2 and oxygen saturation of the hemoglobin are unchanged, but the total amount of oxygen per unit volume of blood is increased towards normal levels.

Hypoxemia stimulates the kidney to release the hormone erythropoietin, which increases red-cell production. This leads to a higher oxygen-carrying capacity but has the adverse effect of increasing blood viscosity and therefore increasing the tendency for thrombus formation.

Shifting of the oxyhemoglobin dissociation curve

It would be extremely advantageous if we as humans could significantly shift the oxyhemoglobin dissociation curve to the left when loading hemoglobin with oxygen and to the right when unloading oxygen. At altitude, there is a shift to the right, which aids unloading. This is caused by an increase in 2,3-diphosphoglycerate as a result of respiratory alkalosis.

Adverse effects of altitude

Low oxygen tensions in the alveoli cause vasoconstriction of the pulmonary vasculature. This leads to hydrodynamic pulmonary hypertension and increased work for the right heart. Because this alters the Starling forces affecting the pulmonary vessels, pulmonary edema may occur (reducing gas exchange). The permeability of capillaries is increased and a high-protein transudate forms.

Diving

Increased pressure applies in underwater situations. When diving, pressure increases because of the weight of the column of water above. The pressure rises by 1 atm (760 mmHg) for every 10 m descended. Solids and liquids are incompressible, and any increased pressure has little effect on these. Gases, however, are compressible and gas contained within a cavity or in solution (Henry's law) is affected by pressure changes.

Thus, on descent, the pressure increases, and a gas is:
- Compressed
- Forced into solution.

On ascent gas may:
- Expand (which if enclosed in a cavity or sinus could rupture the surrounding structure)
- Come out of solution.

The different types of dive are discussed briefly below.

Single-breath dive

A single-breath dive is short enough to be accomplished on the air inhaled at the surface. The diver holds his breath and submerges. The air in the diver's lung is subjected to increased pressure, increasing the PO_2 and PCO_2. Oxygen supply is increased, but so is carbon dioxide, stimulating the chemoreceptors: the diver soon must return to the surface. The dive can be prolonged by hyperventilation before submerging, but this can be dangerous on ascent because, as the ambient pressure falls, so the PO_2 falls to levels at which the diver may become unconscious. Standard advice is that four maximum breaths are allowed.

The ratio of total lung volume to residual volume theoretically limits the depth of the dive ($6.0/1.5 = 4$ atm—i.e., 40 m).

Snorkel dive

A snorkel dive is carried out at a shallow depth, so that connection with the air can be maintained by a tube. The maximum lung pressure that the inspiratory muscles can generate is about 100 mmHg, equivalent to a depth of about 1.2 m. This pressure cannot be maintained for more than a few minutes, thus the length of the snorkel is reduced to approximately 40 cm, reducing the dead space in the tube.

Conventional and SCUBA dives

Conventional dives involve being enclosed within a chamber while breathing compressed gases.

During SCUBA (self-contained underwater breathing apparatus) dives, gas is breathed through a regulated valve system from a pressure tank carried by the diver. The pressure of gas breathed is ambient, eliminating problems of lung mechanics. There are problems with conventional and SCUBA dives at depths over 50 m (5 atm) because of:
- Increased density of the inhaled gas, increasing the work of breathing
- Nitrogen narcosis
- Decompression sickness.

Nitrogen narcosis

Nitrogen has high solubility in fat and this solubility increases with increasing pressure. Nitrogen acts like a general anesthetic, expanding the lipid components of cell membranes, leading to the distortion of membrane proteins, including ion channels that are responsible for neural signaling. It is believed this property leads to narcosis. Symptoms of nitrogen narcosis include:

- Euphoria
- Mental confusion
- Impaired neuromuscular coordination (clumsiness)
- Loss of consciousness.

Effects are detectable at 4atm; serious impairment of performance occurs at 10atm; full surgical anesthesia occurs at 30atm.

Decompression sickness

Under normal atmospheric pressure, the solubility of nitrogen is low and body tissues contain little nitrogen in solution: 9ml nitrogen dissolved per liter of body water; 50ml of nitrogen dissolved per liter of body fat. As we descend during a dive, ambient pressure increases, thus increasing the partial pressure of nitrogen and forcing nitrogen into solution (especially in adipose tissue).

On ascending, the nitrogen comes out of solution. If ascent is rapid, there is inadequate time for the nitrogen to reach the lungs and be blown off. Instead it comes out of solution and forms bubbles (like formation of bubbles on opening a bottle of soda). Bubbles obstruct the circulation, especially in tissues with a high fat content, leading to bends (bubble formation in the joints) and chokes (bubble formation in the pulmonary vessels).

Drugs and the respiratory system

Overview

Many drugs are used to treat diseases of the respiratory system. Some are considered under the relevant diseases in Chapter 7; however, some important categories of drugs are introduced here. These categories are:

- Drugs used in asthma
- Respiratory stimulants
- Drugs used in allergies and anaphylaxis
- Mucolytics
- Cough preparations
- Drugs used in smoking cessation.

We have not included a review of antibiotics here. You should ensure that you understand the mechanisms of action and main indications of common antibiotics used in respiratory medicine.

In addition, a number of drugs have side effects on the respiratory system; drugs that cause respiratory depression are considered below.

Drugs used in the treatment of asthma

Drugs used in the treatment of asthma can be divided into two main categories:

- Relievers (bronchodilators)
- Preventers (corticosteroids, leukotriene receptor antagonists, cromolyn sodium).

The "step-wise" approach to using these drugs to treat asthma is described in Chapter 7.

Relievers

Bronchodilators

Bronchodilators can be split into four groups:

- Short-acting β_2 agonists
- Anticholinergics
- Long-acting β_2 agonists
- Xanthines.

Short-acting β_2 agonists Bronchial smooth muscle contains numerous β_2 receptors, which act through an adenylate cyclase/cAMP second-messenger system to cause smooth muscle relaxation and hence bronchodilation (Fig. 6.14).

Examples of short-acting β_2 agonists are:

- Albuterol
- Metaproterenol.

These drugs are usually inhaled, either as an aerosol, a powder, or as a nebulized solution. They can also be given intravenously, intramuscularly, and subcutaneously. They are used for acute symptoms and act within minutes, producing effects lasting 4–5 hours.

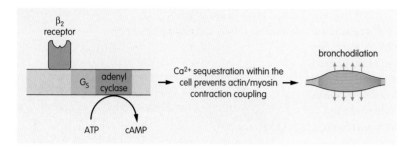

Fig. 6.14 Mechanisms of action of β_2 agonists—relaxation of bronchial muscle (which leads to bronchodilation) and inhibition of mast-cell degranulation (β receptors on mast cell).

The β_2 agonists are not completely specific and have some β_1 agonistic effects, especially in high doses.

Side effects of β_2 agonists include:

- Tachycardia
- Fine tremor
- Nervous tension
- Headache.

At the doses given by aerosol, these side effects seldom occur. Tolerance may occur with high repeated doses.

Anticholinergics Anticholinergics are competitive antagonists of muscarinic acetylcholine receptors. They therefore block the vagal control of bronchial smooth muscle tone in response to irritants and reduce the reflex bronchoconstriction. Ipratropium bromide and oxitropium bromide are both anticholinergics; they have two mechanisms of action:

- Reduction of reflex bronchoconstriction (e.g., from dust or pollen)
- Reduction of mucous secretions.

These drugs reach their maximum effect within 60–90 minutes and act for between 4–6 hours. They are poorly absorbed orally; they must, therefore, be given by aerosol.

Because anticholinergics affect only the vagally mediated element of bronchoconstriction, they are not the first-choice bronchodilator in asthma treatment. There is some evidence that these drugs are effective when given together with a β_2 agonist in severe asthma. However, their main use is in COPD that does not respond to β_2 agonists.

Side effects are rare but may include:

- Dry mouth
- Urinary retention
- Constipation.

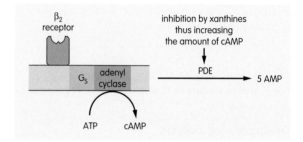

Fig. 6.15 Xanthines. The inhibition of phosphodiesterase (PDE) leads to an increase in cellular cyclic AMP, which leads to bronchodilation as in Fig. 6.1.

Long-acting β_2 agonists Like the short-acting β_2 agonists, these drugs also relax bronchial smooth muscle. They differ from the short-acting drugs in that:

- Their effect lasts for much longer (up to 12 hours)
- Full effect is achieved only after regular administration of several doses and generally less desensitization occurs.

For these reasons long-acting β_2 agonists should be used on a regular basis rather than to treat acute attacks.

The main long-acting β_2 agonists are:

- Salmeterol
- Eformoterol
- Bambuterol.

Xanthines Xanthines appear to work by inhibiting phosphodiesterase, thereby preventing the breakdown of cAMP (Fig. 6.15). The amount of cAMP within the bronchial smooth muscle cells is therefore increased, which causes bronchodilation in a similar way to β_2 agonists.

These drugs are metabolized in the liver and there is a considerable variation in half life between individuals. This has important implications because there is a small therapeutic window. Factors altering theophylline clearance are shown in Fig. 6.16.

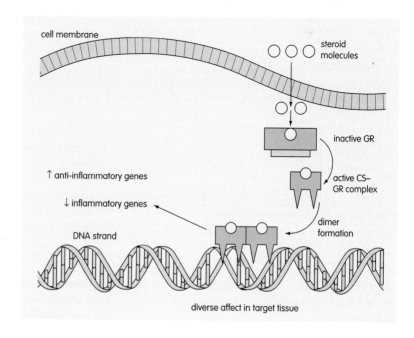

Tobacco shortens the half-life of theophylline (due to enzyme induction), and clearance can remain enhanced for up to 3 months after a patient has stopped smoking.

Theophylline can be given intravenously in the form of aminophylline (theophylline with ethylenediamine) but must be administered very slowly (over 20 minutes to administer dose). Aminophylline is given in cases of severe asthma attacks that do not respond to β_2 agonists and in acute asthma.

Prophylactic therapy
Glucocorticosteroids

Steroids reduce the formation, release, and action of many different mediators involved in inflammation. Their mode of action is complex and involves gene regulation (Fig. 6.17) after binding to steroid receptors in the cytoplasm of cells. This has a number of effects including:

- Downregulation of proinflammatory cytokines
- Production of anti-inflammatory proteins.

One of these anti-inflammatory proteins is thought to reduce the activity of phospholipase A_2 which itself plays a role in the release of arachidonic acid from membrane phospholipids (Fig. 6.18).

Steroids in treatment of asthma may be topical (inhaled) or systemic (oral or parenteral).

Inhaled steroids   These include:
- Flunisolide
- Triamcinolone acetonide
- Beclomethasone dipropionate

Factors altering theophylline clearance	
Increased clearance	**Decreased clearance**
Smoking	Liver disease
Alcohol	Pneumonia
Rifampicin	Cimetidine
Childhood	Clarythromycin lerythromycin, etc.)
	Old age
i.e. P450 enzyme induction	i.e. P450 enzyme inhibition

Fig. 6.16 Factors altering theophylline clearance.

Fig. 6.17 Mechanism of action of steroids. Steroid molecules diffuse across cell membrane and bind to steroid receptors forming CS–GR complexes. These complexes may bind to DNA as dimers and modulate the output of many different gene products. Alternatively, CS–GR monomers may block induction of inflammatory genes by exogenous stimuli.

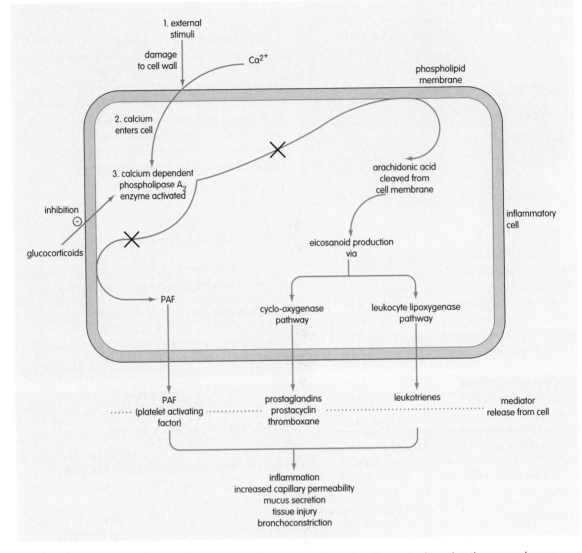

Fig. 6.18 Inhibition of inflammatory mediator cascade (i.e., cross through pathways to show that they are no longer active). PAF is a proinflammatory, bronchoconstrictor substance derived from membrane phospholipids. (From D. Seaton in *Crofton and Douglas's Respiratory Diseases*, 2000. London, Blackwell Science Ltd., Vol. 1, p. 261.)

- Fluticasone propionate
- Budesonide.

Side effects of inhaled steroids in adults are relatively minor (primarily hoarseness and oral candidiasis). Inhaled steroids have been associated with an increased risk of cataracts. They may have a short-term effect on growth in children.

Oral steroids The primary oral steroid is prednisolone. Side effects of systemic steroids include:

- Adrenal suppression
- Effects on bones (including growth retardation)
- Diabetes mellitus
- Increased susceptibility to infection
- Weight gain
- Effects on skin (e.g., bruising and atrophy)
- Mood changes.

Leukotriene receptor antagonists
Cysteinyl leukotrienes are eicosanoids (arachidonic acid metabolites) that cause bronchoconstriction.

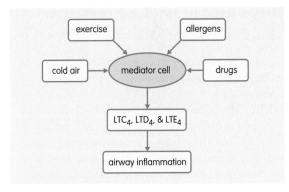

Fig. 6.19 Overview of cysteinyl leukotriene release.

Their proinflammatory actions (Fig. 6.19) center on their ability to:
- Increase vascular permeability
- Cause influx of eosinophils.

Leukotriene receptor antagonists (or leukotriene modifiers), therefore, have anti-inflammatory and bronchodilatory effects. The exact mode of action is unclear.

The two key leukotriene receptor antagonists are montelukast and zafirlukast. Montelukast is used in prophylaxis of exercise-induced asthma and in patients with mild-to-moderate asthma whose symptoms are not well controlled by other asthma drugs.

Cromolyn sodium

The mode of action of cromolyn sodium is not completely understood. It is known to stabilize mast cells, possibly by blocking transport of calcium ions. It cannot be used to treat an acute attack but is given for prophylaxis, especially in patients with atopy. The route of administration is by inhalation.

Its mechanism of action is to:
- Prevent mast-cell degranulation and hence mediator release
- Reduce C fiber response to irritants, therefore reducing bronchoconstriction
- Inhibit platelet-activating factor (PAF)-induced bronchoconstriction.

In addition to its use in allergen-mediated asthma, sodium chromoglycate is effective in non-allergen-mediated bronchoconstriction (e.g., in exercise-induced asthma), and continued use results in reduced bronchial hyperactivity. It is often used in pediatrics. Nedocromil sodium is a drug with similar actions.

Respiratory stimulants

A respiratory stimulant (analeptic) such as doxapram can be used for patients with chronic obstructive pulmonary disease in type II respiratory failure. However, mechanical ventilation and a high incidence of side effects have reduced their use. Doxapram stimulates carotid body chemoreceptors and must be given intravenously.

Side effects of doxapram are:
- Tachycardia
- Palpitations
- Nausea
- Sweating
- Tremor.

Contraindications to the use of doxapram are:
- Epilepsy
- Hypertension
- Hyperthyroidism.

Drugs used for allergies and anaphylaxis

H_1 histamine antagonists

These drugs are used in the treatment of allergies, such as hay fever. Examples of these drugs are:
- Promethazine
- Trimeprazine.

The mechanism of action is to block H_1 receptors. These drugs cross the blood–brain barrier and have a general depressant action (sedative); in high doses, this action can cause respiratory depression.

Newer drugs such as fexofenadine do not readily cross the blood–brain barrier and therefore do not cause respiratory depression.

Anaphylaxis

Anaphylactic shock is a systemic allergic reaction which is a life-threatening condition. The features of anaphylactic shock are:
- Severe hypotension
- Laryngeal spasm
- Bronchoconstriction.

The treatment of anaphylaxis must therefore be rapid:

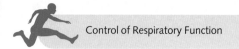

- Secure the airway
- Maintain blood pressure by laying the patient flat and raising his or her legs.

Drug therapy is as follows:
- Subcutaneous or intravenous adrenaline (epinephrine)
- 100% oxygen
- Second-line therapy may include diphenhydramide, methylprednisolone, inhaled beta$_2$ agonists, intravenous aminophylline, or vasopressors (noradrenaline (norepinehrine) or dopamine hydrochloride).

Mucolytics

Mucolytics (e.g., guaifenesin, DNase, and N-acetyl cysteine) are designed to reduce the viscosity of sputum, thereby aiding expectoration. The indications for use have been in:
- Chronic bronchitis
- Chronic asthma
- Cystic fibrosis
- Bronchiectasis.

Some mucolytics may be of benefit in treating acute exacerbations in COPD.

Cough preparations

The cough reflex is a protective mechanism to eliminate particulate matter and mucus from the respiratory tree. Inhibition of this reflex may have a deleterious effect, causing build up of secretions and the risk of infection, especially in patients with chronic bronchitis and bronchiectasis. They may have some use in a dry cough or a nonproductive cough found in bronchial carcinoma.

Typical drugs used are weak opioids, which suppress the cough reflex. Examples are:
- Codeine
- Dextromethorphan.

Codeine inhibits the cough reflex centrally. A side effect is the inhibition of ciliary activity, which reduces the clearance of secretions. It also causes constipation.

Dextromethorphan is a synthetic, non-narcotic, nonanalgesic, and nonaddictive opioid. It has a similar efficacy to codeine but does not have the side effects. It should be noted that both drugs in large doses cause respiratory depression.

Drugs used in smoking cessation

There are two main classes of drugs used in smoking cessation:
- Nicotine replacement therapy (NRT)
- Bupropion (amfebutamone).

NRT products (gums, patches, and nasal sprays) are classified as over-the-counter medicines and have been shown to be effective in treating tobacco withdrawal and dependence. They should not be used in patients with severe cardiovascular disease (including immediately after myocardial infarction).

Bupropion is an antidepressant also licensed for use as an adjunct to smoking cessation. The main side effects are a dry mouth and difficulty sleeping. The drug should not be used if there is a history of epilepsy or eating disorders.

In addition to pharmacologic methods, a number of other interventions have been shown to be effective in helping smokers quit:
- Simple advice and/or brief counselling from primary care providers
- Group counseling at smoking cessation clinics.

Respiratory depressants

If a drug has a depressant action on the central nervous system, large enough doses of it will cause respiratory depression. The most notable of the drugs which cause respiratory depression are the opioid analgesics.

Other drugs that may also cause respiratory depression are listed below:
- Barbiturates
- Benzodiazepines
- H$_1$ histamine antagonists
- Alcohol.

Opioids and barbiturates depress central chemoreceptor activity, and this contributes to the respiratory depression they cause.

Opioid analgesics

These drugs are in very common use in clinical medicine and include:
- Morphine
- Hydrocodone
- Codeine.

In high doses, these drugs cause respiratory and cardiovascular depression, which can be lethal. These drugs bind to opioid receptors in the spinal cord, pons, and midbrain and mimic the action of endogenous opioid.

Overdose is usually iatrogenic in origin or from illicit drug abuse (heroin and prescription opioids such as oxycodone). The effects of overdose can be reversed by administration of an opioid-receptor antagonist (e.g., naloxone).

Overdose may occur in the newborn if the mother has been given opioids during a cesarean section because the drug crosses the placenta. This can cause respiratory depression in the neonate. The infant is injected with naloxone and resuscitation commenced immediately.

Signs of overdose are varied state of consciousness, respiratory depression, and pin-point pupils.

Other main side effects of opioids are:
• Nausea and vomiting
• Constipation
• Difficulty in micturition
• Drowsiness.

Contraindications to opioid analgesics are respiratory depression and acute alcoholism.

Barbiturates

All barbiturates have a depressant activity on the central nervous system. They are used as induction agents for general anesthesia (thiopental), for treatment of grand mal epilepsy (phenobarbital), and for sedation.

The mechanism of action of barbiturates is enhancement of GABA-mediated inhibition of the central nervous system. These drugs prolong the opening of individual chloride channels by a given GABA stimulus.

Barbiturates cause respiratory and cardiovascular depression when administered at 10–100 times the clinical dose.

Benzodiazepines

Benzodiazepines are extensively used as anxiolytics, hypnotics, and for sedation. Their use has become unfashionable because of tolerance and withdrawal effects, which develop after about 2–4 weeks of use.

Their mechanism of action is the same as that of the barbiturates, although benzodiazepines bind to a different site on the $GABA_A$ receptor complex.

Normally, even high orally administered doses of benzodiazepines do not cause severe respiratory depression. However, intravenous or oral administration either to elderly patients or to patients with underlying pulmonary disease can cause respiratory depression.

Respiratory support

Patients with respiratory disease who are hypoxemic and/or hypercapnic often require a form of respiratory support. This support may range from oxygen given briefly via a face mask in a patient with mild hypoxemia to mechanical ventilation in respiratory failure. The two basic categories of respiratory support are considered below:

Oxygen therapy

Assisted ventilation (noninvasive or mechanical).

Oxygen therapy

Oxygen therapy aims to correct hypoxemia. Progress is monitored, and the amount of oxygen adjusted, according to pulse oximetry and arterial blood gas analysis.

Oxygen can be delivered either by:
• Nasal cannula
• Face mask.

Nasal cannulas

These allow the patient to talk and eat while receiving oxygen. Air is humidified to avoid discomfort from nasal crusting. Oxygen is delivered at rates of 1–4L/min, which, when diluted with inspiratory air, equates to oxygen concentrations of 25–30%.

Delivery through nasal prongs is also used in long-term oxygen therapy (LTOT)—for example, in patients with COPD who have a home oxygen supply.

Face masks

These fit over the nose and mouth and are used with higher-flow oxygen (e.g., 6L/min or an oxygen concentration of 60%). Remember that high concentrations of oxygen should not be given to patients with acute-on-chronic respiratory failure (see p. 96).

Assisted ventilation

In some cases even high-flow oxygen is not sufficient to restore blood gases to adequate levels. A patient with COPD for example , may maintain near normal blood gases until an infection adds to the workload; some form of ventilatory support is then indicated in order to:

- Offload the respiratory muscles and reduce the work of breathing
- Improve gas exchange.

> Remember that excessive load is a major problem in acute-on-chronic respiratory failure. Taking away some of the work with assisted ventilation will help correct the vicious circle in which lung disease increases work which consumes oxygen which increases work requirement.

Noninvasive ventilation (NIV)

In noninvasive ventilation, respiratory support is given via the patient's upper airway and intubation is avoided. This method, therefore, is suitable only if a patient can protect his or her own airway but has the advantage of reducing the risks of a hospital-acquired infection. The patient breathes spontaneously, and the lungs are expanded by a volume of gas delivered, usually at a positive pressure. This decreases the work of the respiratory muscles, particularly the diaphragm.

NIV is particularly effective in patients with acute hypercapnic respiratory failure, particularly in COPD. Lung volumes in these patients do not return to baseline after expiration so that greater pressures are needed to expand the lungs (i.e., there is an intrinsic positive end expiratory pressure or iPEEP). The positive pressure of the gas given via the mask therefore reduces the extra work generated by air trapping.

Two basic types of noninvasive ventilation are considered here:

- Continuous positive airway pressure (CPAP)
- Bilevel positive airway pressure (BiPAP).

As the name implies, CPAP delivers a continuous positive air pressure throughout the respiratory cycle. BiPAP is an example of intermittent positive pressure ventilation (IPPV). BiPAP also reduces the work of breathing but differs in that it senses when inspiration is occurring and delivers a higher pressure during the inspiratory part of the cycle.

Noninvasive ventilation may be used in acute situations or on a long-term basis in patients with COPD; it is also used in weaning from conventional, intubated ventilators.

Mechanical ventilation

True mechanical ventilation links the patient to the ventilator by means of an endotracheal tube (usually inserted via the nose) or, if ventilation is likely to be prolonged, via tracheostomy. An airtight seal is created and gas is delivered either at constant pressure or at PEEP. Indications for mechanical ventilation include:

- Protection of airway in unconscious patients
- Severe hypoxemia (e.g., in ARDS)
- Controlling hypercapnia in ventilatory failure (i.e., type 2 respiratory failure) when NIV is inappropriate.

Complications of respiratory support

There are several important complications of respiratory support; most, including those presented by intubation and difficulties in weaning the patient, are outside the scope of this book.

Oxygen toxicity

The use of high-concentration oxygen therapy can have adverse effects on the respiratory system. This is especially evident after prolonged use.

Oxygen intoxication was first recognized by Paul Bert in 1878. He noticed that breathing oxygen at 1 atm for as little as 12 hours can lead to pulmonary congestion (reducing vital capacity), pulmonary edema, exudation (reducing gaseous exchange), and damage to the pulmonary epithelium.

In the premature infant, administration of high-concentration oxygen can also cause retrolental fibroplasia. Fibrous tissue forms behind the lens and can lead to permanent blindness. This is thought to be caused by vasoconstriction, secondary to a high partial pressure of oxygen. This can be avoided by keeping a low PO_2.

Respiratory distress can occur because of absorption atelectasis.

Absorption atelectasis

Absorption atelectasis is the collapse of an alveolus due to blockage. When breathing 100% O_2, the oxygen in the alveolus is quickly absorbed because there is a huge partial pressure difference between the alveolar gas and the partial pressure of gases in the venous blood. This results in collapse of the alveolus. It is then difficult to open the collapsed alveoli because of high surface-tension effects.

Absorption atelectasis also occurs in airway occlusion when breathing a normal air mixture. The rate of absorption is much slower as the driving force (the partial pressure difference between venous blood and alveolar gas) is much lower. There is still a partial pressure difference driving diffusion because the fall in oxygen tension from arterial to venous blood is greater than the rise in carbon dioxide tension. Collapse can be avoided by adding even small concentrations of nitrogen. Nitrogen is poorly absorbed because of its poor solubility and therefore remains in the alveoli delaying or preventing collapse.

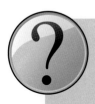

- Describe what is meant by feedback and feed-forward control.
- Discuss the central control of breathing with reference to the pontine respiratory group, and the dorsal and ventral respiratory groups of the medulla.
- List the different types of receptors involved in control.
- What factors stimulate central and peripheral chemoreceptors?
- Outline the responses of the respiratory system to changes in carbon dioxide concentration, oxygen concentration, and pH.
- Discuss the mechanisms thought to influence the control of ventilation in exercise.
- Discuss the changes that occur in response to high altitude.
- What types of respiratory support might a patient with COPD receive?
- Outline the treatment of a patient with an acute asthma attack.
- Explain the mechanism of action of the β_2 agonists.
- Outline the drugs used to prevent asthma attacks.
- List the classes of drugs used to treat diseases of the respiratory system.
- List the treatment measures for management of anaphylaxis.
- Describe the drugs that have an adverse effect on the respiratory system.
- Describe absorption atelectasis.

7. Disorders of the Lungs

Introduction

A large number of lung disorders are covered in this chapter; they are grouped mainly according to the "surgical sieve" approach, that is, in categories reflecting the type of disorder (e.g., congenital) or underlying pathology (e.g., infection). The aim is to provide a clear structure for review, allowing the disorders to be worked through in a logical fashion. However, this may make it difficult to see which are the common or important diseases. Therefore, set out below is a list of key disorders; this is necessarily brief but includes some of the diseases commonly seen in clinical practice plus others that illustrate an important pathologic process.

The surgical sieve can be a tool for fomulating a differential diagnosis, making sure that no possible cause has been forgotten. A number of mnemonics exist for the categories. One is TIN CAN BED PAN: trauma, inflammatory, neoplastic, congenital, arteriovenous, neurologic, blood, endocrine, drugs, psychogenic, allergic, not known.

The key disorders

Asthma
- A chronic inflammatory disorder of the airways, characterized by symptoms that are intermittent and have a diurnal variation (p. 139).

Chronic obstructive pulmonary disease (COPD)
- Chronic bronchitis and emphysema in the same patient, who is almost always a smoker (p. 135).

Lung cancer
- Accounts for 20% of all cancers; the risk is directly related to tobacco exposure (p. 157).

Pneumonia
- An infection of peripheral lung tissue associated with significant morbidity and mortality worldwide (p. 127).

Pulmonary embolism
- The most serious complication of venous thrombosis; prophylaxis is important in high-risk patients (p. 147).

Bronchiectasis
- Permanent dilatation of the bronchi secondary to chronic infection (p. 142).

Cystic fibrosis
- An autosomal recessive condition predisposing to chronic lung infection and bronchiectasis (p. 143).

Pneumothorax
- Air in the pleural space; the tension type is a medical emergency (p. 166).

Pleural effusion
- Fluid in the pleural space; a complication of several common lung disorders (p. 165).

Pulmonary fibrosis
- End point of many different lung diseases and an example of the basic pathology of restrictive disorders (p. 151).

Sarcoidosis
- A multisystem disorder; pulmonary features include bilateral hilar lymphadenopathy (p. 153).

Occupational lung diseases
Certain disorders with common themes are dealt with separately under the surgical sieve approach.

One category that is important, and that you should consider as a whole, is that of occupational lung disorders. More details on this group of diseases are given in Chapter 9 (see Fig. 9.1).

Congenital abnormalities

Congenital cysts

The respiratory system is an outgrowth of the ventral wall of the foregut. Bronchogenic cysts may result from abnormal budding of the tracheobronchial tree. They are lined by bronchial elements: cartilage, smooth muscle, and ciliated respiratory epithelium. Cysts are classified according to position:

• Central (mediastinal)—85%
• Peripheral (intrapulmonary)—15%.

Cysts are usually single, spherical or oval, unilocular masses. They are mainly asymptomatic and can present at any age, although they are more common in men. Surgical excision is recommended. Radiologically, it is impossible to differentiate between a bronchogenic cyst and malignancy (Fig. 7.1).

Lobar sequestrations

Lobar sequestrations are masses of pulmonary tissue that do not communicate anatomically with the tracheobronchial tree (Fig. 7.2).

Vascular abnormalities

Vascular abnormalities include absent pulmonary artery trunk, absent unilateral pulmonary artery, pulmonary artery stenosis, pulmonary arteriovenous malformations, anomalous origin of the left pulmonary artery, and anomalous pulmonary venous drainage.

Congenital lobar emphysema

Lobar emphysema is an overdistension of a lobe (usually an upper lobe) caused by intermittent bronchial obstruction. Symptoms in early life are caused by pressure effects. Pathogenesis includes defects in the bronchial cartilage, mechanical causes of bronchial obstruction and idiopathic causes. Prognosis is good.

Agenesis and hypoplasia
Agenesis

Agenesis is a complete absence of one or both lungs with no trace of bronchial or vascular supply.

Hypoplasia

In hypoplasia, the bronchus is fully formed but reduced in size; there is failure of alveolar development. Hypoplasia is associated with other congenital abnormalities such as Potter's syndrome and diaphragmatic hernia.

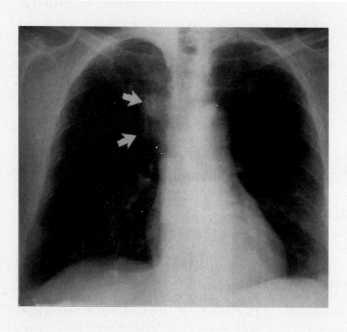

Fig. 7.1 Radiograph of a bronchogenic cyst. There is a right paratracheal mass (arrows). (Courtesy of Dr D. Sutton and Dr J.W.R. Young.)

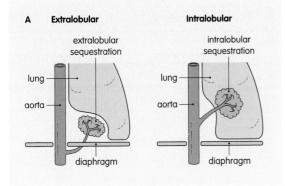

B	Comparison between intralobular and extralobular sequestrations	
	Intralobular	Extralobular
incidence	more common	less common
male-to-female ratio	1:1	4:1
side of thorax	60% left	90% left
arterial supply	70% thoracic aorta	40% thoracic aorta
venous drainage	pulmonary veins	systemic
position	within normal lung and its pleural covering	separate from normal lung in its own pleural cover
other congenital defects	uncommon	frequent

Fig. 7.2 (A and B) Differences between extralobular and intralobular sequestrations.

Abnormalities of trachea or bronchi

Abnormalities of trachea or bronchi include tracheal agenesis, tracheoesophageal fistula, tracheal stenosis, tracheal narrowing caused by extrinsic pressure, tracheomalacia, and tracheobronchomegaly.

Atelectasis

Atelectasis (from the Greek *ateles*, meaning imperfect, and *ektasis*, meaning expansion) is classified as primary or secondary:
- Primary—lung fails to expand at birth
- Secondary—caused by obstruction or compression (Fig. 7.3).

Obstructive atelectasis

Obstruction is the most common cause of atelectasis; this is also known as resorptive atelectasis (Fig. 7.4).

Obstructive atelectasis follows an acute and complete obstruction of a large bronchus. Air in the collapsed area of the lung is absorbed and secretions distal to the obstruction accumulate; subsequently, these bronchial secretions become infected and suppurate. Distal to the blockage, the bronchi mechanically distend.

If the collapse has been present for some time, irreversible pulmonary fibrosis occurs. Pulmonary artery branches may have narrowed lumens.

Compressive atelectasis

In compressive atelectasis, bronchial obstruction does not occur; therefore, bronchial secretions are free to drain up the bronchial tree. As such, the collapsed lung does not become seriously infected.

Compressive atelectasis results from external compression of the lung. Causes of compression include pleural effusion, hemothorax, empyema, pneumothorax, space-occupying intrathoracic lesion, and abdominal distension.

Hemodynamic and vascular changes occur. High inflation pressures on inspiration are required to overcome retractive forces. Re-expansion of the lung usually occurs after compression is resolved.

Patchy atelectasis

Depending on the cause, atelectasis may occur in a patchy or diffuse distribution.

Infections of the lung

Pneumonia

Pneumonia is defined as an infection of peripheral lung parenchyma (as opposed to infection of the central conducting airways—bronchitis). Clinically, pneumonia is an acute illness in which there are signs of consolidation in the chest or new changes on chest x-ray. In the U.S. pneumonia is responsible for approximately 65000 deaths a year.

127

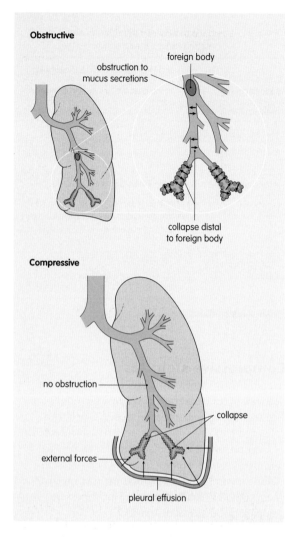

Fig. 7.3 Obstructive and compressive atelectasis.

Pneumonia can be classified on the basis of:
- The setting or circumstances in which it originated (community- or hospital-acquired or pneumonia in immunocompromised hosts)
- Anatomy (lobar or bronchopneumonia)
- Organisms (bacterial, atypical, viral, fungal, protozoal).

It is now common to use the first classification because it has more clinical significance (while the anatomic site is of limited use in guiding treatment and the organism may never be known).

Comparison of acute and chronic obstruction	
Acute	**Chronic**
inhalation and impaction of foreign bodies	tumors
mucus plugging of bronchi (e.g. after anesthesia)	lymphadenopathy
after tracheostomy	aneurysm
lung infections	

Fig. 7.4 Causes of acute and chronic obstruction.

The anatomic classification for pneumonia is not used here, but if you come across it elsewhere: lobar pneumonia occurs when organisms widely colonize alveolar spaces, whereas bronchopneumonia occurs when organisms colonize bronchi and extend into alveoli.

Community-acquired pneumonia
Pathogenesis
Organisms enter the lungs usually having been inhaled from the environment or nasopharynx. These organisms may be eliminated by the lung's defense mechanisms (see Chapter 3), or they may survive and multiply. Factors that undermine the lung's defenses, therefore, increase the risk of pneumonia. These factors include:
- Alcohol excess
- Cigarette smoking
- Chronic heart and lung diseases
- Bronchial obstruction
- Immunosuppression
- Drug abuse.

The pathogen stimulates host defenses and alveolar airspaces become filled with eosinophilic edematous fluid containing neutrophil polymorphs. The edema transports organisms through the pores of Kohn into the alveoli.

In days 2–4, a red hepatization occurs; there is accumulation in alveolar spaces of polymorphs, lymphocytes, and macrophages. The alveolar

Causes and features of community acquired pneumonia		
Organism	Features of pneumonia	% cases
Streptococcus pneumoniae	Gram-positive alpha-hemolytic; polysaccharide capsule determines virulence and is detectable serologically; responsible for a high mortality (especially in the setting of bacteremia) unless treated appropriately; vaccine available	55–75
Mycoplasma pneumoniae	epidemics every 3–4 years usually in young patients; 50% have cold agglutinins; associated with many extrapulmonary manifestations; penicillin ineffective as no bacterial cell wall	5–18
Influenzo	epidemics common; affects patients with underlying lung disease; can be severe; S. aureus, S. pneumoniae, H. influenzae occur secondarily; a vaccine is available	8
Legionella pneumophila	gram-negative; found in cooling towers and air-conditioning; causes very severe pneumonia with high mortality and is frequently associated with extrapulmonary features; antigen may help in diagnosis	2–5
Chlamydia pneumoniae	headache very common; usually serological diagnosis	2–5
Haemophilus influenzae	gram-negative rod; more commonly associated with exacerbations of COPD	4–5
Viruses other than influenza		2–8
Staphylococcus aureus	gram-positive coccus; often follows flu; alcoholics and patients with mitral valve disease are susceptible; often causes severe, often cavitating pneumonia; commonly fatal	1–5
Klebsiella pneumoniae	gram-negative; seen in alcoholics; severe and often cavitates	1

Fig. 7.5 Organisms causing community-acquired pneumonia.

exudate contains a fine network of fibrin and large numbers of extravasated red cells. The lung is red, solid, and airless. Red hepatization corresponds to an area of edema and hemorrhage.

In days 4–8, a gray hepatization occurs. Fibrinous pleurisy is present. Alveolar spaces are microscopically distended and filled by a dense network of fibrin-containing neutrophil polymorphs. Gray hepatization represents a zone of advanced consolidation with destruction of red and white blood cells. The lung is gray or brown and solid.

Resolution occurs after 8–10 days in untreated cases. When bacteria have been eliminated, macrophages enter and replace granulocytes. The exudate is liquefied by fibrinolytic enzymes and coughed up or absorbed. There is preservation of the underlying alveolar wall architecture.

Etiology
Figure 7.5 shows the key pathogens in CAP. *S. pneumoniae* is the causative organism in 55–75% of cases. Note, however, that in around a third of cases, no cause is found.

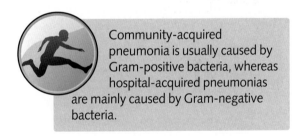

Community-acquired pneumonia is usually caused by Gram-positive bacteria, whereas hospital-acquired pneumonias are mainly caused by Gram-negative bacteria.

Clinical features
The common respiratory symptoms are shown in Fig. 7.6. Note that the presence of confusion is a poor prognostic factor (see below).

On examination the patient is typically pyrexial, tachycardic, and tachypneic. Lung expansion is reduced and signs of consolidation are found (see Chapter 9). Coarse crackles may be heard as the infection resolves.

Typical clinical features of bacterial pneumonia	
Clinical feature	Incidence (%)
respiratory features	
cough	90
sputum	70
dyspnea	70
chest pain	65
upper respiratory tract symptoms	33
hemoptysis	13
nonrespiratory features	
vomiting	20
confusion	15
diarrhea	15
rash	5
abdominal pain	5
signs	
fever	80–90
tachypnea	80–90
tachycardia	80–90
abnormal chest signs	80–90
hypotension	20
confusion	15
herpes labialis	10

Fig. 7.6 Typical clinical features of bacterial pneumonia.

If you suspect pneumonia, ask about alcohol intake and comorbidities (especially chronic heart and lung disease and diabetes mellitus); foreign travel (i.e., risk of legionella) and upper respiratory tract infection are so common that positive answers are unlikely to narrow down the list of possible organisms.

Complications

The key complications are:
- Respiratory failure
- Parapneumonic effusions
- Empyema
- Lung abscess
- Pulmonary fibrosis, after resolution.

Laboratory tests

- Sputum—culture and Gram stain
- Blood—full blood count, blood culture (low sensitivity, high specificity)
- Pleural fluid—culture and Gram stain

- Chest radiography
- Bronchoscopy with BAL if diagnosis uncertain
- Assessment of oxygenation
- Other specific tests—*Mycoplasma*, *Legionella*, and *Chlamydia* antibodies; pneumococcal antigen testing by counter-immunoelectrophoresis (CIE) of the sputum, urine, and serum.

Management

Antibiotic treatment should be started immediately, without waiting for microbiology results.

For most cases use:
- Empirical treatment with macrolide, doxycycline, or fluoroquinolone (outpatients)
- Fluoroquinolone or an extended-spectrum cephalosporin in combination with a macrolide (hospitalized patients)
- Ceftriaxone, cefotaxime, ampicillin-sulbactam, or piperacillin-tazobactam combined with a fluoroquinolone or macrolide (ICU patients)
- Pathogen-specific therapy when the pathogen is identified.

In addition, pleuritic pain should be relieved with simple analgesia and oxygen therapy administered if appropriate.

Prognosis

It is important to assess the severity of CAP as this impacts on prognosis and therefore treatment planning. Prognosis may range from full recovery to death. The key adverse prognostic features are:
- New mental confusion
- Urea > 7 mmol/L.
- Respiratory rate ≥ 30/min
- Systolic blood pressure < 90 mmHg or diastolic ≤ 60 mmHg.

Patients with two or more of these features are at high risk of mortality and should be managed aggressively.

Hospital-acquired pneumonia

Hospital-acquired or nosocomial pneumonia refers to a new lower respiratory tract infection at least two days after hospital admission. It occurs in 1–5% of admissions and is a serious cause of morbidity and mortality.

Etiology

In addition to the risk factors discussed above, factors predisposing to hospital-acquired infections are:

- Intubation
- Suppressed cough leading to aspiration (e.g., postoperatively)
- Reduced host defenses
- Long stays in hospital, with associated exposure to pathogens.

Pathogens
Gram-negative bacteria (e.g., *Escherichia*, *Klebsiella*, and *Pseudomonas* spp.) are the cause of hospital acquired pneumonia in many cases, although *Staphylococcus aureus* (particularly drug-resistant strains) is also common.

Clinical features and laboratory tests
These are similar to those described above under CAP.

Management
Good Gram-negative coverage is achieved with an aminoglycoside plus antipseudomonal penicillin or a third-generation cephalosporin. Most hospital-acquired pneumonia is serious, and these drugs are frequently given intravenously.

Pneumonia in the immunocompromised patient

Pneumocystis carinii pneumonia
Pneumocystis carinii pneumonia (PCP) is a fungal infection that is largely confined to the lung. It is the most common opportunistic infection in the immunocompromised. Infection occurs by inhalation of the organism. The patient presents with an insidious or abrupt onset of dry cough, fever, and dyspnea.

Pleural effusions are rare.

Pathology   There is an interstitial infiltrate of mononuclear cells and alveolar airspaces are filled with foamy eosinophilic material.

Diagnosis   Bilateral pneumonia in an immunocompromised patient should raise suspicion of PCP. Diagnosis in 90% of cases is by staining using Giemsa, methanamine–silver, Papanicocoau, or Gram–Weigert stains with monoclonal antibodies.

Chest radiography shows diffuse bilateral alveolar and interstitial shadowing, beginning in peripheral regions and spreading in a butterfly pattern.

Treatment   Trimethoprim-sulfamethoxazole is given, intravenously at first. Prophylaxis is recommended in patients with low CD4 counts or where previous infection has occurred. Mortality of untreated patients is 100%; in treated patients, mortality is 20–50%.

Cytomegalovirus
Cytomegalovirus (CMV) is a DNA virus in the herpes group. Of patients with AIDS, 90% are infected with CMV. CMV also occurs in recipients of bone marrow and solid organ transplants. Only occasionally does CMV cause pneumonia.

Usual symptoms are a nonproductive cough, dyspnea, and fever. Disseminated infection occurs, causing encephalitis, pneumonitis, retinitis, and diffuse involvement of the gastrointestinal tract.

Pathology   Features in the pathology of CMV infection include:
- Interstitial inflammatory infiltrate of mononuclear cells
- Scattered alveolar hyaline membranes
- Protein-rich fluid in alveoli
- Intranuclear inclusion bodies found in alveolar epithelial cells.

Diagnosis   CMV infection can be diagnosed by the identification of characteristic intranuclear owl's eye inclusions in tissues and by direct immunofluorescence.

Treatment   Treatment is by intravenous or oral ganciclovir.

Aspergillus
Four pulmonary diseases are caused by the fungus *Aspergillus fumigatus*:
- Allergic aspergillosis
- Mucoid impaction
- Aspergilloma
- Invasive aspergillosis.

Invasive aspergillosis   Invasive aspergillosis occurs in immunocompromised individuals with severe neutropenia or T-lymphocyte deficiency. It may present as a necrotizing pneumonia, lung abscess, or solitary granuloma. Microabscesses contain the characteristic fungal filaments. Aspergillosis becomes invasive when it spreads to other parts of the body via the circulation.

Recovery may occur after vigorous treatment with intravenous amphotericin. Prognosis is generally poor.

Cryptococcus
Cryptococcus is a budding, yeast-like fungus that may disseminate to all organs. Pulmonary lesions may

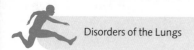

not be clinically apparent but can commonly involve the lower lobes. Other pulmonary manifestations include:

- Cavitation within lung nodules
- Calcification
- Pneumonitis
- Pleural effusions
- Intrathoracic lymph node enlargement.

Meningeal involvement is the most common form of cryptococcosis.

Varicella zoster

Varicella zoster is an uncommon cause of pneumonia. The associated pustular rash confirms diagnosis. Treatment is with acyclovir.

Kaposi's sarcoma

Kaposi's sarcoma is included here because it may be a differential diagnosis in the immunocompromised host. It is a multifocal neoplastic condition typically seen in patients with AIDS. Lesions of the pleura, parenchyma, lymph nodes, and airways occur. Overall prognosis is poor.

Lung abscess

Lung abscess is a localized area of infected parenchyma, with necrosis and suppuration.

Etiology

A lung abscess may occur due to:

- Aspiration of infected material (e.g., in alcoholism, unconscious patients)
- Complications of pneumonia
- Infection of cavities in bronchiectasis or TB
- Bronchial obstructions (e.g., tumors or foreign body)
- Pulmonary infarction.

Clinical features

Onset may be acute or insidious, depending on the cause of the abscess. Acute symptoms include malaise, anorexia, fever, and a productive cough. Copious foul-smelling sputum is present, caused by the growth of anaerobic organisms.

In large abscesses there may be dullness to percussion. Pallor is common, caused by anemia. Clubbing is a late sign.

Complications

Abscesses can heal completely leaving a small fibrous scar. Complications include empyema,

bronchopleural fistula, pyopneumothorax, pneumatoceles, hemorrhage caused by erosion of a bronchial or pulmonary artery, meningitis, and cerebral abscess.

Tests

- Diagnosis must exclude necrosis in a malignant tumor or cavitation caused by tuberculosis; bronchosopy may be indicated to sample cells or exclude an obstruction. Chest radiography shows a walled cavity with fluid level.
- Sputum culture may identify a causative organism.
- Blood culture and complete blood count show that the patient is often anemic with a high erythrocyte sedimentation rate. Patients usually have mild to moderate leukocytosis.

Treatment

Follow disease carefully with regular chest radiographs and sputum collections. Resolution of disease is prompt after institution of appropriate antibiotics. Postural drainage should be used. Surgery is not usually indicated.

Tuberculosis

Tuberculosis is the world's leading cause of death from a single infectious disease. It is a reportable disease, and the prevalence is increased by the human immunodeficiency virus (HIV). In the U.S., 15 000 new cases occur per year, with the highest incidence among immigrants. The discussion below deals only with pulmonary tuberculosis and does not consider the extrapulmonary effects.

The causative agent in most cases of tuberculosis is *Mycobacterium tuberculosis*. Patients with pre-existing lung disease or immunosuppression may also be infected by opportunistic mycobacteria. These are also known as atypical mycobacteria or nontuberculous mycobacteria and include:

- *Mycobacterium kansasii*
- *Mycobacterium avium* complex (MAC).

Transmission and dissemination

Transmission is through the air or from direct contact. The pulmonary or bronchial focus ulcerates into an airway. A cough, sneeze, or exhalation then discharges droplets of viable mycobacterium. The droplet nuclei are then inhaled by an uninfected person and can lodge anywhere in the lungs or airways. Initial infection usually occurs in childhood.

Primary tuberculosis

The initial lesion is usually solitary, 1–2cm in diameter, and subpleural in the middle or upper zones of the lung. The focus of primary infection is called a Ghon complex. The primary infection has two components:

- The initial inflammatory reaction
- Resultant inflammation in lymph nodes draining the area.

Within 3–8 weeks, the process becomes a tubercle, a granulomatous form of inflammation. The granulomatous lesion commonly undergoes necrosis in a process called caseation and is surrounded by multinucleated giant cells and epithelioid cells (both derived from macrophage). The caseous tissue may liquefy, empty into an airway, and be transmitted to other parts of the lung. Lymphatic spread of mycobacterium occurs. The combination of tuberculous lymphadenitis and the Ghon complex is termed the primary complex.

In most cases, the primary foci will organize and form a fibrocalcific nodule in the lung with no clinical sequelae.

Secondary tuberculosis (postprimary tuberculosis)

Secondary tuberculosis results from reactivation of a primary infection or re-infection. Any form of immunocompromise may allow reactivation. The common sites are posterior or apical segments of the upper lobe or the superior segment of the lower lobe. Tubercle follicles develop and lesions enlarge by formation of new tubercles. Infection spreads by lymphatics and a delayed hypersensitivity reaction occurs.

In secondary tuberculosis, the lesions are often bilateral and usually cavitated. Most lesions are connected to fibrocalcific scars.

Progressive tuberculosis

Progressive tuberculosis may arise from a primary lesion or may be caused by reactivation of an incompletely healed primary lesion or re-infection. Tuberculosis progresses to widespread cavitation, pneumonitis, and lung fibrosis. Early symptoms are seldom diagnostic.

Miliary tuberculosis

In miliary tuberculosis, an acute diffuse dissemination of tubercle bacilli occurs through the bloodstream. Numerous small granulomas form in many organs, with the highest numbers found in the lungs. These granulomas often contain numerous mycobacteria and are usually the result of a delay in diagnosis or commencement of treatment.

Miliary tuberculosis may be a consequence of either primary or secondary tuberculosis and is universally fatal without treatment.

The pathology of tuberculosis is shown in Fig. 7.7; complications are shown in Fig. 7.8.

Clinical features

Primary tuberculosis is usually asymptomatic but may cause a mild febrile illness, with or without erythema nodosum. If the illness follows the progressive course, other symptoms then appear either immediately or gradually over weeks or months. Symptoms range from tiredness, anorexia, and malaise to bronchopneumonia with fever, cough, dyspnea, and respiratory distress. Sputum is purulent, mucoid, or blood-stained.

A pleural effusion or pneumonia may be the presenting complaint; often the disease is discovered due to an abnormal chest radiograph in an asymptomatic patient.

Diagnosis

Chest radiographs show upper zone shadows and fibrosis. Sequential sputum samples are taken:

- Stain with Ziehl–Neelson stain for acid-fast and alcohol-fast bacilli
- Culture on Lowenstein–Jensen medium, which takes up to 8 weeks.

Bronchoscopy is useful if no sputum is available. Biopsies from pleura, lymph nodes, and solid lesions within the lung may be necessary.

Prevention

BCG (bacille Calmette–Guérin) vaccination is a vaccine made from nonvirulent tubercle bacilli. The BCG vaccination is not recommended for general use in the U.S., where the risk of infection with *Mycobacterium tuberculosis* is low, except in children continually exposed to ineffectively treated adults and in healthcare workers in settings where infection is likely.

Treatment

Most patients are treated on an outpatient basis with combination therapy, involving four drugs: isoniazid, rifampin, pyrazinamide, and ethambutol.

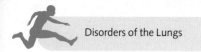

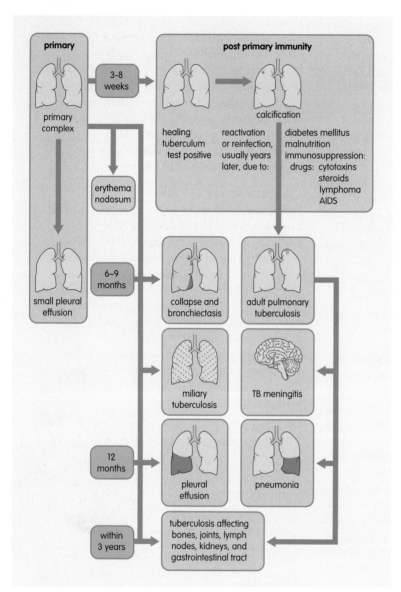

Fig. 7.7 Pathology of tuberculosis. Note the different routes from primary systems (via progression, reactivation, or re-infection). (From *Clinical Medicine*, 3rd ed., by P. Kumar and M. Clark. Baillière Tindall, 1994.)

Early and late complications of tuberculosis	
Early	**Late**
pneumonia	bronchiectasis
empyema	mycetomas in cavities
hemoptysis	colonization of fibrotic lung with a nontuberculous mycobacterium
laryngitis	extra-pulmonary disease
pneumothorax	

Fig. 7.8 Complications of tuberculosis.

Treatment lasts 6 months and is in two phases:
- Initial phase lasting 2 months (usually rifampin, isoniazid, pyrazinamide plus ethambutol)
- Continuation phase lasting 4 or 7 months (usually isoniazid and rifampin).

Specific treatment regimens are complicated, and algorithms for specific drugs and doses are followed.

Patients should be regularly followed up because lack of compliance is a major reason for treatment failure. Drug toxicity is a problem in a minority of cases.

Disorders of the airways

Obstructive and restrictive defects
Obstructive defects
Airway obstruction and resultant airflow limitation may be caused by local or diffuse lesions; examples include asthma and COPD. Airways are widened distal to the diseased airway. Symptoms include coughing, wheezing, and dyspnea.

Pulmonary function tests show the following results:
- Increased residual volume and total lung capacity
- Reduced vital capacity, FEV_1, peak expiratory flow rate and $FEV_1:FVC$ ratio.

Restrictive defects
Examples of defects that restrict normal lung movement during respiration include pulmonary fibrosis, pleural disease, and consolidation. Patients' breathing is shallow and rapid.

Characteristically, all lung volumes are reduced. $FEV_1:FVC$ ratio is normal, but vital capacity is decreased.

Chronic obstructive pulmonary disease
Chronic obstructive pulmonary disease (COPD) is a gradually progressive disease of the lungs involving airway obstruction. Unlike in asthma, the airway obstruction does not change over several months and is only partially reversible (e.g., with a bronchodilator). COPD is a very common disease and is a leading cause of death in the U.S. (120000 deaths per year). The disease is strongly associated with cigarette smoking.

Two disorders comprise COPD—chronic bronchitis and emphysema. Although by definition both are present in a patient with COPD, they differ in pathology and site and are dealt with separately below. Clinical presentation varies widely, depending on which of the two diseases predominates; two clinical groups of patient can be identified, although these represent the two ends of a spectrum of illness and in practice most patients will fall between the two (Fig. 7.9).

Etiology
Cigarette smoking is the major etiologic factor; all others are minor in comparison. Cigarette smoking has three major effects:
- Impairs ciliary movement

'Pink puffers' and 'blue bloaters'		
	Pink puffer	Blue bloater
body size	thin	obese
chest hyperinflation	marked	present
predominant disease	emphysema	chronic bronchitis
postmortem finding	panacinar emphysema	centrilobular emphysema
cor pulmonale	absent	present
secondary polycythemia	absent	present
cyanosis	absent	centrally
blood gases	low P_aCO_2	raised P_aCO_2

Fig. 7.9 "Pink puffers" and "blue bloaters."

- Causes mucus gland hypertrophy
- Alters the structure and function of alveolar macrophages.

Atmospheric pollution, occupational exposure, and recurrent bronchial infections are also implicated. Recurrent bronchial infections are frequent causes of acute exacerbations; their role in development rather than progression of the condition is less clear. Genetic abnormalities play a small role in the etiology of emphysema (see below) but a genetic component of COPD is likely since only 15% of smokers will develop the disease.

Diagnosis
A diagnosis of COPD is based on:
- History of chronic symptoms, without intervening periods when the patient is well
- Exposure to risk factors (primarily smoking)
- Evidence of airways obstruction (preferably using spirometry) that is not completely reversible.

Clinical features depend on the severity of the disease but can be summarized as:
- Productive cough
- Breathlessness, with or without wheeze
- Recurrent low-grade infective exacerbations.

Typical signs found on examination are shown in Chapter 9 (Fig. 9.42).

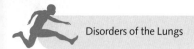

Complications of COPD
Exacerbations
An acute worsening of the patient's condition is usually due to infection, which can be viral (e.g., influenza) or bacterial (commonly *H. influenzae*). A mild exacerbation may require only an increase in medication at home. If the exacerbation is severe, the patient may deteriorate rapidly and require hospitalization.

Respiratory failure
In severe exacerbations the patient may be unable to maintain normal blood gases. This state is known as respiratory failure and is discussed in more detail elsewhere. Respiratory failure is the leading cause of death in patients with COPD and is often hypercapnic (type II).

Cor pulmonale
Mortality increases in patients with COPD who develop cor pulmonale, or right ventricular enlargement secondary to disorders affecting the lungs. In COPD it is pulmonary hypertension that causes the right ventricle to hypertrophy and eventually fail. Further details are found under pulmonary hypertension below.

Laboratory tests
Lung function tests show an obstructive pattern. Transfer factor/diffusing capacity is low (note that it is normal in asthma). Exercise testing assesses the extent of disability.

Chest radiography typically shows hyperinflation or flat hemidiaphragms, reduced peripheral vascular markings, and bullae. Alternatively, radiographs may appear normal.

Full blood counts may show secondary polycythemia, but blood gas tests are often normal. Alpha$_1$ antitrypsin levels should be measured.

Treatment
The most important intervention is to encourage smoking cessation, thus reducing the rate of deterioration. Self-administration of inhaled drugs is the key to management of COPD: patients must be taught correct inhaler technique. Treatment options include:
- Bronchodilators—long-term treatment with long-acting β_2 agonists
- Xanthine (e.g., theophylline)—but remember the narrow therapeutic window

- Corticosteroids—only if there is a documented spirometric response or if FEV$_1$ is < 50% of predicted or best. Clinical trials show limited efficacy in stable COPD
- Antibiotics—shorten exacerbations and should always be given in acute episodes
- Vaccine—annual flu vaccine
- Long-term oxygen therapy—recommended when PaO_2 is 55 mmHg or less or when oxygen saturation is less than 88% during sleep. Arterial oxygen saturation needs to be above 90%
- Surgery—may be indicated to remove emphysematous lung.

In addition, severe exacerbations may be treated by:
- Oxygen by mask
- Ventilatory support if pH < 7.6 and P_aCO_2 is rising (intubation or NIV).

Chronic bronchitis
Chronic bronchitis is defined clinically as a persistent cough with sputum production for at least 3 months of the year for 2 consecutive years.

Pathology
Hyperplasia and hypertrophy occur to the mucus-secreting glands found in the submucosa of the large cartilaginous airways. Mucous gland hypertrophy is expressed as gland–wall ratio or by the Reid index (normally, <0.4). Hyperplasia of the intraepithelial goblet cells occurs at the expense of ciliated cells in the lining epithelium. Regions of epithelium may undergo squamous metaplasia.

Small airways become obstructed by intraluminal mucus plugs, mucosal edema, smooth muscle hypertrophy and peribronchial fibrosis. Secondary bacterial colonization of retained products occurs (Fig. 7.10).

The effect of these changes is to cause obstruction, increasing resistance to airflow. A mismatch in ventilation:perfusion occurs, impairing gas exchange.

Emphysema
Emphysema is a permanent enlargement of the air spaces distal to the terminal bronchiole accompanied by destruction of their walls. As alveolar walls are destroyed, bullae form which may rupture causing pneumothorax. Destruction of the parenchyma increases compliance of the lung and causes a mismatch in ventilation:perfusion.

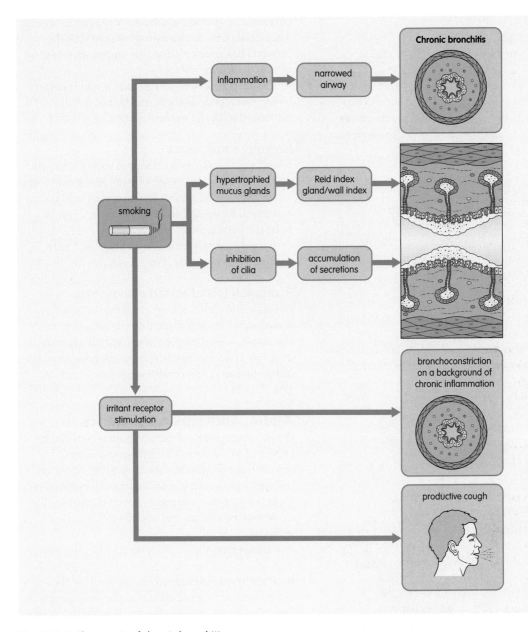

Fig. 7.10 Pathogenesis of chronic bronchitis.

Classification of emphysema is based on anatomic distribution (Fig. 7.11). The two main types are centriacinar and panacinar.

Centriacinar (centrilobular) emphysema

This is the form of emphysema that is associated with chronic bronchitis in COPD ("blue bloater"); it occurs predominantly in male smokers. As the name suggests, damage (i.e., septal destruction and

dilatation) is limited to the center of the acinus, around the terminal bronchiole. The upper lung lobes are affected more commonly than the lower lobes (Fig. 7.11B). Respiratory bronchiolitis is frequently present.

Panacinar (panlobular) emphysema

Panacinar (panlobular) emphysema is a characteristic lesion of α_1 antitrypsin deficiency. Loss of lung

137

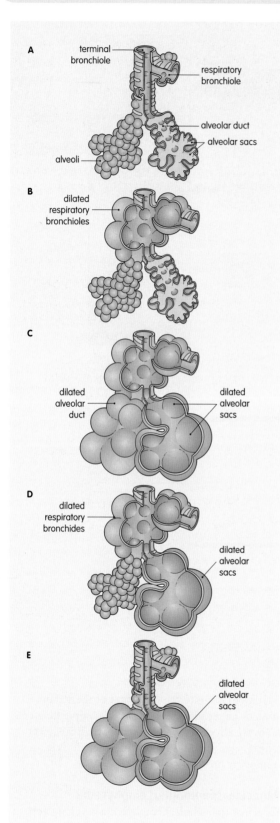

parenchyma, including pulmonary capillaries, occurs. The whole of the acinus is involved distal to the terminal bronchioles. Panacinar emphysema usually affects the lower lobes.

Enlarged air spaces may become cystic and form bullae. This form of emphysema is not usually associated with chronic bronchitis (Fig. 7.11C).

Irregular emphysema

Irregular emphysema is associated with scarring and damage affecting lung parenchyma, commonly found around old healed tuberculosis scars in the lung apices. Air trapping caused by fibrosis is thought to be the pathogenesis.

Irregular emphysema overlaps clinically with paraseptal emphysema (Fig. 7.11D).

Paraseptal (distal acinar) emphysema

In paraseptal (distal acinar) emphysema, alveolar wall destruction is restricted to the periphery of the acinus, with the upper lobes more frequently affected. If dilated airspace measures more than 10 mm in diameter, the condition is termed bullous (Fig. 7.11E).

Alpha$_1$ antitrypsin deficiency

Alpha$_1$ antitrypsin is an acute-phase serum protein produced in the liver, which functions as an antiprotease and inhibits the action of:

- Neutrophil elastase—an enzyme released during an inflammatory response, which is capable of destroying alveolar cell wall tissue
- Trypsin
- Collagenase.

In α_1 antitrypsin deficiency, serum levels of the enzyme are reduced. This is an autosomal dominant condition, in which homozygous individuals develop severe panacinar emphysema.

Alpha$_1$ antitrypsin deficiency develops at an early age (before 40 years of age) with equal distribution between sexes. The homozygous state has an incidence of 1:3630 in Caucasians but is rarer in dark-skinned people.

Fig. 7.11 Main types of emphysema. (A) Normal distal lung acinus; (B) centriacinar emphysema; (C) panacinar emphysema; (D) irregular emphysema; (E) paraseptal emphysema.

Asthma

Asthma is a chronic inflammatory disorder of the lungs characterized by variability in symptoms and lung function.

Prevalence

Five per cent of the adult population are receiving therapy for asthma at any one time. Prevalence of asthma in the Western world is rising, particularly in children; up to 20% have symptoms at some time in their childhood.

Classification

Bronchial asthma may be categorized into two groups on the basis of atopy: extrinsic or intrinsic (Fig. 7.12). Extrinsic asthma is also known as allergic asthma. Intrinsic asthma may be classified into such categories as occupational asthma and exercise-induced asthma. Precipitating factors are described in Fig. 7.13.

Occupational asthma is increasing; currently there are over 200 materials encountered at the workplace that are implicated (Fig. 7.14). Occupational asthma may be classified as:

Fig. 7.12 Classification of asthma.

Asthma		
	Extrinsic asthma	**Intrinsic asthma**
underlying abnormality	immune reaction (atopic)	abnormal autonomic regulation of airways
onset	childhood	adulthood
distribution	60%	40%
allergens	recognized	none identified
family history	present	absent
predisposition to form IgE antibodies	present	absent
association with chronic obstructive pulmonary disease	none	chronic bronchitis
natural progression	improves	worsens
eosinophilia	sputum and blood	sputum
drug hypersensitivity	absent	present

Precipitating factors for asthma					
Allergens	**Occupational sensitizers**	**Viral infections**	**Atmospheric factors**	**Drugs**	**Other factors**
house dust mite (*Dermatophagoides pteronyssius*)	rosin fumes (from soldering)	para influenza	cigarette smoke	β-blockers	cold air
flour	isocyanates (from polyurethane varnishes)	respiratory syncytial virus	ozone	nonsteroidal anti-inflammatory drugs	emotion
animal danders	acid anhydrides (from industrial coatings)	rhinovirus	sulfur dioxide		fumes
grain					exercise

Fig. 7.13 Precipitating factors for asthma.

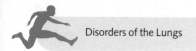

Factors implicated in occupational asthma	
Agents	**Workers at risk include:**
High-molecular-weight agents	
cereals	bakers, millers
animal-derived allergens	animal handlers
enzymes	detergent users, pharmaceutical workers, bakers
gums	carpet makers, pharmaceutical workers
latex	health professionals
seafoods	seafood processors
Low-molecular-weight agents	
isocynates	spray painters, insulation installers, etc.
wood dusts	forest workers, carpenters
anhydrides	users of plastics, expoxy resins
fluxes	electronic workers
chloramine	janitors, cleaners
acrylate	adhesive handlers
drugs	pharmaceutical workers, health professionals
metals	solderers, refiners

Fig. 7.14 Factors implicated in occupational asthma. (From *Pulmonary Physiology* by G. Criner and G. D'Alonzo. Fence Creek Publishing, 1999, p. 213.)

- Allergic (immunologically mediated with a latent period between exposure and symptoms)
- Nonallergic (immediate response after exposure, e.g., to toxic gases).

> Take a full history, including occupational history. Do symptoms improve at the weekend or on vacation? If so, there may be an occupational cause.

Pathogenesis of asthma

Pathogenesis of asthma is very complex. Airway inflammation (Fig. 7.15) causes:
- Smooth muscle constriction
- Thickening of the airway wall (smooth muscle hypertrophy and edema)
- Basement membrane thickening
- Mucus and exudate in the airway lumen.

Microscopically, the viscid mucus contains:
- Desquamated epithelial cells
- Whorls of shed epithelium (Curshmann's whorls)
- Charcot–Leyden crystal (eosinophil cell membranes)
- Infiltration of inflammatory cells, particularly $CD4^+$ T lymphocytes.

Inflammatory mediators

Inflammatory mediators play a vital role in the pathogenesis of asthma. Inflammatory stimuli activate mast cells, epithelial cells, alveolar macrophages, and dendritic cells resident within the airways, causing the release of mediators that are chemotactic for cells derived from the circulation—secondary effector cells (eosinophils, neutrophils, and platelets).

Mediators that are thought to be involved in asthma include (Fig. 7.16):
- Preformed mediators—present in cytoplasmic granules ready for release. Associated with human lung mast cells and include histamine, neutral proteases, and chemotactic factors for neutrophils and eosinophils

Fig. 7.15 Mechanisms of airway narrowing in asthma.

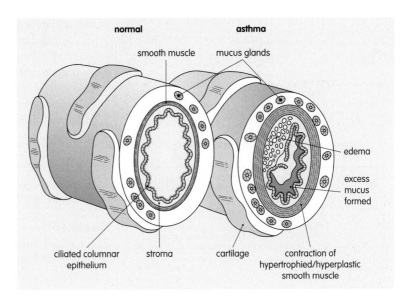

- Newly generated mediators—manufactured secondary to the initial triggering stimulus after release of preformed mediators. Some of these mediators are derived from the membrane phospholipid and are associated with the metabolism of arachidonic acid (e.g., prostaglandins and leukotrienes). The production of inflammatory cytokines and chemokines is important in the activation and recruitment of inflammatory cells.

Early and late responses
Two patterns of response can be considered; in practice most asthmatics show evidence of both responses, although either may be absent.

Immediate (early) reaction The release of preformed mediators causes maximal airway narrowing within 10–15 minutes of challenge with a return to baseline within 1–2 hours.

Late reaction The influx of inflammatory cells and release of additional inflammatory mediators causes airway narrowing after 3–4 hours and is maximal after 6–12 hours. This is much more difficult to reverse than the immediate reaction and there is an increase in level of airway hyperreactivity.

Clinical features
Symptoms (breathlessness, chest tightness, cough, wheeze) classically show a diurnal variation often being worse at night. For example, nocturnal coughing is a common presenting symptom, especially in children.

Clinical features vary according to the severity of asthma (classified from mild to severe and either intermittent or persistent). Acute severe asthma in adults is diagnosed if:
- Patient cannot complete sentences in one breath
- Respiration rate ≥ 25 breaths/min
- Pulse ≥ 110 beats/min
- Peak expiratory flow rate (PEFR) $\leq 50\%$ of predicted or best.

Life-threatening asthma is characterized by the following:
- PEFR $< 33\%$ of predicted or best
- Silent chest and cyanosis
- Bradycardia or hypotension
- Exhaustion, confusion, or coma
- $P_aO_2 < 60$ mmHg.

Tests
Investigations include:
- Lung function tests—FEV_1/FVC is reduced, RV may be increased; tests demonstrate an improvement in FEV_1 of more than 15% after bronchodilator administration
- Peak expiratory flow rate—morning and evening measurements. Useful in the long-term assessment of asthma; a characteristic morning dipping pattern is seen in poorly controlled asthma
- If PEFR $< 50\%$, arterial blood gases should be tested
- Exercise laboratory tests

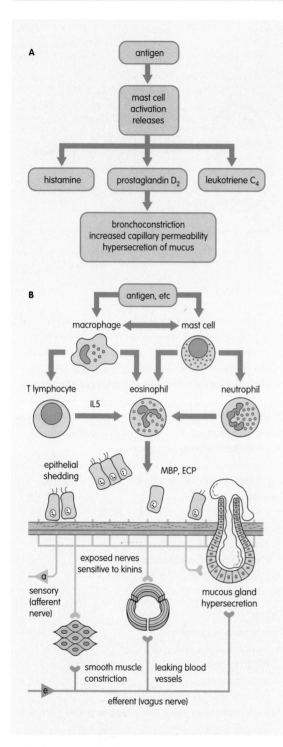

Fig. 7.16 Pathogenesis of asthma. (A) Preformed mediators and formation of arachidonic acid products; (B) additional newly generated mediators. IL5, interleukin 5; MBP, major basic protein; ECP, eosinophil cationic protein.

- Bronchial provocation tests—performed rarely in normal clinical practice, using histamine or methacholine to demonstrate bronchial hyperreactivity
- Chest radiography—no diagnostic features of asthma on chest radiograph; use to rule out a diagnosis of allergic bronchopulmonary aspergillosis
- Skin prick tests—allergen injections into the epidermis of the forearm, which are used to identify extrinsic causes. Look for weal development in sensitive patients.

Treatment

Identify and avoid extrinsic factors. Follow the NHLBI guidelines with a stepwise approach to drug treatment:
- Occasional use of short-acting bronchodilators
- Regular inhaled anti-inflammatory agents: inhaled corticosteroid (low-dose) or cromolyn or nedocromil. Sustained-release theophylline or leukotriene modifiers may also be considered. Short-acting bronchodilator (inhaled β2 agonists) as needed for symptoms
- Inhaled corticosteroid (medium-dose) or inhaled corticosteroid (low- to medium-dose) plus a long-acting bronchodilator for night time symptoms (inhaled β2 agonist, sustained-release theophylline, or long-acting oral β2 agonist). If needed, combined therapy with inhaled corticosteroid and long-acting bronchodilator, with short-acting bronchodilator (β2 agonist) as needed
- High-dose inhaled steroids, regular bronchodilators (long-acting inhaled β2 agonist, sustained-release theophylline, and/or β2 agonist tablets or syrup), and corticosteroid tablets or syrup. Inhaled short-acting β2 agonist as needed for symptoms.

Drugs used in treating asthma are discussed in Chapter 6.

Bronchiectasis

Bronchiectasis is defined as an abnormal and permanent dilatation of the bronchi and is associated with chronic infection. Most cases arise in childhood, and the disease is rare.

Etiology

Bronchiectasis can either be acquired or, less commonly, congenital.

Acquired bronchiectasis

Bronchiectasis is usually caused by a severe childhood infection (e.g., bronchopneumonia, measles, or whooping cough). Inflammation can damage and weaken the bronchial wall, leading to dilatation. It may also be caused by bronchial obstruction (e.g., by a foreign body, tuberculous lymph nodes, or tumor) followed by infection in the lung distal to the obstruction.

Congenital bronchiectasis

Congenital abnormalities that interfere with ciliary function (e.g., primary ciliary dyskinesia, Kartagener's syndrome, and Young's syndrome) impair the transport of mucus and cause recurrent infection. Kartagener's syndrome, which is a rare cause, is also associated with dextrocardia and sinusitis. The viscous mucus and recurrent infections of cystic fibrosis may also lead to bronchiectasis. Recurrent infections are also a feature of immunoglobulin deficiencies (e.g. IgA); therefore these are also associated with bronchiectasis.

Pathology

Infection leads to obstruction, dilation of bronchi, and often loss of cilia. Destruction of the alveolar walls and fibrosis of lung parenchyma occur and pulmonary hemodynamic changes can take place. The dependent portions of the lungs, usually the lower lobes, are affected most commonly.

Symptoms

Cough is the most common symptom; this is often persistent and accompanied by sputum which may be mucopurulent or copious, purulent, and foul-smelling. Systemic features of infection such as fever and malaise also occur.

Hemoptysis may be present and can be massive. Clubbing occurs and coarse inspiratory crackles are heard on auscultation.

Complications

Complications of bronchiectasis include:
- Pneumonia
- Pneumothorax
- Empyema
- Meningitis
- Metastatic disease (e.g., in brain)
- Amyloid formation (e.g., in kidney).

Tests

Bronchiectasis can be investigated through:
- Radiology—chest radiograph may be normal or show bronchial wall thickening. If disease is advanced, cystic spaces may be seen
- High-resolution CT—the investigation of choice to detect bronchial wall thickening
- Sputum tests—Gram stain, anaerobic and aerobic culture, and sensitivity testing are vital during an infective exacerbation. Major pathogens include *Staphylococcus aureus*, *Pseudomonas aeruginosa*, *Haemophilus influenzae*, and anaerobes
- Tests for cystic fibrosis where appropriate (cystic fibrosis sweat test)
- Lung function spirometry (may show an obstructive pattern).

Treatment

Aims of treatment are twofold:
- Control of infection
- Removal of secretions.

Infections should be eradicated with antibiotics if progression of the disease is to be halted. Antibiotic regimens depend on infecting organism. Secretions are removed by postural drainage for 10–20 minutes, two to four times a day. Patients are trained in the method by respiratory therapists.

Bronchodilators are useful if demonstrable airflow limitation exists. Surgery is of limited value but may be indicated in a young patient with adequate lung function, if disease is localized to one lung or segment.

Cystic fibrosis

Cystic fibrosis is a disorder characterized by the production of abnormally viscid secretions by exocrine glands and mucus-secreting glands, such as those in the pancreas and respiratory tract. Impaired mucociliary clearance in the airways leads to recurrent infections and bronchiectasis.

Cystic fibrosis is the most common fatal genetically transmitted disease in Caucasians. It is an autosomal recessive condition occurring in 1:3000 Caucasian live births. One in 15000 African Americans and 1 in 31000 Asian Americans are affected. The gene has been identified on the long arm of chromosome 7.

Etiology

The most common mutation is a specific gene deletion in the codon for phenylalanine at position

508 in the amino-acid sequence (ΔF508). This results in a defect in a transmembrane regulator protein known as the cystic fibrosis transmembrane conductive regulator (CFTR). Mutation causes a failure of opening of the chloride channels in response to elevated cAMP in epithelial cells, leading to:

- Decreased excretion of chloride into the airway lumen
- Increased reabsorption of sodium into the epithelial cells
- Increased viscosity of secretions.

Pathology

The thick secretions produced by the epithelial cells cause:

- Small airway obstruction, leading to recurrent infection and ultimately bronchiectasis
- Pancreatic duct obstruction, causing pancreatic fibrosis and ultimately pancreatic insufficiency.

Clinical features

Presentation depends on age. Usually, the condition presents in infancy with gastrointestinal manifestations (Fig. 7.17).

Stools are bulky, greasy, and offensive in smell. Respiratory signs are normal and symptoms are nonspecific:

- Lungs are normal at birth
- Frequent infections with cough and wheeze as the child gets older
- Clubbing and dyspnea occur.

Almost all men with cystic fibrosis are infertile; females may be subfertile.

Tests

Family history is sought (e.g., affected siblings). Genetic screening is available for couples with a family history.

Prenatal diagnosis is available by chorionic villous sampling or amniocentesis.

Tests include:
- Sweat chloride test
- DNA testing
- Fecal fat testing
- Upper GI and small bowel series
- Pancreatic function tests.

The complications of cystic fibrosis are described in Fig. 7.18.

Treatment

Treatment (Fig. 7.19) is based on:
- Respiratory therapy
- Antibiotics (see below)

Complications of cystic fibrosis	
Respiratory complications	Other complications
allergic aspergillosus bronchiectasis cor pulmonale hemoptysis lobar collapse nasal polyps pneumothorax sinusitis wheezing	abdominal pain biliary cirrhosis delayed puberty diabetes mellitus gall stones growth failure male infertility portal hypertension rectal prolapse

Fig. 7.18 Complications of cystic fibrosis.

Summary of treatment	
Respiratory	Gastrointestinal
drain secretions, postural drainage	pancreatic enzyme supplements with all meals and snacks
prevent infection where possible	high-energy, high-protein diet
exercise encouraged	do not restrict fat in diet
regular sputum cultures	vitamin A, D, and E supplements
immunization against measles and influenza	

Fig. 7.19 Summary of treatment of cystic fibrosis.

Cystic fibrosis	
Respiratory manifestations	Gastrointestinal manifestations
recurrent bronchopulmonary infection bronchiectasis	meconium ileus rectal prolapse diarrhea failure to thrive malabsorption

Fig. 7.17 Manifestations of cystic fibrosis.

- DNase (see below)
- Anti-inflammatory drugs (steroids)
- Nutritional support.

IV antibiotics may be given at home (e.g., through implantable venous access devices) to reduce hospital admissions and improve patient independence.

Human DNase has been cloned, sequenced, and expressed by recombinant techniques. This is:
- Capable of degrading DNA
- Shown to improve FEV_1
- Expensive.

Heart–lung and liver transplantations are possible in severely affected patients.

Prognosis

Prognosis is improving: currently, mean survival is 29 years. Death is caused mainly by respiratory complications.

Disorders of the pulmonary vessels

Pulmonary congestion and edema

Pulmonary edema is defined as an abnormal increase in the amount of interstitial fluid in the lung. The two main causes are:
- Increased venous hydrostatic pressures
- Injury to alveolar capillary walls or vessels, leading to increased permeability.

Less common causes are blockage of lymphatic drainage and lowered plasma oncotic pressure.

High-pressure pulmonary edema

High-pressure or hemodynamic pulmonary edema is cardiogenic; it may occur acutely as a result of a myocardial infarction or chronically in aortic and mitral valve disease.

Fluid movement between intravascular and extravascular compartments is governed by Starling forces (see Fig. 5.11). Net fluid flow through a capillary wall (out of the blood) is governed by:
- Hydrostatic pressure in the capillary; hydrostatic pressure in the interstitium opposes outflow
- Capillary permeability
- Oncotic pressure exerted by plasma proteins (mainly albumin) opposes flow; interstitial oncotic pressure promotes outflow.

Net filtration of fluid out of the blood is more likely at the arteriolar end of the capillaries, while reabsorption of interstitial fluid is more likely at the venular end, due to the drop in hydrostatic pressure within the capillary along its length.

Imbalances in Starling forces and a reduced plasma oncotic pressure will cause expansion of the interstitial spaces.

No pathologic conditions cause a local reduction of plasma protein concentration within the lung capillaries. However, many conditions (e.g., left ventricular failure) cause an elevation of hydrostatic pressure. If left atrial pressure rises, so do pulmonary venous and capillary pressures, thereby raising hydrostatic pressure and causing edema formation. Pulmonary edema occurs only after the lymphatic drainage capacity has been exceeded. Lymphatic drainage can increase 10-fold without edema formation. However, if lymphatic drainage is blocked (e.g., in cancer), edema occurs more readily.

Edema due to hemodynamic causes has a low protein content.

Edema caused by microvascular injury

This is the noncardiogenic form of pulmonary edema.

Capillary blood is separated from alveolar air by three anatomic layers:
- Capillary endothelium
- Narrow interstitial layer
- Alveolar epithelium.

Damage to capillary endothelium

Normal alveolar capillary endothelial cells are joined by tight junctions containing narrow constrictions. Many conditions can damage the pulmonary capillary endothelium, resulting in movement of fluid and a transcapillary leak of proteins. Interstitial oncotic pressure rises; thus, a natural defense against edema formation is disabled.

After damage, fibrinogen enters and coagulates within the interstitium. Interstitial fibrosis subsequently occurs, leading to impaired lymphatic drainage. Edema caused by microvascular damage characteristically has a high protein content.

Progression of pulmonary edema

Fluid first accumulates in loose connective tissue around the bronchi and large vessels. Fluid then

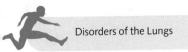

distends the thick, collagen-containing portions of the alveolar wall. The final stage of pulmonary edema is accumulation of fluid within the alveolar spaces. If pulmonary edema is chronic, recurrent alveolar hemorrhages lead to the accumulation of hemosiderin-laden macrophages along with interstitial fibrosis.

Clinical features

Clinical features of edema are as follows:

- Acute breathlessness
- Wheezing
- Anxiety
- Tachypnea
- Profuse perspiration
- Production of pink sputum while coughing
- Peripheral circulatory shutdown
- Tachycardia
- Basal crackles and wheezes heard on auscultation
- Respiratory impairment with hypoxemia
- Overloaded lungs predispose to secondary infection.

Treatment

Acute pulmonary edema is a medical emergency. The patient should be placed in a sitting position and O_2 administered, initially by mask. Intubation may be required. Intravenous diuretics give an immediate and delayed response. Nitrates and diuretics are the initial pharmacologic therapy if the patient is hemodynamically stable. Morphine sedates the patient and produces systemic vasodilation; it should not be used if systemic arterial pressure is low.

Underlying causes should be quickly determined and treated appropriately. Inhaled beta-adrenergic agonists or IV aminophylline may be required to treat bronchospasm.

Adult respiratory distress syndrome (ARDS)

Adult respiratory distress syndrome (ARDS) is noncardiogenic pulmonary edema defined as diffuse pulmonary infiltrates, refractory hypoxemia, stiff lungs, and respiratory distress (Fig. 7.20). ARDS forms part of a systemic inflammatory reaction.

Etiology

Causes are as follows:

- Gram-negative septicemia
- Trauma or shock
- Infection (e.g., pneumonia)

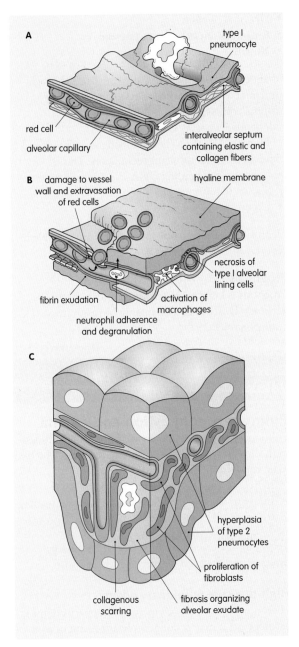

Fig. 7.20 Cell types in adult respiratory distress syndrome. (A) Normal alveolar wall; (B) acute phase of ARDS; (C) organization phase of ARDS.

- Pancreatitis
- Gastric aspiration
- Perforated viscus
- Narcotic abuse
- Disseminated intravascular coagulation
- Oxygen toxicity

- Gas inhalation
- Ionizing radiation.

The underlying insult is damage to the alveolar capillary wall, leading to diffuse alveolar damage.

Precipitating mechanisms of ARDS
Mechanisms include pulmonary capillary hypoxemia, microembolism, and loss of surfactant caused by pulmonary epithelium damage.

Pathology
As noted above, the key feature of ARDS is noncardiogenic pulmonary edema. Pulmonary venous and capillary engorgement occurs, leading to interstitial edema. Pulmonary epithelium damage also occurs.

Pulmonary hypertension is common; hypoxic vasoconstriction redirects blood to better areas of oxygenation.

A protein-rich intra-alveolar hemorrhagic exudate promotes formation of hyaline membranes that line alveolar ducts and alveoli.

In longstanding cases, pulmonary fibrosis ensues and the alveolar walls become lined by metaplastic cuboidal epithelium (see Fig. 7.20).

Resolution
Resolution occurs as follows:
- Resorption of edema
- Ingestion of red cells and hyaline membranes by alveolar macrophages
- Regeneration of type II pneumocytes.

Clinical features
Features change during the progression of ARDS. Patients with ARDS present with:
- Tachypnea, often unexplained
- Dyspnea
- Pulmonary edema—fine crackles throughout both lung fields
- Arterial hypoxemia, refractory to oxygen therapy.

Chest radiography shows bilateral diffuse shadowing.

Management
- Treat underlying condition and provide supportive measures
- Treat as for pulmonary edema: the aim is to achieve a negative fluid balance
- Provide cardiovascular support and mechanical ventilation (e.g., positive end expiratory pressure).

Prognosis
Prognosis is dependent upon cause, but mortality is generally greater than 50%. With septic shock, mortality is 90%. With fat embolism, mortality is 10%. Prognosis is poor in the elderly. Death is caused by cardiac arrhythmias with sepsis, usually from Gram-negative organisms.

Embolism, hemorrhage, and infarction
Vascular disease of the lungs can be caused by:
- Vessel obstruction
- Vessel wall damage
- Intravascular pressure variations.

Obstruction: pulmonary embolism
An embolus is an abnormal mass of material that is transported in the bloodstream from one part of the circulation to another and which impacts finally in the lumen of a vessel which has a caliber too small to allow passage. The end result of an embolus derived from venous thrombus is impaction in the pulmonary arterial tree. Most thrombi originate in the deep veins of the calf or pelvis.

This is a common condition: incidence of pulmonary emboli at autopsy has been reported to be 12%.

Pulmonary emboli rarely have a cardiac cause and are very rare in children.

Predisposing factors
Predisposing factors are:
- Immobilization (e.g., prolonged bed rest)
- In women, the oral contraceptive pill—minor risk factor, increased by cigarette smoking
- Malignancy, especially of pancreas, uterus, breast, and stomach
- Cardiac failure
- Chronic pulmonary disease
- Postoperative recovery
- Fractures of the pelvis or lower limb
- Hypercoagulable states (e.g., pregnancy).

 When a patient presents postoperatively with sudden-onset chest pain, pulmonary embolism should be at the top of the list of differential diagnoses.

Clinical features
Common symptoms are:
- Dyspnea
- Tachypnea
- Pleuritic pain
- Apprehension
- Tachycardia
- Cough
- Hemoptysis
- Leg pain/clinical DVT.

Symptoms are related to the size of the embolus and the corresponding volume of lung tissue deprived of blood in addition to the presence or absence of congestion in the pulmonary circulation at the time of impaction.

Pulmonary embolism can be classified as massive, moderate, or small.

Massive pulmonary embolism
A massive pulmonary embolism is a clinical emergency. The embolus is typically derived from a thrombus that occludes a long venous segment in the lower limb. The caliber of the main pulmonary arteries is greater than the iliac and femoral veins; therefore, thrombi must loosely bundle together to block the pulmonary arteries (as seen in a saddle embolus, which occurs at the bifurcation of the left and right pulmonary arteries).

Within normal human lung, occlusion of more than 50% of the pulmonary vascular bed is necessary for a massive pulmonary embolism to prove fatal.

Clinical features
This is a clinical emergency presenting as sudden-onset severe chest pain and dyspnea. Often onset occurs when straining during defecation. Classically, a massive pulmonary embolism occurs a week or more after operation.

There are signs of shock: tachycardia, low blood pressure. Right ventricular heave, gallop rhythm, and a prominent a-wave in the jugular venous pulse may also be noted. Sudden death can occur.

Small or medium-sized pulmonary embolism
Moderate pulmonary embolism is caused by occlusion of a lobar or segmental artery. Perfusion of a segment may be reduced producing an area of localized necrosis.

An area of necrosis secondary to ischemia is known as an infarct.

Clinical features
Pulmonary infarction presents with sudden-onset pleuritic chest pain. Cough with hemoptysis and dyspnea are other symptoms.

Multiple microemboli
Multiple small emboli can occlude arterioles, but this process is usually clinically silent. Gradual occlusion of the pulmonary arterial bed leads to pulmonary hypertension. This is a rare condition characterized by exertional dyspnea, tiredness, and syncope. Basal crackles are heard on auscultation.

Other forms of emboli
Fat embolism
Fat embolism results from massive injury to subcutaneous fat or fracture of bones containing fatty marrow. Globules of lipid enter the torn vessels.

Air embolism
Air embolism arises during childbirth or abortion or after chest wall injury. These microemboli can cause tiny infarcts in several organs.

Tumor embolism
Tumor cells, like other particulate matter, become trapped in the pulmonary capillary bed. This is an important mechanism in the development of metastases.

Amniotic fluid embolism
Amniotic fluid embolism can occur during childbirth or abortion and may be fatal. Small fragments of trophoblast are commonly found in lungs of pregnant women at autopsy but do not cause any symptoms.

Investigations in suspected pulmonary emboli
Chest radiography is usually unremarkable but valuable in excluding other causes.

Electrocardiography may show signs of right ventricular strain (deep S waves in lead I, Q waves in lead III, and inverted T waves in lead III).

Arterial blood gases show arterial hypoxemia and hypocapnia.

Radioisotope ventilation:perfusion scans demonstrate ventilated areas of lung and filling defects on the corresponding perfusion scans; these are assessed on the basis of probability of pulmonary embolism (see Chapter 10). In nondiagnostic scans, pulmonary angiography should be performed in the acutely ill patient or leg ultrasound if the patient is stable.

Treatment
Treatment is based on:
- Supportive measures (e.g., analgesia, oxygen)
- Anticoagulation
- Thrombolysis.

Anticoagulation
Further emboli should be prevented (patients with a pulmonary embolism have a 30% chance of developing further emboli). Heparin is administered intravenously, carefully regulating the dose with the aim of achieving maximal effect within 24 hours.

Oral anticoagulants are given after 48 hours, and heparin is reduced. Oral anticoagulants are continued for between 6 weeks and 6 months.

Thrombolysis
Thrombolysis is indicated in patients who are hemodynamically unstable (e.g., hypotensive). It is possible to break down thrombi by:
- Intravenous streptokinase
- Intravenous tissue plasminogen activator (TPA).

Thrombolytics are contraindicated in:
- Pregnancy
- Recent stroke
- Recent surgery
- Bleeding disorders.

Surgery is performed only on massive pulmonary emboli in patients who fail to respond to thrombolysis.

Prevention
This is by avoidance of deep vein thromboses:
- Early mobilization of patients after operation
- Use of tight elastic stockings
- Leg exercises
- Prophylactic anticoagulation.

Pulmonary infarction
Less than 10% of pulmonary emboli cause infarction within the lung. Lung infarcts are more common in the lower lobes; infarction is less common in the lungs than in other organs because of the lungs' dual blood supply.

Pulmonary infarction is usually a consequence of a moderate pulmonary embolism. Pulmonary infarction is rare in young people.

Predisposing factors
Predisposing factors for infarction include:
- Rise in pulmonary venous pressure

- Mitral stenosis or left ventricular failure
- Bronchial occlusion
- Pleural effusion
- Infection.

Pathology
A wedge-shaped section of the lung downstream from the blockage becomes necrotic. The base of the wedge is situated toward the pleural aspect of the lung. Pleural inflammation over the infarcted area is common. Organization of pulmonary infarcts proceeds rapidly.

Clinical features
Clinical features include sudden-onset pleuritic chest pain and dyspnea.

Tests
Blood tests show increases in erythrocyte sedimentation rate and lactate dehydrogenase (LDH) levels. Polymorphonuclear leucocytosis is present.

Arterial blood gas measurement reveals hypoxemia but normal PCO_2.

Ventilation:perfusion scans show mismatching.

Pulmonary hypertension and vascular sclerosis
Pulmonary hypertension occurs when blood pressure in the pulmonary circulation exceeds 30 mmHg (Fig. 7.21).

Pulmonary hypertension can be caused by:
- Increased vascular resistance in the pulmonary circulation

Pulmonary hypertension	
Etiology	Vascular lesion
Cardiac disease	Precapillary (e.g. left-to-right shunt)
Hypoxia	Capillary (e.g. hypoxia)
Fibrosis	Postcapillary (e.g. left ventricular failure)
Miscellaneous	
Idiopathic (primary)	

Fig. 7.21 Classification of pulmonary hypertension. Note that pulmonary arterial changes depend on etiology of the pulmonary hypertension.

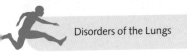

- Increased pulmonary venous pressure
- Increased pulmonary blood flow.

The increase in vascular resistance is of most interest in respiratory medicine. This can occur due to:
- Chronic hypoxia
- Obstruction of pulmonary vessels
- Pulmonary fibrosis.

Chronic hypoxia

Chronic airflow obstruction or living at high altitude can lead to chronic hypoxia. This is also seen in Pickwickian syndrome, in which pulmonary hypertension is caused by poor respiration associated with gross obesity. Because insignificant intimal fibrosis occurs, the condition is largely reversible.

Obstruction of pulmonary vessels

This is seen in primary pulmonary hypertension, a rare condition of unknown etiology, predominantly seen in women aged 20–30 years. The condition may be familial.

Pulmonary fibrosis

Early changes of pulmonary vasculature are initially muscular in type and reversible. Obliterative fibrosis of pulmonary arteries and arterioles occurs later, with irreversible increases in pulmonary vascular resistance.

The other causes of pulmonary hypertension (those due to increased pulmonary venous pressure and increased pulmonary blood flow) are primarily cardiac and are not considered here.

Pathology

Effects of pulmonary hypertension include:
- Enlarged proximal pulmonary arteries
- Right ventricular hypertrophy
- Right arterial dilatation
- Necrotizing arteritis.

Clinical features

Clinical features are as follows:
- Symptoms of the underlying cause
- Chest pain and exertional dyspnea
- Syncope and fatigue
- Prominent a-wave in jugular venous pulse
- Right ventricular heave
- Loud pulmonary component to second heart sound
- Midsystolic ejection murmur.

Tests

When investigating pulmonary hypertension, a possible cause should be sought.

A complete blood count may show secondary polycythemia. Chest radiography may reveal right ventricular enlargement, pulmonary artery dilatation, or oligemic peripheral lung fields.

Electrocardiography may indicate right ventricular hypertrophy, right-axis deviation, a prominent R wave in V1, or inverted T waves in the right precordial leads.

Radioisotope lung scans and echocardiography may also be useful.

Treatment

Treatment is dependent upon cause. Primary pulmonary hypertension is treated with anticoagulation therapy.

If the underlying cause of hypertension is untreatable, the patient will progress to cor pulmonale and death. Continuous oxygen therapy is beneficial in patients with cor pulmonale. Diuretics are used to treat fluid overload.

Heart–lung transplantation is recommended in young patients.

Prognosis is poor: 5-year survival rate is 40%.

Cor pulmonale

Cor pulmonale is a major complication of pulmonary hypertension. It is defined as right heart failure secondary to lung disease and occurs as a result of any disorder that leads to pulmonary hypertension. Of most interest here is its presence in lung disease. As noted above, lung disease that causes chronic hypoxia may lead to pulmonary hypertension and therefore cor pulmonale. The main respiratory diseases associated with cor pulmonale are:
- COPD
- Severe, chronic asthma
- Bronchiectasis
- Pulmonary emboli
- Pulmonary fibrosis.

The principal signs are those of the underlying disease in addition to edema, raised JVP, and atrial gallop rhythm. Arterial blood gases show hypoxemia with or without hypercapnia.

Disorders of the lung interstitium

Disorders of the lung interstitium can cause confusion because many different synonyms are used. The diseases themselves can be referred to as diffuse parenchymal lung diseases (DPLD), acknowledging that it is not just the interstitium that is affected. There are several synonyms for idiopathic pulmonary fibrosis (see below), pneumoconioses are also known as industrial dust diseases, and extrinsic allergic alveolitis is the same as hypersensitivity alveolitis or pneumonitis.

Remember that the interstitium is the space between the alveolar epithelium and capillary endothelium (see Fig. 3.12, p. 32).

Pulmonary fibrosis

Pulmonary fibrosis is the end result of many respiratory diseases (Fig. 7.22) and is characterized by scar tissue in the lungs which decreases lung compliance, i.e., the lungs become stiffer.

The pathogenesis of pulmonary fibrosis is complex, involving many factors (Fig. 7.23).

The main features are:
- A lesion affecting the alveolar–capillary basement membrane
- Cellular infiltration and thickening by collagen of the interstitium of the alveolar wall
- Fibroblasts proliferate, leading to further collagen deposition.

The end stage is characterized by a honeycomb lung, a nonspecific condition in which cystic spaces develop in fibrotic lungs with compensatory dilatation of unaffected neighboring bronchioles.

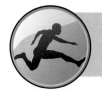

The end stage of chronic interstitial lung disease is termed honeycomb lung.

Note from Fig. 7.23 that the initial injury to the alveolar–capillary basement membrane may be caused by several different mechanisms. Some (e.g., dusts) are considered below.

Clinical features

Patients become progressively breathless and develop a dry, nonproductive cough. On examination, lung expansion is reduced and end-inspiratory crackles are heard.

Tests

Chest x-ray may show fine reticular, nodular, or reticulonodular infiltration in the basal areas. High-resolution CT (HRCT) or biopsy may be used to aid diagnosis. Lung function tests demonstrate a restrictive pattern along with a decreased transfer factor.

The pneumoconioses

The pneumoconioses are a group of disorders caused by inhalation of mineral or biologic dusts. The incidence is decreasing as working conditions continue to improve.

Causes of pulmonary fibrosis					
Dusts		Inhalants	Infection	Iatrogenic causes	Other causes
Mineral	Biological				
coal	avian protein	oxygen	postpneumonic infection	cytotoxic drugs	sarcoidosis
silica	*Actinomyces*	sulfur dioxide	tuberculosis	noncytotoxics	connective-tissue disease
asbestos	*Aspergillus*	nitrogen dioxide	—	radiation	chronic pulmonary edema

Fig. 7.22 Causes of pulmonary fibrosis.

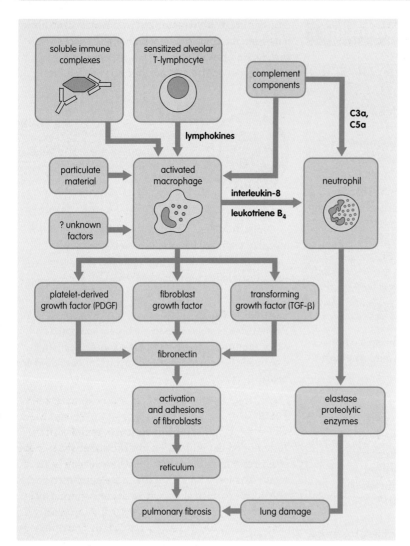

Fig. 7.23 Pathogenesis of pulmonary fibrosis. Macrophages can be activated by several factors (e.g., soluble immune complexes and sensitized T-lymphocytes), resulting in the release of various cytokines leading to fibrosis. (From *Clinical Medicine*, 3rd ed., by P. Kumar and M. Clark. Baillière Tindall, 1994.)

Four types of reaction occur:
- Inert (e.g., simple coal-worker's pneumoconiosis)
- Fibrous (e.g., asbestosis)
- Allergic (e.g., extrinsic allergic alveolitis)
- Neoplastic (e.g., mesothelioma).

Distribution of lung disease depends on the dust involved: particles measuring less than 2–3 μm in diameter reach the distal alveoli. Dust particles that are phagocytosed by alveolar macrophages drain into peribronchial lymphatics and hilar lymph nodes.

Radiologic appearances are related to the degree of associated fibrosis and atomic number of dust particles involved.

Coal-worker's pneumoconiosis

The incidence of coal-worker's pneumoconiosis (black lung disease) is related to total dust exposure: it is highest in men who work at the coal face. Two syndromes exist: simple pneumoconiosis and an advanced form, progressive massive fibrosis.

Simple pneumoconiosis

Simple pneumoconiosis is the most common type of pneumoconiosis, reflecting coal dust deposition within the lung. It is asymptomatic and diagnosis is made on the basis of chest x-rays. Opacities on chest radiographs are mainly in the upper zone and are graded as follows:

1. A few small, round opacities are present.
2. Numerous small, round opacities are present. Normal lung markings are visible.
3. Very numerous small, round opacities are present. Normal lung markings are partially or totally obscured.

Of patients with category 3 simple pneumoconiosis, 30% will develop progressive massive fibrosis.

Progressive massive fibrosis

In progressive massive fibrosis, large, round fibrotic nodules measuring more than 10mm in diameter are seen, usually in the upper lobes. Scarring is present. Nodules may show central liquefaction and become infected by tuberculosis. The associated emphysema is always severe.

Symptoms include dyspnea, cough, and sputum production (which may be black as cavitating lesions rupture). Lung function tests show a mixed restrictive and obstructive pattern.

The disease may progress once exposure has ceased (unlike simple coal-worker's pneumoconiosis), and there is no specific treatment.

Caplan's syndrome

Caplan's syndrome (rheumatoid pneumoconiosis) is the association of coal-worker's pneumoconiosis and rheumatoid arthritis.

Rounded lesions, measuring 0.5–5.0cm in diameter, are seen on x-ray.

Asbestosis

Asbestosis is a diffuse fibrosis which is caused by the inhalation of asbestos. Asbestos is a mixture of silicates of iron, nickel, magnesium, aluminum, and cadmium. It is mined in Southern Africa, the former Soviet Union, and Canada. Several types of asbestos exist: amphiboles are the fibers that cause pulmonary disease in humans, of which crocidolite (blue asbestos) is the most important.

Blue asbestos exists in straight fibers measuring 50μm in length and 1–2μm in width; they are resistant to macrophage and neutrophil enzyme destruction.

Asbestos fibers may become coated in acid mucopolysaccharide and encrusted with hemosiderin to form the drumstick-shaped asbestos bodies. Histology shows features of pulmonary fibrosis and honeycomb lung, affecting the lower lobes more commonly.

A considerable time lag exists between exposure and disease development. The first clinical symptoms are dyspnea and a dry cough; signs include clubbing. Bilateral end inspiratory crackles indicate significant diffuse pulmonary fibrosis.

No treatment is available.

You might be forgiven for thinking that asbestosis is yet another synonym. But it does not simply mean exposure to asbestos (this in itself may not cause symptoms), nor is it a synonym for pleural plaques (you can have asbestosis with or without plaques), and mesothelioma is different again (see below).

Sarcoidosis

Sarcoidosis is a multisystem granulomatous disorder of unknown etiology. Sarcoidosis is a common cause of interstitial lung disease, with only lymph nodes involved more commonly than the lungs. Women are more likely to develop the condition, which has a peak incidence in patients aged 20–40 years.

Prevalence in the U.S. is estimated to be 1–40 in 100000. A geographical distribution shows that it is common in the U.S. and rare in Japan. The disease is more common and its course more severe in African Americans.

Clinical features

Sarcoidosis is asymptomatic in 30% of patients. The most common presentation is with respiratory symptoms or radiographic abnormalities, notably bilateral hilar lymphadenopathy. Other symptoms include mild fever, malaise, arthralgia, and erythema nodosum.

Pulmonary infiltration

Pulmonary infiltration occurs as noncaseating granulomas distributed along the lymphatics and the walls of small airways and blood vessels. These granulomas usually heal with minimal fibrosis. In 10–20% the disease progresses and an interstitial fibrosis develops. If untreated, pulmonary fibrosis leads to progressive dyspnea and cor pulmonale.

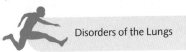
Extrapulmonary manifestations

Extrapulmonary manifestations are as follows:

- Skin sarcoidosis (e.g., erythema nodosum)
- Eye manifestations (e.g., anterior uveitis)
- Metabolic manifestations (e.g., hypercalcemia)
- Central nervous system involvement (e.g., cranial nerve palsies)
- Bone and joint involvement (e.g., arthralgia)
- Hepatosplenomegaly
- Cardiac involvement (e.g., cor pulmonale).

Sarcoidosis is diagnosed on histologic evidence of widespread noncaseating epithelioid granulomas in more than one organ.

History taking in these diseases should include a detailed evaluation of systemic features such as fever, rashes, eye signs, etc.

Tests

Chest radiography can be useful:

- Bilateral hilar lymphadenopathy is a characteristic feature
- Reticular shadows typically appear in upper lobes after fibrosis starts.

Complete blood count can show mild normochromic normocytic anemia and raised erythrocyte sedimentation rate. Serum biochemistry can reveal hypercalcemia. The tuberculin skin test is negative or depressed in most cases.

Lymph node transbronchial biopsy, which has superseded the Kveim test, gives positive results in 90% of cases of pulmonary sarcoidosis.

Serum ACE levels are two standard deviations above their normal mean value in 75% of patients. This test is nonspecific and is therefore of no diagnostic value but can help to monitor response to treatment.

Treatment

If the patient has hilar lymphadenopathy and no lung involvement, then no treatment is required.

If infiltration has occurred for more than 6 weeks treat with corticosteroids (20–40mg per day for 4–6 weeks then reduced dose for up to one year).

Prognosis

Mortality is low in all ethnic groups but 16 times higher in African Americans than in Caucasians.

Extrinsic allergic alveolitis

Hypersensitivity pneumonitis is also known as extrinsic allergic alveolitis. The condition is a widespread diffuse inflammatory reaction caused by a type III hypersensitivity reaction and results from the individual being already sensitized to the inhaled antigen. Antigens that can cause allergic lung disease include:

- Moldy hay (e.g., farmer's lung)
- Bird feces (e.g., in bird fancier's lung)
- Cotton fibers (e.g., byssinosis)
- Sugar cane fibers (e.g., bagassosis).

Clinical features are acute and severe if there is exposure to large doses of the antigen. Onset is more insidious in long-term exposure to small amounts.

Farmer's lung

In farmer's lung, a fungus present in moldy hay is inhaled and a type III immune complex reaction follows if the individual is already sensitized. Initial infiltration of small airways and alveolar walls with neutrophils occurs. Lymphocytes and macrophages then infiltrate, leading to the development of noncaseating granulomas, which may resolve or organize leading to pulmonary fibrosis.

Clinical features consist of fever, malaise, cough, and dyspnea developing several hours after initial exposure to the antigen. Coarse end-inspiratory crackles are heard on auscultation.

Tests include polymorphonuclear leukocyte count, precipitating antibodies (evidence of exposure not disease), lung function tests, and bronchoalveolar lavage.

Prevention is the aim of treatment. Corticosteroids help prevent onset of pulmonary fibrosis.

Idiopathic pulmonary fibrosis

Also known as fibrosing alveolitis or cryptogenic fibrosing alveolitis, idiopathic pulmonary fibrosis is a rare, progressive chronic pulmonary fibrosis of unknown etiology. It has a peak incidence in patients aged 45–65 years.

Clinical features

Clinical features of idiopathic pulmonary fibrosis include progressive breathlessness and a dry cough.

Fatigue and considerable weight loss can occur. There is progression to cyanosis, respiratory failure, pulmonary hypertension, and cor pulmonale over time.

Clubbing occurs in two-thirds of patients; chest expansion is reduced and bilateral, fine, end-inspiratory crackles are heard on auscultation.

> Interstitial lung diseases provide an opportunity for a board examiner's favorite—questions about clubbing. Note that clubbing occurs in idiopathic fibrosing alveolitis and asbestosis, but not in other interstitial diseases.

Pathology

The alveoli walls are thickened because of fibrosis, predominantly in the subpleural regions of the lower lobes. An increased number of chronic inflammatory cells are in the alveoli and interstitium. This pattern is termed "usual interstitial pneumonitis" and is a progressive condition.

Patterns of disease also include:
- Desquamative interstitial pneumonitis
- Bronchiolitis obliterans.

Idiopathic pulmonary fibrosis has been reported with a number of other conditions: connective-tissue disorders, celiac disease, ulcerative colitis, and renal tubular acidosis.

Tests

Several investigations are made:
- Transbronchial or open lung biopsy to confirm histological diagnosis
- CT scan
- Blood gases may show arterial hypoxemia
- Complete blood count may show raised erythrocyte sedimentation rate
- Lung function test shows a restrictive pattern
- Bronchoalveolar lavage shows increased numbers of neutrophils
- Autoantibody tests
- Antinuclear factor is positive in one-third of patients. Rheumatoid factor is positive in one-half of patients.

Prognosis

Of patients with the condition, 50% die within 4–5 years.

Treatment

About 50% of patients respond to immunosuppression. Conventional therapy may include:
- High-dose prednisone or prednisolone for 2–4 months, then tapered
- Azathioprine or cyclophosphamide is used in steroid nonresponders or when steroids are contraindicated.

Single lung transplantation may be attempted where necessary.

Supportive treatment includes oxygen therapy.

Diffuse pulmonary hemorrhage syndromes
Goodpasture's syndrome

Goodpasture's syndrome is characterized by glomerulonephritis and respiratory symptoms. It usually begins with an upper respiratory tract infection. Goodpasture's syndrome is thought to be a type II hypersensitivity reaction.

Clinical features

Clinical features include hemoptysis, hematuria, and anemia caused by massive bleeding.

Most patients have antiglomerular basement membrane antibody circulating in their blood, which causes glomerulonephritis and also acts on alveolar membranes, causing pulmonary hemorrhage. The course of the disease is variable: some patients resolve completely, others proceed to renal failure. There is an association with influenza virus A_2.

Treatment

Treatment is by corticosteroids or plasmapheresis to remove antibodies.

Idiopathic pulmonary hemosiderosis

Idiopathic pulmonary hemosiderosis is a rare condition, typically occurring in children aged under 7 years. An association with sensitivity to cow's milk has been suggested.

Clinical features

Patients present with hemoptysis because of recurrent episodes of intra-alveolar hemorrhage, cough, and dyspnea.

Pathology

The more acute form of idiopathic pulmonary hemosiderosis shows evidence of diffuse alveolar damage and type II pneumocyte hyperplasia. Hemosiderin-containing macrophages are found in the sputum.

Treatment

Treatment is by corticosteroids and azathioprine. Prognosis is poor.

Pulmonary eosinophilia

Pulmonary eosinophilia is a group of syndromes characterized by abnormally high levels of eosinophils in the blood, or in the case of acute eosinophilic pneumonia, in lung lavage fluid. The severity of these diseases can range from mild to fatal (Fig. 7.24).

Bronchiolitis obliterans

In bronchiolitis obliterans, characteristic histological appearance shows:

- Polypoid masses of organizing inflammatory exudates
- Granulation tissue extending from alveoli to bronchioles.

Etiology is unknown, although an association with a number of clinical conditions exists:

- Viral infections (e.g., respiratory syncytial virus)
- Aspiration
- Inhalation of toxic fumes
- Extrinsic allergic alveolitis
- Pulmonary fibrosis
- Collagen or vascular disorders.

Bronchiolitis obliterans is sensitive to corticosteroid treatment.

Collagen disorders and vascular disorders

Rheumatoid diseases

The respiratory system is affected in 10–15% of patients with rheumatoid disease; respiratory disease may occur before other systemic features. Patients characteristically have severe seropositive rheumatoid disease.

Diffuse pulmonary fibrosis can occur. Small-airway disease shows bronchiolitis obliterans or follicular bronchiolitis with lymphoid aggregates and germinal centers. Rheumatoid nodules are rare in the lung, and when they do occur, they usually cavitate. The pleura may show fibrosis, and chronic unilateral pleural effusions are common.

Pulmonary eosinophilia						
Disease	Etiology	Symptoms	Blood eosinophils (%)	Multisystem involvement	Duration	Outcome
simple	passage of parasitic larvae through lung	mild	10	none	<1 month	good
prolonged	unknown	mild/moderate	<20	none	>1 month	good
asthmatic	often type 1 hypersensitivity to *Aspergillus*	moderate/severe	5–20	none	years	fair
tropical	hypersensitivity reaction to filarial infestation	moderate/severe	>20	none	years	fair
hypereosinophilic syndrome	unknown	severe	>20	always	months/years	poor
Churg-Strauss syndrome	possibly immune complex vasculitis	severe	>20	always	months/years	poor/fair

Fig. 7.24 Causes of pulmonary eosinophilia.

Systemic lupus erythematosus

In patients with systemic lupus erythematosus (SLE), pleurisy may develop, with or without an effusion. When present, effusions are small and bilateral.

Basal pneumonitis may be present and diffuse pulmonary fibrosis is rare.

Desquamative interstitial pneumonitis

Desquamative interstitial pneumonitis is found in patients with fibrosing alveolitis. It is more diffuse than usual interstitial pneumonitis. A proliferation of macrophages in the alveolar airspaces occurs, along with interstitial thickening by mononuclear inflammatory cells. Lymphoid tissue and a small amount of collagen are sometimes present.

Desquamative interstitial pneumonitis has a distinctly uniform histologic pattern. The alveolar walls show relatively little fibrosis.

Corticosteroids may be beneficial, and prognosis is good.

Alveolar proteinosis

Alveolar proteinosis is a rare condition, also known as alveolar lipoproteinosis. The etiology is unknown in the majority of cases, and pathogenesis is uncertain. It has been hypothesized that there is increased destruction or decreased clearance of type II cells and accumulation of eosinophilic material within the alveoli. Alveolar proteinosis is associated with a high incidence of concomitant fungal infections and may complicate other interstitial disease (e.g. desquamative interstitial pneumonitis).

The main symptoms of alveolar proteinosis are dyspnea and cough. Chest pain and hemoptysis are rare.

The course of the disease is variable, but the majority of patients enjoy spontaneous remission.

Neoplastic disease of the lung

Bronchial carcinoma

Bronchial carcinoma accounts for 95% of all primary tumors of the lung and is the most common malignant tumor in the Western world. Bronchogenic carcinoma affects men more than women (M:F ratio = 3.5:1), but incidence has risen in women and it is now the most common cancer in both sexes. Typically patients are aged 40–70 years at presentation; only 2–3% occur in younger patients.

Risk factors in lung cancer	
Factor	Relative risk
nonsmoker	1
smoker, 1–2 packs/day	42
ex-smoker	2 to 10
passive smoke exposure	1.5 to 2
asbestos exposure	5
asbestos plus tobacco	90

Fig. 7.25 Risk factors in lung cancer. (Adapted from *Pulmonary Physiology* by G. Criner and G. D'Alonzo. Fence Creek Publishing, 1999, p. 303.)

Etiology

Risk factors are summarized in Fig. 7.25. Cigarette smoking is the largest contributory factor:

- It is related to the amount smoked, duration, and tar content
- The rise in incidence of lung cancer correlates closely to the increase in smoking over the past century
- In nonsmokers, the incidence is less than 5 cases per 100000
- The risk in those who give up smoking decreases with time
- Passive smoking also increases risk.

Environmental and occupational factors include:
- Radon released from granite rock
- Asbestos
- Air pollution (e.g., beryllium emissions).

Histologic types

There are four main histologic types of bronchogenic carcinoma:

- Non-small-cell carcinomas (70%):
  - Squamous cell carcinoma (52%)
  - Adenocarcinoma (13%)
  - Large-cell carcinoma (5%)
- Small-cell carcinomas (30%).

The different types of tumor are summarized in Fig. 7.26.

Tumors may occur as discrete or mixed histological patterns; the development from the initial malignant change to presentation is variable:
- Squamous cell carcinoma: 8 years

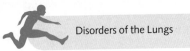

Fig. 7.26 Summary of tumor types.

Tumor types				
	Non-small-cell tumors			Small cell
	Squamous cell tumor	Adenocarcinoma	Large cell	
incidence (%)	52	13	5	30
male/female incidence	M > F	F > M	M > F	M > F
location	hilar	peripheral	peripheral/central	hilar
histological stain	keratin	mucin	—	—
relationship to smoking	high	low	high	high
growth rate	slow	medium	rapid	very rapid
metastasis	late	intermediate	early	very early
treatment	surgery			chemotherapy
prognosis	2-year survival = 50%			3 months if untreated; 1 year if treated

- Adenocarcinoma: 15 years
- Small-cell carcinoma: 3 years.

Squamous cell carcinoma

Squamous cell carcinoma arises from squamous epithelium in the large bronchi. A strong association between cigarette smoking and squamous cell carcinoma exists. Males are affected most commonly, with a mean age at diagnosis of 57 years.

Squamous cell carcinomas are histologically well differentiated and are associated with keratinization. The cancer commonly produces a substance similar to parathyroid hormone (PTH), which leads to hypercalcemia (see Fig. 7.29).

The major mass of the tumor may occur outside the bronchial cartilage and encircle the bronchial lumen, producing obstructive phenomena. The tumors are almost always hilar and are prone to massive necrosis and cavitation, with upper lobe lesions more likely to cavitate. Of squamous cell carcinomas, 13% show cavitation on chest radiographs. Peripheral lesions tend to be larger than those seen in adenocarcinomas.

If squamous carcinoma occurs in the apical portion of the lung, it may produce Pancoast's syndrome (see below).

Squamous cell carcinoma is the least likely type to metastasize, and untreated it has the longest patient survival of any of the bronchogenic carcinomas.

Adenocarcinoma of the lung is usually a peripheral tumor.

Adenocarcinoma

Adenocarcinomas are most common in:
- Nonsmoking elderly women
- The Far East.

Adenocarcinomas are associated with diffuse pulmonary fibrosis and honeycomb lung. Bronchogenic tumors associated with occupational factors are mainly adenocarcinomas. Ninety per cent of adenocarcinomas occur between 40–69 years of age, with the mean age for diagnosis being 53.3 years. Two-thirds of adenocarcinomas are found peripherally. Usually, tumors measure more than 4 cm in diameter.

Adenocarcinoma arises from glandular cells such as mucus goblet cells, type II pneumocytes, and clara cells. Histologically, they are differentiated from other bronchogenic tumors by their glandular configuration and mucin production. The gland structure may be acinar or papillary.

Clinically, two growth patterns are seen:
- Discrete nodule in the periphery with pleural tethering (most common)
- Multifocal and bilateral diffuse tumor (so-called bronchoalveolar cell carcinoma).

Because the tumor is commonly in the periphery, obstructive symptoms are rare, so the tumor tends to be clinically silent. Symptoms include coughing, hemoptysis, chest pain, and weight loss. A wide range of paraneoplastic syndromes are seen (see below). Malignant cells are detected in the sputum in 50% of patients, and the most common radiologic presentation is a solitary peripheral pulmonary nodule, close to the pleural surface.

Resection is possible in a small proportion of cases; 5-year survival rate is less than 10%. Invasion of the pleura and mediastinal lymph nodes is common, as is metastasis to the brain and bones.

Metastasis in the gastrointestinal tract, pancreas, or ovaries must be excluded after having made a diagnosis.

Large-cell anaplastic carcinomas lack features of differentiation.

Large-cell anaplastic tumor

Large-cell anaplastic tumors are diagnosed by a process of elimination. No clear-cut pattern of clinical or radiologic presentation distinguishes them from other malignant lung tumors.

Under light microscopy, findings include:
- Pleomorphic cells with large, darkly staining nuclei
- Prominent nucleoli, abundant cytoplasm, and well-defined cell borders
- Abundant mitoses.

Large-cell anaplastic tumors are variable in location but are usually centrally located. Peripherally located lesions are larger than adenocarcinomas. The point of origin of the carcinoma influences symptomatic presentation of the disease: central lesions present earlier than peripheral lesions because they cause obstruction.

The tumor causes coughing, sputum production, and hemoptysis. When a tumor occurs in a major airway, obstructive pneumonia can occur. Sputum cytology and bronchoscopy with bronchial biopsy are the basis for diagnosis.

On electron microscopy, these tumors turn out to be poorly differentiated variants of squamous cell carcinoma and adenocarcinoma; they are extremely aggressive and destructive lesions. Early invasion of blood vessels and lymphatics occurs, and treatment is by surgical resection whenever possible.

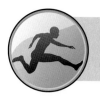

Squamous cell carcinoma is the most common cause of bronchogenic carcinoma.

Small-cell carcinoma

Small-cell carcinomas arise from endocrine cells—Kulchitsky cells, members of the amine precursor uptake decarboxylase (APUD) system.

The incidence of this carcinoma is directly related to cigarette consumption and it is considered to be a systemic disease. Small-cell carcinomas are the most aggressive malignancy of all the bronchogenic tumors.

Most small-cell anaplastic tumors originate in the large bronchi and obstructive pneumonitis is frequently seen. Several histologic subgroups of this carcinoma exist and all have:
- Cell size: 6–8µm
- High nucleus:cytoplasm ratio
- Hyperchromatism of the nuclei.

When almost no cytoplasm is present, and the cells are compressed into an ovoid form, the neoplasm is called an oat-cell carcinoma. On radiography, the oat-cell carcinoma does not cavitate.

There is a high occurrence of paraneoplastic syndromes associated with this type of tumor, so presentation may be varied. The most frequent presenting complaint is coughing. Spread is rapid, and metastatic lesions may be the presenting sign. Small-cell carcinomas metastasize through the lymphatic route.

Chest radiography may help in diagnosis, although the diagnosis must be confirmed by histologic or cytologic means.

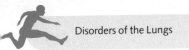

Prognosis is very poor, with a mean survival time for untreated patients with small-cell carcinoma of 7 weeks after diagnosis. Death is generally caused by metastatic disease.

Small-cell carcinoma is the only bronchial carcinoma that responds to chemotherapy.

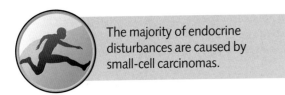

The majority of endocrine disturbances are caused by small-cell carcinomas.

Mixed tumors

A number of mixed tumor types exist that are commonly seen in resection material at autopsy.

Many pathologists base their diagnosis on the prominent cell type present because the predominant cell type predicts prognosis of the condition.

Clinical features

Features specific to the histologic types have already been introduced above. There are no specific signs of bronchogenic carcinoma. Diagnosis always needs to be excluded in cigarette smokers who present with recurrent respiratory symptoms:

- Persistent cough—most common presentation; may be productive if obstruction leads to infection
- Hemoptysis—occurs at some stage in disease in 50%
- Dyspnea—rarely at presentation but occurs as disease progresses
- Chest pain—often pleuritic caused by obstructive changes
- Wheezing—monophonic, due to obstruction.

Unexplained weight loss is also a common presenting complaint. Other symptoms may be present due to complications decribed below.

In 10–30% of patients finger clubbing is present on examination.

Complications
Local complications
Symptoms may be caused by:

- Ulceration of bronchus; occurs in up to 50% of patients and produces hemoptysis in varying degrees

Effects of local spread	
Site of spread	**Symptoms**
pleura/ribs	pain on respiration/pathological fractures
brachial plexus	shoulder pain and small muscle wasting of the hand
sympathetic ganglia	ipsilateral Horner's syndrome
recurrent laryngeal nerve	hoarse voice and bovine cough
superior vena cava	facial congestion; distended neck veins

Fig. 7.27 Effects and symptoms of local spread.

- Bronchial obstruction. The lumen of the bronchus becomes occluded; distal collapse and retention of secretions subsequently occur. This clinically causes dyspnea, secondary infection, and lung abscesses
- Central necrosis. Carcinomas can outgrow their blood supply leading to central necrosis. The main complication is then the development of a lung abscess.

Figure 7.27 summarizes the effects of local spread.

Pancoast's syndrome

Pancoast's syndrome can be caused by all types of bronchogenic carcinoma, although two-thirds originate from squamous cells. As the tumor grows outward from the pulmonary parenchymal apex, it encroaches on anatomical structures, including:

- Chest wall
- Subpleural lymphatics
- Sympathetic chain.

As noted above, Pancoast's tumor can affect the sympathetic chain, resulting in loss of sympathetic tone and an ipsilateral Horner's syndrome. Intractable shoulder pain occurs when the upper rib is involved. The subclavian artery and vein may become compressed. Destruction of the inferior trunk of the brachial plexus leads to pain in the ulnar nerve distribution and may lead to small-muscle wasting of the hand.

Pancoast's tumor is diagnosed by percutaneous needle aspiration of the tumor.

Paraneoplastic disorders associated with lung cancer			
	Mechanism	Clinical features	Lung cancer association
SIADH: syndrome of inappropriate ADH	excess scretion of ADH	headache, nausea, muscle weakness, drowsiness, confusion, eventually coma	small cell
ectopic ACTH	adrenal hyperplasia and secretion of large amounts of cortisol	Cushings: polyuria, edema, hypokalemia, hypertension, increased pigmentation	small cell or carcinoid
hypercalcemia	ectopic PTH secretion	lethargy, nausea, polyuria, eventually coma	squamous cell (but may be due to bone metastases)
hypertrophic pulmonary osteoarthropathy	unknown	digital clubbing and periosteal inflammation	adenocarcinoma, squamous cell
gonadotrophins	ectopic secretion	gynecomastia, testicular atrophy	large cell

Fig. 7.28 Paraneoplastic disorders associated with lung cancer.

Metastatic complications
Local metastases to lymph nodes, bone, liver, and adrenal glands occur.

Metastases to the brain present as:
- Change in personality
- Epilepsy
- Focal neurologic lesion.

Paraneoplastic syndromes
Paraneoplastic syndromes (Fig. 7.28) cannot be explained by direct invasion of the tumor. They are caused by production by tumor cells of polypeptides that mimic various hormones. Paraneoplastic syndromes are commonly associated with small-cell lung cancer.

Tests
Tests are performed to confirm diagnosis and assess tumor histology and spread.

Chest radiography
Good posteroanterior and lateral views are required. Seventy per cent of bronchial carcinomas arise centrally, and chest radiography demonstrates over 90% of carcinomas. The mass needs to be between 1–2 cm in size to be recognized reliably. Lobar collapse and pleural effusions may be present.

CT scan
CT scan gives good visualization of the mediastinum and is good at identifying small lesions. Valuable to assess extent of tumor and the operability of the mass. Lymph nodes >1.5 cm are pathologic.

Scan should include brain, liver, and adrenals to identify distant metastases.

Fiberoptic bronchoscopy
Confirms central lesion, assesses operability, and allows accurate cell type to be determined. Used to obtain cytological specimens. Mucus secretions plus sputum examined for presence of malignant cells.

If carcinoma involves the first 2 cm of either main bronchus, the tumor is inoperable.

Transthoracic fine-needle aspiration biopsy
In transthoracic fine-needle aspiration biopsy, the needle is guided by x-ray or CT. Direct aspiration of peripheral lung lesion takes place through the chest wall; 25% of patients suffer pneumothorax due to the procedure.

Implantation metastases do not occur.

Staging
Small-cell and non-small-cell cancers are staged differently. Small-cell is staged as either limited or extensive while the TNM system (Fig. 7.29) is used for non-small-cell cancer.

Treatment
Surgery
The only treatment of any value in non-small-cell carcinoma is surgery; however, only 15% of cases are operable at diagnosis.

Surgery can only be performed after:

Staging in non-small-cell lung cancer

Primary tumor

T1	<3 cm—no evidence of invasion proximal to a lobar bronchus
T2	≥3 cm or any site involving pleura or hilum; within a lobar bronchus or at least 2 cm distal to the carina
T3	any size extending into the chest wall, diaphragm, pericardium (not involving great vessels etc.)
T4	inoperable tumor of any size with invasion of the mediastium or involving heart, great vessels, trachea, esophagus, vertebral body or carina or malignant pleural effusion

Regional lymph nodes		**Distant metastases**	
N0	no nodal involvement	M0	no metastases
N1	peribronchial and/or ipsilateral hilar nodes	M1	distant metastases
N2	ipsilateral mediastinal and sub-carinal lymph nodes		
N3	inoperable contralateral node involvement		

Fig. 7.29 Staging in non-small-cell lung cancer.

- Lung function tests show the patient has sufficient respiratory reserve
- CT scan shows no evidence of metastases.

Radiation therapy

Treatment of choice if tumor is inoperable. Good for slowly growing squamous carcinoma.

Radiation pneumonitis develops in 10–15%, and radiation fibrosis occurs to some degree in all cases.

Chemotherapy

Only effective treatment for small-cell carcinoma but is not undertaken with intent to cure. Platinum compounds can achieve good results.

Terminal care

Endoscopic therapy and transbronchial stenting are used to provide symptomatic relief in patients with terminal disease. Daily prednisolone may improve appetite. Opioid analgesia is given to control pain, and laxatives should be prescribed to counteract the opioid side effects. Candidiasis is a common treatable problem.

Both patient and relatives require counseling.

Prognosis

Overall prognosis is poor. Only 6–8% survive 5 years, and mean survival is less than 6 months.

Rarer types of lung tumors
Malignant tumors
Bronchoalveolar cell carcinoma

A distinctive type of adenocarcinoma occurring in the distal portions of the pulmonary parenchyma accounting for 3% of all primary neoplasms of lung. The carcinoma affects males and females equally, and the incidence is not related to cigarette consumption.

Unifocal point of origin within the lung with the major bulk of the tumor seen in the alveoli rather than the bronchi. The lesion grows very slowly and spreads by the bronchial route to implant on other portions of the respiratory epithelium. The lesion may be stable for 5–10 years.

Associated with profuse mucoid sputum production.

In the early stage, radiography may show a nonspecific peripheral coin lesion. Diagnosis of the disease is based on histological examination of tissue obtained by transbronchial or open lung biopsy.

Surgical resection may be curative, although surgical intervention is useless once dissemination has occurred.

Bronchial carcinoid

Low-grade malignant tumor accounting for 1% of tumors found in the lungs. It affects males and females equally and presents <40 years.

Bronchial carcinoids are locally invasive, highly vascular tumors that cause recurrent hemoptysis. The tumor grows slowly, eventually blocking a bronchus.

Rarely gives rise to the carcinoid syndrome and the 5-year survival is >80%.

Malignant mesenchymal tumors (sarcomas) are extremely rare.

Primary pulmonary lymphomas

Rare tumors composed of small B lymphocytes arising from the bronchus and bronchiole-associated lymphoid tissue. Monotypic immunoglobulin may be secreted into the blood.

Benign tumors
Adenomas

Arise from bronchial mucous glands. They present as polypoid or sessile lesions and symptoms are related to obstruction.

Benign mesenchymal tumors

Arise anywhere that mesenchyme occurs. The lesion is probably a hamartoma, it is a well-circumscribed, round lesion of 1–2cm, composed of cartilage and found in the periphery of the lung. Rarely arises from a major bronchus and presents as an isolated coin lesion on radiographs.

Metastatic malignancy to the lung

Metastases to the lung are a common clinical and radiologic finding. Metastases are more likely to be multiple than solitary. Most hematogenous metastases are sharply circumscribed with smooth edges, and the appearance of multiple smoothly circumscribed nodules is highly suggestive of metastatic disease. Cavitation is unusual in metastatic lesions.

Solitary pulmonary metastases do occur as sarcomas of soft tissue or bone, carcinoma of the breast, colon, and kidney.

Multinodular lung metastases may be of varying sizes (Fig. 7.30):

- Very large dimensions—cannonball pattern
- Many small nodules—snowstorm pattern.

Diseases of iatrogenic origin

Drug-induced lung disease

Pulmonary disease caused by medication is a growing problem. The mechanisms of drug-induced lung damage are either immunologic or cytotoxic, and the type of adverse reaction can be either:

- Predictable if caused by a dose-related effect
- Unpredictable if caused by the development of hypersensitivity reactions.

There are no specific clinical, functional, or radiologic findings in drug-induced pulmonary disease. The most common symptoms include dyspnea and cough (Fig. 7.31).

Examples of drug-induced lung diseases include:

- Bleomycin—the development of bleomycin-induced pulmonary disease is dose-dependent. Bleomycin causes oxygen-radical-induced lung damage. Incidence is approximately 3%, with a mortality rate of 1–2%
- Amiodarone—a class III antiarrhythmic drug, which can cause fatal interstitial pneumonitis. Lung damage has its onset several months after

Metastatic malignancy of lung and the resulting radiological appearance		
Multinodular patterns		**Solitary nodule**
Cannonball	**Snowstorm**	
salivary gland	breast	breast
kidney	kidney	kidney
bowel	bladder	bowel
uterus/ovarian	thyroid	
testis	prostate	

Fig. 7.30 Metastatic malignancy of lung and the resulting radiologic appearance.

Pulmonary manifestations of adverse drug reactions	
Adverse reaction	**Examples**
diffuse alveolar damage	bleomycin, methotrexate, amiodarone, radiotherapy
interstitial pneumonitis	methotrexate, busulphan, amiodarone, gold
eosinophilic pneumonia	bleomycin, naproxen, sulfasalazine
bronchiolitis obliterans	methotrexate, gold, mitomycin
pulmonary hemorrhage	amphotericin B, anticoagulants, hydralazine
pulmonary edema	codeine, methadone, naloxone, salicylates
pleural effusions and fibrosis	amiodarone, hydralazine, bleomycin, bromocriptine

Fig. 7.31 Summary of pulmonary manifestations of adverse drug reactions.

commencement of amiodarone treatment. Incidence of toxicity is 1–2%. The condition responds well to corticosteroid treatment
- Beta blockers—β blockers are contraindicated in patients with asthma because they also block airway β receptors, thus precipitating bronchoconstriction
- Aspirin—may induce asthma, either through decreased prostaglandin production or by increased leukotriene production. Recovery is usual on discontinuation of the drug.

Complications of radiotherapy

The lungs are very sensitive to radiation. Clinical effects depend on the dose given, volume of lung irradiated, and length of treatment. Pulmonary response to radiation is characterized by:
- Acute phase of radiation pneumonitis
- Chronic phase of healing or fibrosis.

Acute radiation pneumonitis

Acute radiation pneumonitis is defined as an acute infiltrate precisely confined to the radiation area and occurring within 3 months of radiotherapy. Acute radiation pneumonitis rarely produces symptoms within the first month after therapy. Symptoms have an insidious onset and include nonproductive cough, shortness of breath on exertion, and low-grade fever.

Diffuse alveolar damage occurs, consisting of a proteinaceous exudate of material in the alveolar air spaces associated with hyaline membranes, especially in alveolar ducts. Endothelial damage, loss of normal respiratory epithelium, and hyperplasia of type II pneumocytes also occur.

Radiation pneumonitis results in a restrictive lung defect and corticosteroids should be given in the acute phase.

Chronic fibrosis

Acute radiation pneumonitis can resolve spontaneously or progress to pulmonary fibrosis. The chronic fibrosing state is usually asymptomatic. Proliferation and fragmentation of elastic fibers occurs, and bronchiolitis obliterans and bronchial fibrosis may be present.

Chronic fibrosis is not precisely confined to irradiated areas.

Lung transplantation

Single lung transplantation is preferred to double transplantation because of donor availability. Bilateral lung transplantation is required in infective conditions to prevent bacterial spill-over from a diseased lung to a single lung transplant.

Patients must have end-stage lung or pulmonary vascular disease with no other treatment options (Fig. 7.32).

Complications

The complications of lung transplantation are described in Fig. 7.33.

Strategies for avoiding rejection

Lung transplantation does not require any significant degree of matching based on tissue type. The main

Lung transplantation	
Indications	Diseases treated by transplantation
age <60 years	pulmonary fibrosis
life expectancy <18 months without transplantation	primary pulmonary hypertension
no underlying cancer	bronchiectasis and cystic fibrosis
no serious systemic disease	emphysema including α_1-antitrypsin deficiency

Fig. 7.32 Indications and diseases treated by lung transplantation.

Complications of lung transplantation	
Complication	Time
hyperacute rejection	seconds/minutes
pulmonary edema	12–72 hours

bacterial lower respiratory tract infection:
    donor-acquired
    recipient-acquired
	
	hours/days
	days/years

acute rejection	day 5/years
airway complications	week 1/months
opportunistic infection	week 4/years
chronic rejection (e.g. bronchiolitis obliterans)	week 6/years

Fig. 7.33 Summary of the complications of lung transplantation.

criteria are compatibility of blood group and size match between organ and recipient.

Suppression of the immune system

All transplant patients require immunsuppression for life. This begins immediately before transplantation; drugs used include:

- Prednisolone
- Azathioprine
- Cyclosporin.

Large doses are given in the initial postoperative period. Lower maintenance doses are achieved after a few months. Rejection episodes are treated with high-dose intravenous corticosteroids.

Prognosis

One-year survival rates are 60–70%.

Diseases of the pleura

Pleural effusions

A pleural effusion is the presence of fluid between the visceral and parietal pleura. Effusions can be categorized as transudative or exudative, depending on the protein concentration (Fig. 7.34).

Transudative pleural effusions (protein <30g/L) occur as a result of an imbalance between hydrostatic and osmotic forces, for example in congestive cardiac failure (hydrothorax). Exudative pleural effusions (protein >30g/L) occur when local factors influencing pleural fluid formation and reabsorption are altered specifically through injury or inflammation. Causes of each type of effusion are shown in Fig. 7.35. Exudative effusions often occur as a complication of pneumonia; these are termed parapneumonic effusions.

Gross appearance

On examination, the pleural fluid may be clear or straw-colored, turbid (signifying infection) or hemorrhagic. If a hemorrhagic effusion exists, neoplastic infiltration, pulmonary infarction, and TB need to be excluded. Leading malignancies that have associated pleural effusions are breast carcinoma, bronchial carcinoma, and lymphomas/leukemia.

Clinical features

Pleural effusions are typically asymptomatic until >500ml of fluid is present. Pleuritic chest pain may develop in addition to dyspnea, which is dependent on the size of effusion.

Signs on examination include stony dull percussion note; see Chapter 9.

Tests

Features on a chest radiograph include blunting of costophrenic angles. Ultrasound is used to detect small effusions not seen on CXR and for guiding aspiration which is performed for microbiological examination or therapeutically.

A pleural biopsy may be necessary if the aspiration is inconclusive.

Treatment

Treat the underlying disease. If the patient is symptomatic, drain the effusion. Drain fluid slowly. Malignant effusions—chemical pleurodesis can provide temporary relief. Use bleomycin/tetracycline.

Pleural effusions			
Transudate		Exudate	
protein	<30 g/L	protein	>30 g/L
lactate dehydrogenase	<200 IU/L	lactate dehydrogenase	>200 IU/L
usually bilateral		unilateral in focal disease; bilateral in systemic disease	

Fig. 7.34 Classification of pleural effusions.

Causes of transudates and exudates	
Transudate	Exudate
left heart failure	bacterial pneumonia
hypoproteinemia	carcinoma bronchus
constrictive pericarditis	pulmonary infarction
hypothyroidism	tuberculosis
cirrhosis	connective-tissue disease

Fig. 7.35 Causes of transudates and exudates.

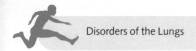

Questions about the cause of exudative and transudative pleural effusions are common in clinical examinations.

Hemothorax	
Degree	Management
minimal (<350 ml)	blood usually reabsorbs spontaneously with conservative treatment
moderate (300–1500 ml)	thoracentesis and tube drainage with underwater seal drainage
massive (>1500 ml)	two drainage tubes inserted; immediate or early thoracotomy may be necessary to arrest bleeding

Fig. 7.36 Management of hemothorax.

Empyema

Also known as a pyothorax, this is a collection of pus within the pleural cavity caused by:

- Complication of thoracic surgery
- Rupture of lung abscess into the pleural space
- Perforation of esophagus
- Mediastinitis
- Bacterial spread of pneumonia.

The empyema cavity can become infected by anaerobes. The patients are feverish and ill. The pus must be removed and appropriate antibiotic treatment should be initiated immediately.

Hemothorax

Blood in the pleural cavity—common in both penetrating and nonpenetrating injuries of the chest. Hemothorax may cause hypovolemic shock and reduce vital capacity through compression. Due to the defibrinating action that occurs with motions of respiration and the presence of an anticoagulant enzyme, the clot may be defibrinated and leave fluid radiologically indistinguishable from effusions of another cause.

Blood may originate from lung, internal mammary artery, thoracicoacromial artery, lateral thoracic artery, mediastinal great vessels, heart, or abdominal structures via diaphragm. See Fig. 7.36 for the management of hemothorax.

Chylothorax

Accumulation of lymph in the pleural space. The most common causes are rupture or obstruction of the thoracic duct due to surgical trauma or neoplasm (e.g., lymphoma). A latent period between injury and onset of 2–10 days occurs. The pleural fluid is high in lipid content and is characteristically milky in appearance. The prognosis is generally good.

Chylous effusion

Caused by the escape of chyle into the pleural space from obstruction or laceration of the thoracic duct.

Chyliform effusion

Results from degeneration of malignant and other cells in pleural fluid.

Pneumothorax

Pneumothorax is the accumulation of air in the pleural space. It may occur spontaneously or following trauma.

Spontaneous

Results from rupture of a pleural bleb, the pleural bleb being a congenital defect of the alveolar wall connective tissue. Patients are typically tall, thin, young males. M:F ratio = 6:1. Spontaneous pneumothoraces are usually apical, affecting both lungs with equal frequency.

Secondary causes of spontaneous pneumothorax occur in patients with underlying disease, such as COPD, TB, pneumonia, bronchial carcinoma, sarcoidosis, and cystic fibrosis.

Patients present with sudden onset of unilateral pleuritic pain and increasing breathlessness.

The main aim of treatment is to get the patient back to active life as soon as possible.

Tests

Chest radiography may show an area devoid of lung markings. May be more clearly seen on the expiratory film.

Management

Small pneumothorax: no treatment, but review in 7–10 days. Admit patients with moderate pneumothorax for simple aspiration.

Tension pneumothorax

This is a medical emergency. The most common causes are:

- Positive pressure ventilation
- Stab wound or rib fracture.

Air escapes into the pleural space, and the rise above atmospheric pressure causes the lung to collapse. At each inspiration intrapleural pressure increases as the pleural tear acts as a ball valve that permits air to enter but not leave the pleural space. Venous return to the heart is impaired as pressure rises and patients experience dyspnea and chest pain. They may also be cyanotic.

Clinically:

- Mediastinum pushed over into contralateral hemithorax. Tracheal deviation
- Hyperresonance, absence of breath sounds
- Intercostal spaces widened on ipsilateral side.

On ECG there is a rightward shift in mean frontal QRS complex, diminution in QRS amplitude, and inversion of precordial T waves. The condition is diagnosed on needle insertion.

Treat with immediate thoracostomy with underwater seal drainage, before requesting chest radiographs. See Fig. 7.37 for a radiograph of a tension pneumothorax. Fig. 7.38 gives a summary of noninflammatory pleural effusions.

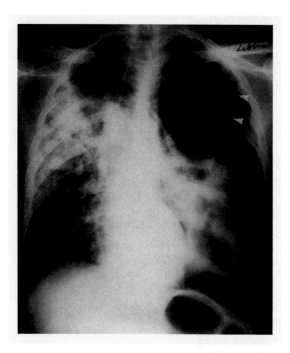

Fig. 7.37 Radiograph of a tension pneumothorax. Tension pneumothorax displacing mediastinum and depressing left hemidiaphragm. Extensive consolidation and cavitation in both lungs is due to tuberculosis. A pleural adhesion (arrowheads) is visible. (Courtesy of Dr D. Sutton and Dr J.W.R. Young.)

A tension pneumothorax should never be diagnosed by chest radiography. It is a clinical diagnosis which requires treatment before requesting a chest x-ray.

Neoplasms of the pleura

Malignant mesothelioma

Malignant mesothelioma is a tumor of mesothelial cells most commonly affecting the visceral or parietal pleura. The incidence of mesothelioma is rising rapidly. In 90% of cases it is associated with occupational exposure to asbestos, especially fibers which are <0.25 μm diameter (e.g., crocidolite and amiosite). The latent period between exposure and death is long, ranging from 15–67 years.

Two histologic varieties exist—50% of mesotheliomas have elements of both:

Noninflammatory pleural effusions		
Disorder	Collection	Cause
hemothorax	blood	chest trauma; rupture of aortic aneurysm
hydrothorax	proteinaceous fluid	congestive cardiac failure
chylothorax	lymph	neoplastic infiltration; trauma
pneumothorax	air	spontaneous; traumatic

Fig. 7.38 Summary of noninflammatory pleural effusions.

- Epithelial: tubular structure
- Fibrous: solid structure with spindle-shaped cells.

The tumor begins as nodules in the pleura and eventually obliterates the pleural cavity.

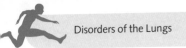

Clinical features
- Initial symptoms are very vague.
- Pain is the main complaint, often affecting sleep and results from infiltration of the tumor into the chest wall with involvement of intercostal nerves and ribs.

Other features include:
- Dyspnea
- Weight loss
- Finger clubbing.

Tests
Features of chest radiograph are:
- Pleural effusions
- Unilateral pleural thickening
- Nodular appearance.

Open lung biopsy may be needed to confirm diagnosis.

Prognosis
No treatment is available, and the condition is universally fatal. Pain responds poorly to therapy.

Metastases are common to hilar and abdominal lymph nodes with secondary deposits arising in lung, liver, thyroid, adrenals, bone, skeletal muscle, and brain. The patient's symptoms become worse until death occurs, usually within 2 years of diagnosis; the cause of death is usually infection, vascular compromise, or pulmonary embolus.

Pleural fibroma
Rare neoplasm of the pleura not related to asbestos exposure which consists of:
- Fibrous connective tissue
- Mesothelial cells.

A solitary mass can grow to be very large, and hypertrophic pulmonary osteoarthropathy is a

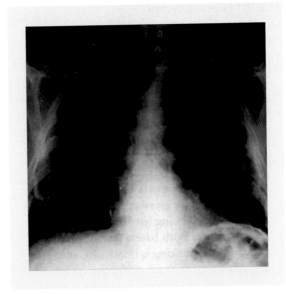

Fig. 7.39 Mesothelioma of the right pleura. The patient had a long history of asbestos exposure and has now developed a large pleural mass. (Courtesy of Professor C.D. Forbes and Dr W.F. Jackson.)

frequent association. Affects females most commonly with a mean age at presentation of 50 years.

The etiology is unknown; most patients are asymptomatic.

Tumors grow slowly and behave generally in a benign fashion, although malignant tumors do exist.

Surgical excision usually results in complete cure.

Up to 80% of localized fibrous tumors arise in relation to the visceral pleura.

Figure 7.39 is a radiograph showing pleural thickening.

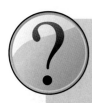

- Describe the two main ways in which atelectasis can occur.
- Classify and give examples of the causes of atelectasis.
- List the causes of pulmonary edema.
- List the multifactoral etiology of adult respiratory distress syndrome.
- List the tests required to diagnose pulmonary embolism.
- Describe the consequences of pulmonary hypertension.
- What are the definitions of chronic bronchitis and emphysema?
- Describe the management of patients with COPD.
- Describe the management of a patient with bronchial asthma.
- What is the pathology of bronchiectasis?
- List the complications of cystic fibrosis.
- Describe the management of a patient with pneumonia.
- What is the pathogenesis of tuberculosis?
- List the common causes of pneumonia in the immunocompromised patient.
- What is the pathogenesis of pulmonary fibrosis?
- Describe the different forms of pneumoconioses.
- What is the relationship between cigarette smoking and bronchogenic carcinomas?
- Describe the differences between small-cell and non-small-cell carcinomas.
- Describe the endocrine manifestations of bronchogenic carcinomas.
- Describe the relationship between asbestos and pleural disease.

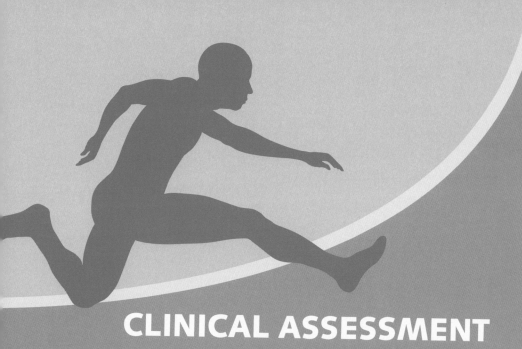

CLINICAL ASSESSMENT

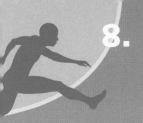

Common presentations

The principal symptoms of respiratory disease (breathlessness, cough, sputum, hemoptysis, wheeze, and chest pain) are common to many different conditions. Clinical findings often overlap considerably and this can make diagnosis seem difficult. However, a good history focusing on the time course and progression of the illness will often reveal recognizable patterns of symptoms and enable you to narrow down the differential diagnoses. Chapter 9 gives a framework for history taking; the main symptoms of respiratory disease and the key details that you should establish are described below.

It is important to remember that extreme lung disease does not necessarily produce clinical signs (e.g., a silent chest is an ominous sign in severe asthma).

Dyspnea

Breathlessness or dyspnea is a difficulty or distress in breathing and is a symptom of many different diseases (Fig. 8.1). Dyspnea is a very common reason for referral to a respiratory clinic.

The patient may describe the symptom in a variety of ways. Common terms used are "out of breath," "can't get enough air," and "feeling suffocated." A number of physiologic factors (Fig. 8.2) underlie this sensation, and sometimes several mechanisms coexist to cause breathlessness. However, understanding the physiologic basis of dyspnea is of limited help clinically; a good history is vital in diagnosing the underlying disease. Key points to establish include the speed of onset of dyspnea (Figs 8.3–8.5), its progression and variability, exacerbating and relieving factors, and response to any treatment. Ask specifically about breathlessness on lying flat (orthopnea), which can occur in severe airflow obstruction or cardiac failure.

The severity of the symptom should be assessed by questioning patients about how it affects their daily life (Fig. 8.6).

Although dyspnea is a subjective sensation, you may be able to see objective evidence of respiratory distress, such as use of accessory muscles of inspiration or obvious tachypnea. See Chapter 9 for more key signs.

Cough

A cough is the most common manifestation of lower respiratory tract disease. The cough reflex is a complex centrally mediated defense reflex, resulting from the appropriate chemical or mechanical stimulation of the larynx and the more proximal portion of the tracheobronchial tree. The basic pattern of a cough can be divided into four components:
- Rapid deep inspiration
- Expiration against a closed glottis
- Sudden glottal opening
- Relaxation of expiratory muscles.

A cough may be voluntary but is usually an involuntary response to an irritant such as:
- Infection (upper or lower respiratory tract)
- Cigarette smoke
- Dusts
- Danders (e.g., from cats).

Common respiratory diseases causing cough are shown in Fig. 8.7. Remember that gastroesophageal reflux or ACE inhibitor therapy can cause a patient to cough. Cough can also be due to paralysis of the vocal cords; this "bovine" cough is low-pitched and occurs

Causes of dyspnea	
physiological	exercise
	high altitude
pathological	respiratory disorders
	cardiac disorders
	obesity
	anemia
psychological	anxiety (hyperventilation)
pharmacological	drug-induced respiratory disorders
	drug-induced cardiac disorders

Fig. 8.1 Causes of breathlessness. (Adapted from *Macleod's Clinical Examination*, 10th ed., edited by J.F. Munro and I.W. Campbell. New York, Churchill Livingstone, 2000.)

Physiology of dyspnea	
Mechanism causing dyspnea	**Responds to:**
chemoreceptors	hypercapnia and to lesser extent hypoxemia
lung receptors (stretch and J receptors)	lung pathology (congestion, etc.)
chest wall receptors	increased work
sense of effort	increased skeletal muscle effort
afferent mismatch	relationship between force generated and lung volume produced; mismatch may lead to dyspnea

Fig. 8.2 Physiology of dyspnea.

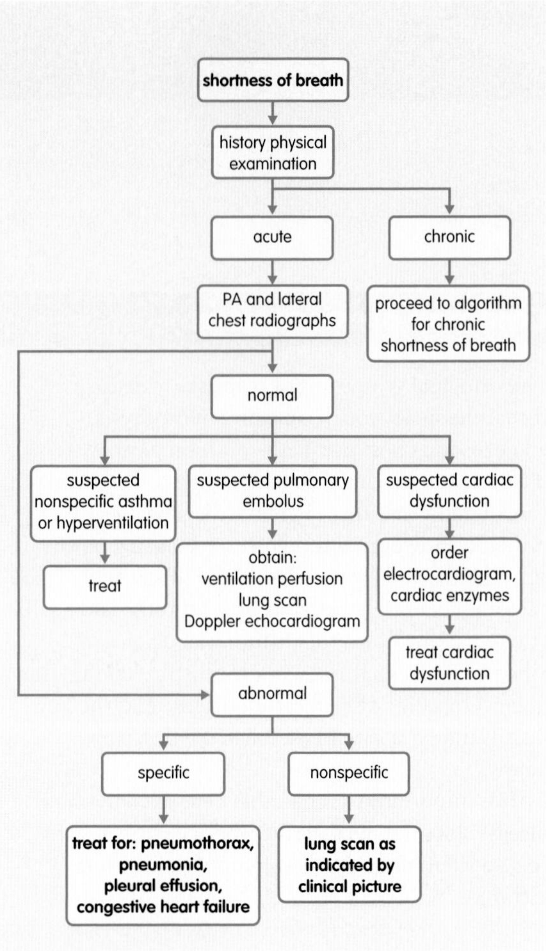

Fig. 8.4 Diagnostic algorithm dyspnea. (Adapted from *Clinical Medicine*, 2nd ed., by H.L. Greene *et al.* St. Louis, Mosby Year Book, 1996.)

Conditions associated with dyspnea, grouped according to onset		
Sudden onset	**Onset occurring over hours**	**Onset occurring over weeks**
pulmonary embolism	pneumonia	chronic obstructive pulmonary disease (COPD)
spontaneous pneumothorax	exacerbation of asthma	pleural effusion
acute pulmonary edema	pulmonary edema	bronchial carcinoma
inhalation of foreign body		pulmonary fibrosis
acute asthma		anemia

Fig. 8.3 Onset of dyspnea.

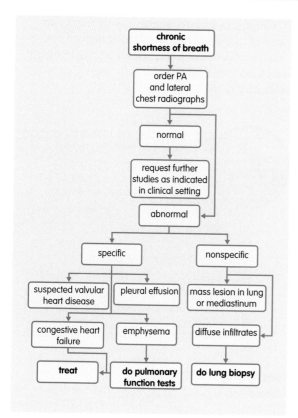

Fig. 8.5 Diagnostic algorithm of chronic dyspnea. (Adapted from *Clinical Medicine*, 2nd ed., by H.L. Greene *et al.* St. Louis, Mosby Year Book, 1996.)

Key questions in assessing dyspnea
How far can you walk upstairs/uphill without stopping?
How far can you walk on level ground without stopping?
Do you feel breathless when washing or dressing?
Do you feel breathless at rest?

Fig. 8.6 Assessing the severity of dyspnea.

Common respiratory causes of cough	
Cause	**Nature**
asthma	worse at night; dry or productive
COPD	worse in morning; often productive
bronchiectasis	related to posture
post-nasal drip	persistent
tracheitis	painful
croup	harsh
interstitial fibrosis	dry

Fig. 8.7 Common respiratory causes of cough.

Patterns of cough in asthma and chronic bronchitis		
	Asthma	**Chronic bronchitis**
timing	worse at night	worse in the morning
chronicity	dry (may be green sputum)	productive
nature	intermittent	persistent
response to treatment	associated wheeze is reversible	associated wheeze is irreversible

Fig. 8.8 Patterns of cough in asthma and chronic bronchitis.

when the recurrent laryngeal nerve is compressed (e.g., by a tumor).

Inquire about the timing of the cough (morning or evening), its chronicity and nature (i.e., productive or nonproductive). Answers to these questions should allow you to differentiate between two common causes of cough: asthma and chronic bronchitis (Fig. 8.8).

Sputum

Everybody produces airway secretions. In a healthy nonsmoker, approximately 100–150ml of mucus is produced every day. Normally, this mucus is transported up the airway's ciliary mucus escalator and swallowed. This process is not normally perceived. However, expectorating sputum is always abnormal and is a sign that excessive mucus has been generated. This can result from irritation of the respiratory tract (commonly caused by cigarette smoking or the common cold) or from infection.

Sputum may be classified as:

- Mucoid: clear, gray, or white
- Serous: watery or frothy
- Mucopurulent: a yellowish tinge
- Purulent: dark green/yellow.

Always try to inspect the sputum and note its volume, color, consistency, and odor. These details can provide clues as to the underlying pathology (Fig. 8.9). A yellow/green color usually means infection and is due to myeloperoxidase produced by eosinophils or neutrophils. However, note that sputum in asthma contains high numbers of eosinophils and is often yellow or green without underlying infection.

Most bronchogenic carcinomas do not produce sputum. The exception is alveolar cell carcinoma, which produces copious amounts of mucoid sputum.

You may have to prompt the patient when investigating the volume of sputum. Does the patient cough up enough to fill a teaspoon, tablespoon, shot glass, or cup?

Chronic bronchitis is a particularly important cause of sputum production. This is defined as a cough productive of sputum for most days during at least three consecutive months for more than two successive years.

Detailed questioning about cough is needed in patients with chronic bronchitis. Useful questions include:

- Do you cough up sputum, spit, or phlegm from your chest on most mornings?
- Would you say you cough up sputum on most days for as much as 3 months a year?
- Do you often need antibiotics in winter?

Hemoptysis

Hemoptysis is coughing up blood; this needs to be differentiated from other sources of bleeding within the oral cavity and hematemesis (vomiting blood). This distinction is usually obvious from the history. Hemoptysis is not usually a solitary event; if possible, the sputum sample should be inspected.

Hemoptysis is a serious and often alarming symptom that requires immediate investigation (Fig. 8.10). A chest radiograph is mandatory in a patient with hemoptysis, and the symptom should be treated as bronchogenic carcinoma until proved otherwise. Despite appropriate investigations, often no obvious cause can be found, and the episode is attributed to a simple bronchial infection.

Important respiratory causes of hemoptysis are:

- Bronchial carcinoma
- Pulmonary infarction
- TB
- Pneumonia (particularly pneumococcal)
- Bronchiectasis
- Acute/chronic bronchitis.

In investigating the cause of hemoptysis, ask about any preceding events, such as respiratory infection or deep vein thrombosis (DVT), and establish the frequency and volume as well as whether the blood is fresh or altered. Figure 8.11 gives some characteristic patterns of hemoptysis and possible diagnoses.

Types of sputum	
Character	**Cause**
pink/frothy	pulmonary edema
yellow/green	infections/eosinophils in asthma
rusty	pneumococcal pneumonia
foul-tasting	anaerobic infection
viscous, difficult to cough up	asthma/infections
large volumes	bronchiectasis
black	cavitating lesions in coal miners
blood-stained	see Figs 8.10 and 8.11

Fig. 8.9 Types of sputum.

Fig. 8.10 Diagnostic algorithm of hemoptysis. (Adapted from *Decision Making in Medicine* by H.L. Greene, W.P. Johnson and M.J. Maricic. St. Louis, Mosby Year Book, 1993.)

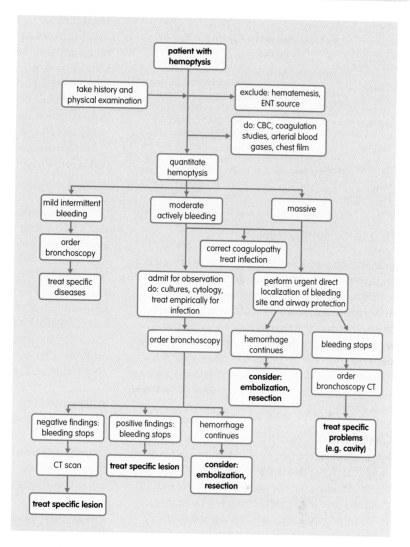

Patterns of hemoptysis	
Pattern	Possible diagnosis
recurrent blood-streaked sputum	bronchial carcinoma
frank, becoming progressively darker over 24/48 h	infarction
recurrent over years, with purulent sputum	bronchiectasis

Fig. 8.11 Patterns of hemoptysis.

Wheeze

Wheezing is a common complaint, complicating many different disease processes. Establish exactly what a patient means by "wheeze"; used correctly the term describes musical notes heard mainly on expiration and caused by narrowed airways.

Wheezes are classified as either polyphonic (of many different notes) or monophonic (just one note). Poylphonic wheezes are common in widespread airflow obstruction; it is the characteristic wheeze heard in asthmatics. A localized monophonic wheeze suggests that a single airway is partially obstructed; this can also occur in asthma (e.g., by a mucus plug) but may be a sign of narrowing due to a tumor.

The symptom of wheezing is not diagnostic of asthma, although asthma and chronic obstructive pulmonary disease are the most common causes and can be difficult to distinguish. You should establish whether the patient wheezes first thing in the

Causes of chest pain	
Structure	**Possible cause of pain**
pleura	pneumothorax, pulmonary infarction
muscle	strain (e.g. from coughing)
bone	rib fracture or tumor
costochondral junctions	Tietze's syndrome
nerves	herpes zoster, Pancoast's syndrome
heart and great vessels	cardiac ischemia/infarction aortic dissection/aneurysm
esophagus	spasm, reflux

Fig. 8.12 Causes of chest pain.

morning (common in chronic bronchitis), at night (common in asthma), or during exercise.

Stridor is an audible *inspiratory* noise and indicates partial obstruction of the upper, larger airways, such as the larynx, trachea, and main bronchus. It is very important that you differentiate between a wheeze and stridor because stridor is a serious sign requiring urgent investigation. Causes of obstruction include tumor and inhalation of a foreign body.

Chest pain

Pain can originate from most of the structures in the chest (Fig. 8.12) and can be classified as central or lateral. As with pain anywhere in the body, inquire about site, mode of onset, character, radiation, intensity, precipitating, aggravating, and relieving factors, and response to any analgesics taken. Make sure you ask specifically about the pain's relationship to breathing, coughing, or movement; if it is made worse by these, it is likely to be pleural in origin. Pleural pain is sharp and stabbing in character and may be referred to the shoulder tip if the diaphragmatic pleura is involved. It can be very severe and often leads to shallow breathing, avoidance of movement, and cough suppression.

The most common causes of pleural pain are pulmonary infarction or infection.

Respiratory causes of central, or retrosternal, chest pain include bronchitis and acute tracheitis. This pain is often made worse by coughing and may be relieved when the patient coughs up sputum.

Other associated symptoms

In addition to the principal presentations, there are several other symptoms that you should note.

Hoarseness

Ask if the patient's voice has changed at all in recent times, and if so, was there anything that preceded the change (e.g., overuse of the voice, thyroidectomy). There may be a simple, benign cause of hoarseness such as:

- Cigarette smoking
- Acute laryngitis as part of an acute upper respiratory tract infection
- Use of inhaled steroids.

However, there may be a more sinister cause: like the bovine cough noted above, hoarseness may be a sign that a lung tumor is compressing the recurrent laryngeal nerve.

Weight loss

Unintentional weight loss is always an important sign, raising suspicion of carcinoma. Establish how much weight the patient has lost, over what period, and whether there is any loss of appetite. Note, however, that it is common for patients with severe emphysema to lose weight.

Ankle swelling

Patients with chronic obstructive pulmonary disease (COPD) may comment that their ankles swell during acute exacerbations. Ask about this, and check for edema as part of your examination; it is an important sign of cor pulmonale.

Acute presentations

Respiratory failure

Respiratory failure is not a presentation seen in isolation but a possible outcome of many different respiratory diseases.

In the initial stages of lung disease, the body may be able to maintain normal blood gases by adapting to increased ventilatory demand. However, if the underlying disease progresses, the ventilatory workload may become excessive. The result is a failure to oxygenate the blood or failure to remove carbon dioxide by ventilation. The patient is said to be in respiratory failure, a state which can be diagnosed on the clinical picture and by blood gas analysis. The patient will usually have signs of underlying disease in addition to the clinical features of respiratory failure, which are principally those of hypoxia (Fig. 8.13).

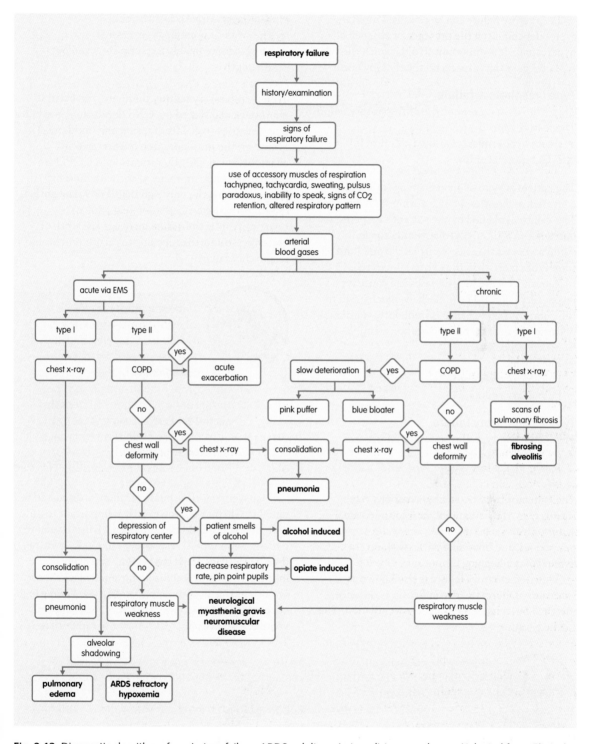

Fig. 8.13 Diagnostic algorithm of respiratory failure. ARDS: adult respiratory distress syndrome. (Adapted from *Clinical Medicine*, 2nd ed., by H.L. Greene *et al.* St. Louis, Mosby Year Book, 1996.)

Respiratory failure can be classified into two types, depending on the presence or absence of hypercapnia. It is important to distinguish the two types because this impacts on the therapy given.

Type I respiratory failure

This is the most common type of respiratory failure. The features are:

- Acute hypoxemia: P_aO_2 low (<60mmHg)
- P_aCO_2 normal or low.

The patient is hypoxic (and becomes cyanotic, confused, and restless) but is normo- or hypocapnic. This can be explained by the patient's response to an initial rise in P_aCO_2. Alveolar ventilation is stimulated, and the excess carbon dioxide (and sometimes more than the excess) is expired.

Almost all acute lung diseases can cause type I respiratory failure. The underlying mechanism for the failure of gas exchange is frequently ventilation: perfusion mismatch. Some common examples are:

- Severe acute asthma
- Pneumonia
- Pulmonary embolism
- Pulmonary edema.

Type II respiratory failure

The features of type II respiratory failure are:

- P_aO_2 low (<60mmHg)
- P_aCO_2 high (>50mmHg).

The patient is hypoxic and hypercapnic. As the P_aCO_2 rises, the patient will develop additional symptoms and signs including headache, warm peripheries, and bounding pulse; with severe hypercapnia a flapping tremor may develop.

Type II respiratory failure is also known as ventilatory failure; the rise in P_aCO_2 is no longer matched by an increase in alveolar ventilation. This can be because:

- Ventilatory drive is insufficient
- The work of breathing is excessive
- The lungs are unable to pump air in and out efficiently.

Type II respiratory failure, therefore, can occur in neuromuscular disorders, CNS depression, or when a lung collapses (e.g., after tension pneumothorax). However, the most common cause is an acute exacerbation of COPD. Patients with COPD are often hypoxemic for many years, with morning headache being the only sign that P_aCO_2 is slightly raised. An acute exacerbation (e.g., due to respiratory infection) then increases the work of breathing still further, leading to "acute-on-chronic" respiratory failure.

If the respiratory failure develops quickly, increased P_aCO_2 leads to a rise in pH: respiratory acidosis. If it develops more slowly, there is time for renal compensation and pH may be normal or near-normal: compensated respiratory acidosis. Always look at bicarbonate levels to see if they have risen in compensation.

Management of respiratory failure is discussed in detail in Chapter 6. However, it is important to note here that you should be cautious in giving oxygen to patients with type II respiratory failure. Respiratory drive in these patients has become relatively insensitive to hypercapnia; hypoxemia plays a more important role in stimulating ventilation. Giving high concentrations of oxygen, therefore, will suppress ventilatory drive and P_aCO_2 may rise rather than fall.

- What are the key differences in presentation between a patient with COPD and a patient with asthma?
- What important facts do you need to establish if a patient complains of coughing up blood?
- Explain the difference between type I and II respiratory failure in terms of blood gases and symptoms.
- What are the three basic mechanisms that contribute to type II respiratory failure?
- Why do you need to exercise caution in administering oxygen to a patient with COPD who is in respiratory failure?

9. History and Examination

Taking a history

In respiratory medicine your skills in history taking will be tested by both:
- Acute presentations—diagnosis must be quick but may be hindered by the patient's condition
- Chronic presentations—documenting the key features in an illness that may span many years.

Each situation has its specific challenges, and in each a good history should tell you the diagnosis.

This section outlines a generic approach to history taking. In practice, you should tailor your history to the possible diagnoses. In a female patient with a suspected deep vein thrombosis (DVT) you will need to ask about pregnancy, oral contraceptive use, recent travel or surgery, and family history of DVT or PE. Obviously, you will need a different set of questions to establish a diagnosis of asthma.

Initial observations

Before you begin, take a few minutes to introduce yourself and to put the patient at ease. Simple observation at the bedside can often give a good clue to the likely diagnosis:
- Inhalers and oxygen bottles
- Emesis trays
- Canes or walkers.

How does the patient appear during the interview? Agitated or distressed? Is there a visible tremor? Is the patient too breathless to speak in full sentences? Is the voice rough or hoarse? Simple observations now will save time later.

Structure of the history
Presenting complaint (PC)

The presenting complaint is a concise statement of the symptoms felt by the patient. Use the patient's own words—this is not a diagnosis. For example, for shortness of breath the patient might use "out of breath" or "can't get any air in."

History of presenting complaint

Build up a picture of the presenting complaint, investigating each symptom as described in Chapter 8. You should establish the following details:
- Onset: acute or gradual
- Pattern: intermittent or continuous
- Frequency: daily, weekly, or monthly
- Duration: minutes or hours
- Progression: better or worse than in the past
- Severity: mild, moderate, or severe
- Character (e.g., is the pain sharp, dull or aching?)
- Precipitating and relieving factors (e.g., are any medications used?)
- Associated symptoms (e.g., cough, wheeze, hemoptysis, dyspnea, chest pain, orthopnea)
- Systemic symptoms (e.g., fever, malaise, anorexia, weight loss).

Has the patient had the problem before? If so, what were the diagnosis, treatment, and outcome?

Ask the patient how disabling the problem is and how it affects daily life. In patients with chronic illness, you should establish exercise tolerance and whether it has declined.

Past medical history

Present the past medical history in chronological order, listing any hospital admissions, surgical operations, and major illnesses.

Take a careful note of anything that might contribute to the presenting complaint. For example:
- Pneumonia—complications include pleural effusion, bronchiectasis
- Asthma or bronchitis as a child—possibly asthma

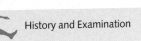
- Severe measles or whooping cough in childhood—may lead to bronchiectasis
- Previous pulmonary embolism (PE) or deep vein thrombosis (DVT)
- Pregnancy—risk of PE
- Recent surgery—PE, hospital-acquired or aspiration pneumonia
- Eczema or hay fever—evidence of atopy.

Has the patient received BCG immunization or experienced tuberculosis contact in the past? Has he or she ever had a chest radiograph? It may be useful for comparison. Note any other factors that might have contributed. For example:

- Recent travel—DVT, legionella
- Recent life events (e.g., moving house)—stress, house dust.

Drug history (DH)

When taking the drug history, list the patient's current intake of both prescription and over-the-counter (OTC) drugs, recording dosage, frequency, and duration of treatment. Ask the patient what each tablet is for and when it is taken; this gives an indication of the patient's understanding of his or her problems and compliance. Remember that some drugs (e.g., beta-blockers or NSAIDs) can make asthma worse. The oral contraceptive pill is a risk factor for pulmonary embolism. ACE inhibitors prescribed for hypertension can cause cough.

Drug allergies

Ask about any allergies. If the patient mentions an allergy, ask what exactly happened and how long ago it happened.

Family history (FH)

When noting a family history, it may help to draw a family tree. Do any members of the family suffer from a respiratory disorder? A family history of premature emphysema or liver cirrhosis may indicate α_1 antitrypsin deficiency. Is there a family history of pulmonary embolism or deep vein thrombosis? Ask about atopy, asthma, eczema, and hay fever. Does anybody in the family smoke?

Social history

Social history is important in respiratory disease, which can be caused, or worsened, by social factors such as housing, occupation, hobbies, or pets.

Home and social situation

Ask who lives with the patient at home and whether they are well. Do they have any additional help around the home?

Ask about accommodation:

- Type: house, apartment (which floor?), or dorm?
- Heating: central heating or other?
- Conditions: damp or dry?
- Number of people living in the accommodation
- Area of town: gives an indication of socioeconomic conditions
- Pets: dogs, cats, or birds.

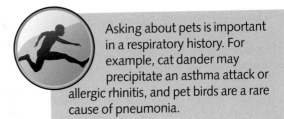

Asking about pets is important in a respiratory history. For example, cat dander may precipitate an asthma attack or allergic rhinitis, and pet birds are a rare cause of pneumonia.

Inquire about diet and exercise.

Smoking and alcohol

A detailed smoking history is essential. You should record:

- Age started
- Age stopped (if applicable)
- Whether cigarettes, cigars, or pipe
- Average smoked per day.

It may help to convert this information into "pack years" (one pack year is 20 cigarettes smoked each day for a year).

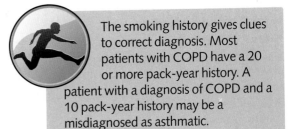

The smoking history gives clues to correct diagnosis. Most patients with COPD have a 20 or more pack-year history. A patient with a diagnosis of COPD and a 10 pack-year history may be a misdiagnosed as asthmatic.

Ask if the patient drinks alcohol. If yes, convert the weekly intake into units if possible. One glass of wine, a beer, or a mixed drink is equivalent to 1 unit. Remember that some forms of pneumonia (*S. aureus* and *Klebsiella*) occur more often in alcoholics.

Occupational causes of lung disease	
Disease	**Area of work**
asbestosis	automobile body workers, ship building, demolition
malignant mesothelioma	as above
byssinosis	textile workers
stannosis	tin mining
farmer's lung	farming (exposure to moldy hay)
coal worker's pneumoconiosis	coal mining
silicosis	mining, quarrying, foundry work, etc.
occupational asthma	see Fig. 7.14
beryllosis	electronic industries

Fig. 9.1 Occupational causes of lung disease.

Occupation

Present the patient's jobs in chronological order starting from the time the patient left school. Some respiratory conditions have a long latent period between time of exposure and presentation.

Inquire about occupational risks (e.g., asbestos exposure is linked to mesothelioma). The length of each job and the job description need to be recorded. Figure 9.1 lists some lung diseases associated with specific occupations. Hobbies may also be relevant.

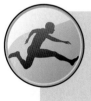

Once you have finished, check that you have not missed anything and then summarize the key points to add clarity and ease presentation.

Communication skills

The sections above outline the information you need to elicit from the patient. Being able to gather all this information in a pleasant but efficient manner is dependent on the rapport you generate with the patient and your ability to communicate.

Communication skills are now an important part of the curriculum at most medical schools and form part of clinical skills assessment exams (CSAs). These skills can take time to develop, but with practice you can improve. Rehearse some communication scenarios with friends and on the wards if you can. Watching "good" and "bad" communicators in action can also be helpful. Some of the basic techniques are discussed below.

Asthma is a favorite with examiners. Practice explaining to an imaginary patient:
- The pathologic basis of the illness (without using jargon)
- How it should be managed
- The difference between medications used to prevent asthma attacks and those used to treat attacks
- How to use an inhaler/peak flow meter.

Verbal skills

How we say things is as important as what we say. Be aware that the tone, pitch, and speed of your speech will have an effect on the consultation. Tailor your language to the patient's understanding and avoid jargon.

Open-ended questions

Effective consultations often begin with an open-ended question, i.e., one that encourages the patient to give a spontaneous account. Allow the patient to speak for a minute or two without interruption before picking up on aspects of their narrative. Open-ended questions can also help to gather information when a new subject is introduced. Examples include:
- What made you come to the hospital today?
- Tell me how your breathing has been.
- Tell me more about the chest pain.

Closed-ended questions

These ask for specific information and can fill in any gaps in the history. Questions such as "Does the pain get worse when you breathe in?" focus the narrative and speed it up. Closed-ended questions can be a useful prompt when patients are reluctant to give specific facts (e.g., how much they are smoking).

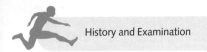

Supplying an answer of "About 2 packs a day?" may elicit a gasp followed by a reasonably truthful answer.

Responses

Your response to the narrative can encourage the patient and confirm your understanding. The appropriate response may:

- Demonstrate empathy and build trust: "That must have been very frightening."
- Show you are actively listening: "Yes, go on ..."
- Pick up on cues from the patient: "You mentioned that your breathing was worse at night."
- Clarify: "What did you mean by ...?"

Nonverbal skills

A large proportion of our communication is nonverbal. Be aware of your own posture, facial expressions, and gestures, and be alert to those of the patient—they may give you clues to their concerns. You should also ensure that you:

- Position yourself so that you face the patient and there is a comfortable distance between you. Sit beside the desk rather than across it.
- Maintain good eye contact, even if the patient doesn't.
- Use nonverbal cues to demonstrate you are listening (e.g., smiling, nodding).
- Try to minimize any irritating habits you may have—other people may be able to point these out to you!

Obstacles to communication

Many factors can provide a barrier to effective communication. The following may help to minimize them.

- Use a quiet exam room or cubicle with reasonable privacy.
- If the patient is in pain, determine whether he or she needs analgesia before the history.
- Be patient and persistent if the history is hindered by a patient's symptoms (e.g., breathlessness).
- Try to minimize language and cultural barriers by having an interpreter or family member present.

Framework for the consultation

A mental checklist can be useful. Examiners will be looking for a "patient-centered" approach; you should explore the patient's ideas, concerns, and expectations and demonstrate an intention to involve them in decisions about their treatment. One such framework is:

- Introduce yourself and explain what you would like to do.
- Find out why the patient has presented to you.
- Establish how much the patient knows about their problem
- What does the patient expect from the consultation?
- Take a history and perform a physical examination.
- Explain your diagnosis clearly.
- Check that the patient understands.
- Ask the patient if he or she has any questions.
- Literature—provide leaflets or written notes to the patient.
- Follow-up. Clarify what the next step is (e.g., appointment for bronchoscopy).

The last four points can be remembered as **CALF**:
- **C**heck that the patient understands.
- **A**sk the patient if he or she has any questions.
- **L**iterature: provide leaflets or written notes to the patient.
- **F**ollow-up. Clarify what the next step is.

Gain some extra marks during clinical skills assessment by running through these at the end.

Physical examination

Overview

As with any examination, it is important that you:

- Introduce yourself if you have not already done so
- Wash your hands before you begin and when you finish the examination
- Explain to the patient what you propose to do and ask if this is acceptable.

The structure of the examination is inspection, palpation, percussion, and auscultation. For a respiratory examination, patients should be fully exposed to the waist, comfortable, and sitting at 45°, with their hands by their sides.

In clinical examinations, purposefully walk to the end of the bed to observe the patient; this emphasizes that you are observing the patient and also gives you thinking time. Give a running commentary of what you are doing. This needs practice as you will be nervous.

General inspection

The initial observation is vital. If you have not already done so as part of the history, stand at the end of the bed and look for sputum cups, inhalers, and charts. Note any IV stands that are present, intravenous lines, or bandages.

Stand back and note the patient's general appearance. Is the patient:

- Obviously unwell or distressed?
- Alert or confused?
- Thin or overweight?

There are some signs (e.g., use of accessory muscles of inspiration or pallor) that you may notice immediately. Does the patient have a cough and, if so, does it sound productive? Is there any abnormality (e.g., hoarseness) in the voice?

Then run through a systematic general inspection. You should look generally at muscle bulk, noting any cachexia (Fig. 9.2,) and then inspect the skin in detail (Fig. 9.3). You may want to inspect the thorax at this point too; these aspects are discussed below.

It is essential that you look closely at how the patient is breathing. In addition to respiratory rate (Fig. 9.4), which is easier to test with the pulse, you should note:

- Signs of dyspnea (e.g., use of accessory muscles of inspiration such as the sternomastoids, patient "fixing" upper body by leaning forward, mouth breathing, nasal flaring)
- Unusual patterns of breathing (Fig. 9.5)
- Any noises you can hear without a stethoscope (e.g., wheeze or stridor).

Hands and limbs
Examination of the hands

The hands can reveal key signs of respiratory disease. Take both the patient's hands and note their temperature. Abnormally warm and cyanosed hands

Cachexia		
Test performed	Signs observed	Differential diagnosis
observe muscle bulk and general condition of the skin	generalized muscle wasting and lack of nutrition; pallor; dry and wrinkled skin	malignant disease bronchial carcinoma chronic disease renal disease hepatic disease cardiac failure tuberculosis other anorexia nervoso malnutrition emotional disturbance

Fig. 9.2 Tests, signs, and differential diagnosis in cachexia.

Inspection of skin		
Test performed	Signs observed	Differential diagnosis
observe the general state of the skin	steroidal skin: shiny excessive bruising thin	prolonged use of corticosteroids: chronic obstructive pulmonary disease asthma fibrosing alveolitis systemic disease (e.g. Crohn's disease)
	generalized dryness and scaling of skin	ichthyosis vulgaris acquired ichthyosis hypothyroidism sarcoidosis
	thin skin	aging Cushing's syndrome topical or systemic steroid use
observe the color of the skin	pale skin	pallor anemia leukemia shock
	light brown colored spots on skin	café-au-lait spots neurofibromatosis tuberous sclerosis

Fig. 9.3 Tests, signs, and differential diagnosis when inspecting the skin.

are a sign of CO_2 retention. Check the fingers for nicotine staining. One important sign of respiratory disease is finger clubbing (Figs 9.6 and 9.7). This is a painless, bulbous enlargement of the distal fingers; it is accompanied by softening of the nail bed and loss of nail bed angle.

Also assess for:
- Muscle wasting (Fig. 9.8)
- Rheumatoid hands (Fig. 9.9)

- Hypertrophic pulmonary osteoarthropathy (HPOA) (Fig. 9.10)
- Hand tremor (Fig. 9.11).

Know the causes of clubbing before any clinical examination. Note that chronic bronchitis does not cause clubbing.

Abnormal ventilation rate		
Test performed	Signs observed	Differential diagnosis
count the respiratory rate while feeling the patient's pulse	12–20 breaths per minute	normal
	>25 breaths per minute (tachypnea)	anxiety pain infection pneumothorax pulmonary embolism
	<12 breaths per minute (bradypnea)	hypothyroidism increased intracranial pressure

Fig. 9.4 Tests, signs, and differential diagnosis when checking the breathing rate.

Abnormal patterns of breathing	
Signs observed	Differential diagnosis
hyperventilation with deep sighing respirations (Kussmaul's respiration)	diabetic ketoacidosis aspirin overdose acute massive pulmonary embolism
increased rate and volume of respiration followed by periods of apnea (Cheyne–Stokes respiration)	terminal disease increased intracranial pressure
prolongation of expiration	airflow limitation
pursed lip breathing	air trapping

Fig. 9.5 Unusual patterns of breathing.

Clubbing		
Test performed	Sign observed	Differential diagnosis

view the nail from the side at eye level; rock the nail from side to side on the nail-bed; look at the nail-bed and nail angle.
 	
place nails back to back; a diamond-shaped area is evident between them if clubbing does not exist.
	increase in the soft tissues of the nail-bed and fingertip, with increased sponginess of the nail-bed
	
	loss of angle between nail and nail-bed
	
	transverse curvature of nail increases
	
	in final stages, whole tip of the finger becomes clubbed
	
	clubbing may also affect the toes
	
	bones are normal
		pulmonary causes:
		  tumor (bronchial carcinoma, mesothelioma)
		  chronic pulmonary sepsis (empyema, lung abscess, bronchiectasis, cystic fibrosis)
		  fibrosing alveolitis asbestosis hypertrophic pulmonary osteoarthropathy
		
		cardiac causes:
		  congenital bacterial endocarditis
		
		other causes:
		  idiopathic causes
		  cirrhosis
		  inflammatory bowel disease

Fig. 9.6 Tests, signs, and differential diagnosis in clubbing.

Examination of the pulse

A normal resting pulse in an adult is between 60–100 bpm. Bradycardia is defined as a pulse rate of less than 60 bpm, and tachycardia is defined as a pulse rate of greater than 100 bpm. Palpate the radial pulse, wait for a moment, and then count for 15 seconds. You can then multiply by four to give a rate per minute. Is the pulse regular? If not, how is it irregular (Fig. 9.12)?

In addition to testing pulse volume and character, which are better assessed from the carotid pulse, you

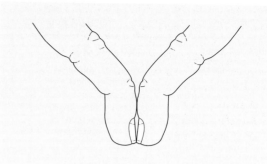

Fig. 9.7 Inspecting for clubbing. Normal fingers: note diamond-shaped area.

Muscle wasting		
Test performed	**Sign observed**	**Differential diagnosis**

look at the dorsal aspect of the hand for any reduction in muscle bulk
 	
always compare both hands together
	muscle wasting: note the distribution and if it is unilateral or bilateral	localized:
		  unilateral
		   —Pancoast's tumor
		  bilateral
		   —disuse atrophy: rheumatoid arthritis
		
		generalized:
		  diabetes
		  thyrotoxicosis
		  anorexia nervosa

Fig. 9.8 Tests, signs, and differential diagnosis in muscle wasting.

Rheumatoid hands		
Test performed	**Sign observed**	**Differential diagnosis**

look at the hands for signs of rheumatoid disease	ulnar deviation of fingers swan-neck or boutonniere deformity Z-deformity of thumb subluxation of proximal phalanx wasting of small muscles	rheumatoid disease, which may affect the lung:
		  pulmonary nodules
		  pleural effusion

Fig. 9.9 Tests, signs, and differential diagnosis in rheumatoid hands.

Hypertrophic pulmonary osteoarthropathy		
Test performed	**Sign observed**	**Differential diagnosis**

apply pressure to the wrist	tenderness on palpation of the wrist; the pain is over the shafts of the long bones adjacent to the joint
	
	arthralgia and joint swelling
		hypertrophic pulmonary osteoarthropathy, a nonmetastatic complication of malignancy—subperiosteal new-bone formation in the long bones of the lower limbs and forearms; clubbing is also present—90% of cases are associated with bronchogenic carcinoma, especially squamous cell carcinoma
		
		other causes:
		  rheumatoid arthritis
		  systemic sclerosis

Fig. 9.10 Tests, signs, and differential diagnosis in hypertrophic pulmonary osteoarthropathy.

187

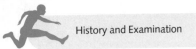

Hand tremor		
Test performed	**Sign observed**	**Differential diagnosis**
ask patient to hold fingers outstretched and spread in front; place a piece of paper on the dorsal aspect of the hands; observe hands at eye level from the side	very fine finger tremor on outstretched fingers; finger tremor is made more obvious by placing a piece of paper on top of the hands	• stimulation of β-receptors by bronchodilator drugs especially nebulized drugs. • thyrotoxicosis
ask patient to hold arm outstretched in front; fully extend the wrists; apply pressure to hands; leave patient like this for 30 seconds	flapping tremor (asterixis) against your hands, which is coarse and irregular in nature; maximum activity at wrist and metacarpophalangeal joints	CO_2 retention hepatic failure encephalopathy metabolic diseases subdural hematoma

Fig. 9.11 Tests, signs, and differential diagnosis in hand tremor.

Abnormal radial pulse	
Sign observed	**Differential diagnosis**
rate <100 beats per minute	normal
rate >100 beats per minute (tachycardia)	pain shock infection thyrotoxicosis sarcoidosis pulmonary embolism drugs, e.g. salbutamol iatrogenic causes
full, exaggerated arterial pulsation (bounding pulse)	CO_2 retention thyrotoxicosis fever anemia hyperkinetic states

Fig. 9.12 Tests, signs, and differential diagnosis when testing the radial pulse.

You will gain points if your examination looks fluent and professional. It is easy to move smoothly from introducing yourself and shaking the patient's hand to examination of the hands to testing the radial pulse. Then you can discreetly test for respiratory rate without the patient realizing and altering his or her breathing.

Examination of the limbs
Examine the axillary lymph nodes as shown in Fig. 9.14. Check the patient's ankles for edema by applying pressure with fingers and thumb for a few seconds. If there is subcutaneous fluid, you may see pitting. Bilateral pitting edema is seen in many conditions, including congestive heart failure, liver failure, and cor pulmonale.

Head and neck
Examination of the face
First, observe the face generally. You may notice:
• Signs of superior vena cava obstruction (Fig. 9.15)
• Cushingoid features (Fig. 9.15).

Look at the mouth for signs of:
• Candida infection—white coating on tongue often seen after steroids or antibiotics
• Central cyanosis (Fig. 9.16).

should also check for the presence of pulsus paradoxus. In normal individuals the pulse decreases slightly in volume on inspiration and systolic blood pressure falls by 3–5mmHg. In severe obstructive diseases (e.g., severe asthma) the contractile force of respiratory muscles is so great that there is a marked fall in systolic pressure on inspiration. A fall of greater than 10mmHg is pathologic. Figure 9.13 shows how to test for this sign.

Fig. 9.13 Tests, signs, and differential diagnosis in pulsus paradoxus.

Pulsus paradoxus		
Test performed	**Sign observed**	**Differential diagnosis**

measure blood pressure using a sphygmomanometer: cuff pressure is reduced and systolic sound is heard; this initially occurs only in expiration; with further reduction of cuff pressure you can hear systole in inspiration as well; the pressure difference between the initial systolic sound in expiration and when it is present throughout the breathing cycle is what is measured	pulse volume decreases with inspiration, the reverse of normal
	
	large fall in systolic blood pressure during inspiration
		severe asthma
		
		other causes:
		  cardiac tamponade
		  massive pulmonary embolism
		
		fall is exaggerated when venous return to the right heart is impaired

Enlarged axillary lymph nodes		
Test performed	**Sign observed**	**Differential diagnosis**
Method 1: face the patient; place the patient's right arm on your right arm; patient's arm must be relaxed; palpate axilla with left hand; place the patient's left arm on your left arm; palpate left axilla	enlarged lymph node (axillary lymphadenopathy)	localized spread of viral or bacterial infection tuberculosis human immunodeficiency virus (HIV) infection actinomycosis cytomegalovirus (CMV) infection measles
Method 2: ask the patient to place hands behind head; palpate axilla by placing your fingers high up in axilla; press tips of fingers against chest wall; move fingers down over ribs		axial lymphadenopathy is often present in breast carcinoma

Fig. 9.14 Tests, signs, and differential diagnosis when examining the axillary lymph nodes.

Then examine the eyes (Figs 9.17 and 9.18) and test for anemia (Fig. 9.19).

Remember that an anemic patient may be dangerously desaturated without appearing cyanotic.

Examination of the neck

Examine tracheal position and measure the cricosternal distance (Figs 9.20 and 9.21). Then make sure the patient is at 45° and test the jugular venous pulse (Figs 9.22 and 9.23). Finally, test for cervical lymphadenopathy from behind (Figs 9.24 and 9.25).

Develop a set system of palpating the lymph nodes of the neck (as mentioned above). Sit the patient up and examine from behind with both hands.

Before a clinical examination, learn the lymph nodes of the neck and into which set of nodes different structures drain.

Observation of the face

Test performed	Sign observed	Differential diagnosis
observe the patient's face	edema cyanosis puffy eyes fixed, engorged neck veins	superior vena cava obstruction: bronchial carcinoma lymphoma mediastinal goitre fibrosis
	features associated with Cushing's syndrome: moon face plethora acne hirsute oral candidiasis	long-term administration of steroids ACTH secretion by small-cell bronchial carcinoma

Fig. 9.15 Tests, signs, and differential diagnosis when observing the face.

Examination of the eyes

Test performed	Sign observed	Differential diagnosis
Look at the eyes, noting the position of the eyelid and pupil size; always compare with the other side.

If an abnormality is present, check that the pupils are reactive to light | Drooping of upper eyelids so that upper part of iris and pupil are covered (ptosis) | Third nerve palsy (with dilated pupil). Horner's syndrome (with small reactive pupil): involvement of the sympathetic chain on the posterior chest wall by an apical bronchial carcinoma; T1 wasting and sensory loss also occur. Idiopathic (usually in young females). Myasthenia gravis (with bilateral ptosis) Dystrophia. Mitochondrial disease (rare) |
| | Small pupil | Old age. Horner's syndrome. Argyll Robertson's pupil: miotic and responsive to accommodation effort, but not to light. Disease in pons. Cerebrovascular accident. Drugs (e.g. opiates) |

Fig. 9.17 Tests, signs, and differential diagnosis when examining the eyes.

Central cyanosis

Test performed	Sign observed	Differential diagnosis
good natural light is needed

ask the patient to stick tongue out

look at the mucous membranes of the lips and tongue | blue discoloration to skin and mucous membrane

central cyanosis cannot be accurately identified in African American and Asian patients | level of deoxygenated hemoglobin >5 g/dl diseases caused by marked ventilation-perfusion mismatch will cause central cyanosis: severe pulmonary fibrosis chronic bronchitis right-left heart shunts pneumonia respiratory failure bronchiectasis chronic obstructive pulmonary disease |

Fig. 9.16 Tests, signs, and differential diagnosis in central cyanosis.

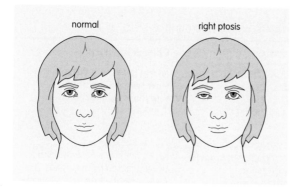

normal   right ptosis

Fig. 9.18 Typical appearance of a patient with ptosis.

Anemia		
Test performed	**Sign observed**	**Differential diagnosis**
ask patient to look up, then evert lower lid of eye note the color of mucous membrane	pale mucous membrane	indication of anemia; however, anemia can only be conclusively diagnosed by measuring hemoglobin levels

Fig. 9.19 Tests, signs, and differential diagnosis in anemia.

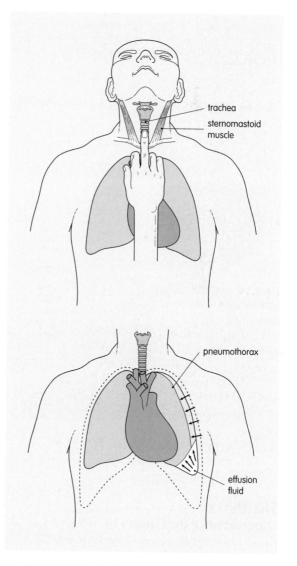

Fig. 9.21 Palpation to determine tracheal position.

Tracheal position and cricosternal distance		
Test performed	**Sign observed**	**Differential diagnosis**
stand at the front of the patient; pressing gently, place one finger on the trachea judge if the finger slides to one side (tracheal deviation gives an indication of the position of the upper mediastinum; however, the only conclusive method of judging the position is chest radiography)	deviation of the trachea away from the midline	pulled to side of collapse pushed away from mass or fluid contralateral side to tension pneumothorax
measure the distance (in finger breadths) between the sternal notch and cricoid cartilage during a full inspiration	three or four finger breadths	normal
	reduced distance	air flow limitation

Fig. 9.20 Tests, signs, and differential diagnosis when checking the trachea.

Jugular venous pressure		
Test performed	**Sign observed**	**Differential diagnosis**
patient must be at 45° looking straight ahead; good light is needed; ask patient to rest head comfortably against a pillow, neck slightly flexed; the patient's neck must be relaxed, as it is impossible to assess jugular venous pressure if the sternomastoid muscles are tensed	elevated jugular venous pressure	resting pressure in thorax is raised: • tension pneumothorax • severe hyperinflation in asthma
a normal jugular pulse becomes visible just above the clavicle between the two heads of sternocleidomastoid; jugular venous pressure is difficult to assess and needs much practice; if the jugular pulse is not seen, try the hepatojugular reflex: apply pressure to the liver, increasing venous return to the heart, and so increasing the jugular venous pressure	elevated nonpulsatile jugular venous pressure	superior vena cave obstruction, usually caused by malignant enlargement of the right bronchus
	elevated pulsatile jugular venous pressure	paratracheal lymph nodes cor pulmonale
time against the contralateral pulse and measure the height of the pulse above the heart (giving a measure of pressure); the normal height of the pulse above the atrium is <4 cm	depressed jugular venous pressure	shock dehydration severe infection

Fig. 9.22 Tests, signs, and differential diagnosis when checking the jugular venous pulse.

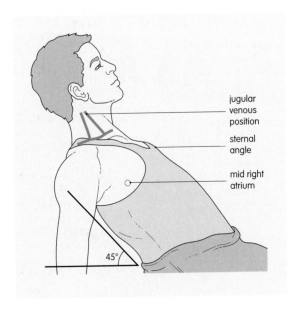

jugular venous position

sternal angle

mid right atrium

45°

Fig. 9.23 Measurement of the height of the jugular venous pulse.

The thorax
Observation of the thorax

As already noted, it is often easier to inspect the thorax as part of your general inspection. In addition to observing chest wall movement, you should note any lesions, thoracic scars (Fig. 9.26), or radiotherapy tattoos (small green or blue dots used as guidance for radiotherapy). Then observe the shape of the thorax from the front, side, and back and look at the curvature of the spine. Chest deformities may be

Fig. 9.24 Tests, signs, and differential diagnosis in cervical lymphadenopathy.

Cervical lymphadenopathy		
Test performed	**Sign observed**	**Differential diagnosis**
examine the cervical chain of lymph nodes from behind the patient; it helps if the neck is slightly flexed; most patients extend neck to try and help you know the nodes which you are feeling using both hands, start at the mandibular ramus, palpate the submandibular nodes then anterior chain nodes, supraclavicular nodes, and posterior chain nodes in a Z-fashion	cervical lymphadenopathy note number of palpable nodes describe as for any lump	infection carcinoma tuberculosis sarcoidosis hard node: calcified soft, matted node: tuberculous

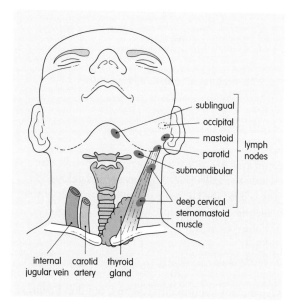

Fig. 9.25 Anatomy of the neck, including lymph node distribution.

Thoracic scars		
Test performed	**Sign observed**	**Differential diagnosis**
look at the thorax for any obvious scars, remembering to look at the front and back of the chest, axilla, and under the breasts	scars present from previous operations	median sternotomy (most open-heart surgery; cardiopulmonary bypass) posteriolateral thoracotomy (ligation of posterior descending artery; lung and esophageal resections) lateral thoracotomy (pneumothorax) left thoracotomy (closed mitral valvotomy)

Fig. 9.26 Tests, signs, and differential diagnosis in thoracic scars.

asymptomatic, or they may restrict the ventilatory capacity of the lungs. Common chest abnormalities and their clinical significance are shown in Figs 9.27 and 9.28.

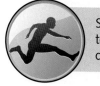

Scoliosis and kyphosis can lead to respiratory failure caused by compressional effects.

Palpation

You should palpate any lumps or depressions you noticed on inspection and test for the symmetry and extent of chest expansion (Fig. 9.29). Chest expansion is tested from the posterior.

193

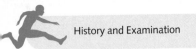

Assessing the chest wall and spine		
Test performed	**Sign observed**	**Differential diagnosis**
look at the sternum and its relationship to the ribs	depressed in pectus excavatum (funnel chest)	benign condition requiring no treatment. On chest radiograph, the heart may be displaced and appear enlarged
	prominent in pectus carinatum (pigeon chest)	may be secondary to severe childhood asthma
observe the patient from the side; ask patient to fold arms and take a deep inspiration	anteroposterior diameter of chest > lateral diameter (barrel chest)	hyperinflation asthma
ask the patient to stand; stand directly behind the patient and look at the curvature of the spine	increased lateral curvature of the spine (scoliosis)	structural abnormality developmental abnormality vertebral disc prolapse
next, stand at the side of the patient and again look at the curvature of the spine	increased forward curvature of the spine (kyphosis)	osteoporosis ankylosing spondylitis

Fig. 9.27 Tests, signs, and differential diagnosis in chest wall abnormalities.

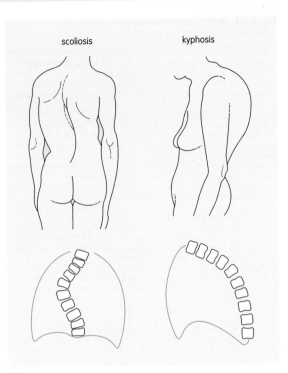

Fig. 9.28 Features of scoliosis and kyphosis.

Test for the position of the apical beat by moving your hand inward from the lateral chest until you feel the pulsation. The apical beat should be in the fifth intercostal space at the midclavicular line. The clinical significance of deviations is shown in Fig. 9.30.

Test for tactile vocal fremitus as shown in Fig. 9.31.

Percussion

The percussion note tells us the consistency of the matter underlying the chest wall, i.e., whether it is air, fluid, or solid. The correct method of percussion is shown in Fig. 9.32. Percuss in a logical order,

comparing one side with other and remember to include the axilla (Fig. 9.33). A normal percussion note is described as resonant. In lung pathology (Fig. 9.34) the percussion note may be:

- Hyperresonant
- Dull
- Stony dull.

Map out any abnormality you find, but don't confuse the cardiac borders or liver edge with lung pathology; they will sound dull normally. The note also sounds muffled in a very muscular or obese patient.

When percussing, remember that the upper lobe predominates anteriorly and the lower lobe predominates posteriorly.

Fig. 9.29 Tests, signs, and differential diagnosis in chest expansion.

Chest expansion		
Test performed	**Sign observed**	**Differential diagnosis**
place the flat of both hands on the pectoral region of the chest; ask the patient to take a deep breath, and note any asymmetry	symmetrical rise of hands as chest expands	normal
	asymmetrical rise	unilateral pathology on the depressed side
put fingers of both hands as far around the chest as possible; bring thumbs together in the midline; keep thumbs off chest wall; ask patient to take a deep breath in; note distance between thumbs; examine both front and back	—	—
place a tape measure around the chest at the nipple line and measure the difference between inspiration and expiration	>4 cm expansion	normal
	<4 cm expansion	reduced expansion

Apical beat	
Sign observed	**Differential diagnosis**
pulsation in fifth intercostal space midclavicular line	normal
deviated pulsation; lower mediastinum displacement	left deviation: cardiomegaly pulmonary fibrosis scoliosis pectus excavatum bronchiectasis
	right deviation: pneumothorax pleural effusion dextracardia

Fig. 9.30 Signs and differential diagnosis in examination of the apical beat.

Tactile vocal fremitus		
Test performed	**Sign observed**	**Differential diagnosis**
place either the ulnar edge or the flat of your hand on the chest wall; ask the patient to repeatedly say '99' or '1, 2, 3'; repeat for front and back, comparing opposite zones the vibrations produced by the maneuver are transmitted through the lung substance and felt by the hand; alterations in disease are the same as for vocal resonance	increased resonance	solid areas of lung with open airways consolidation pneumonia tuberculosis extensive fibrosis
	decreased resonance	feeble voice pleural thickening blocked bronchus

Fig. 9.31 Tests, signs, and differential diagnosis in tactile vocal fremitus.

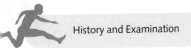
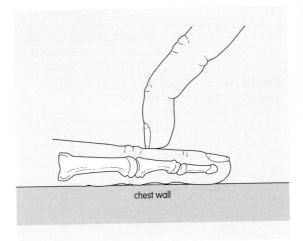

Fig. 9.32 Correct method of percussion (see text for explanation).

Auscultation

Normal breath sounds have a rustling quality heard in inspiration and the first part of expiration. Listen to the patient's chest:

- Using the bell of the stethoscope
- In a logical order, comparing the two sides (as for percussion)
- With the patient taking fairly quick breaths through an open mouth.

You should listen for:

- Diminished breaths (Fig. 9.35)
- Bronchial breathing (Fig. 9.35)
- Added sounds, such as wheezes or stridor (Fig. 9.36), crackles (Fig. 9.37), or pleural rub (Fig. 9.38).

With auscultation always think **BAR** (**B** = Breath sounds; **A** = Added sounds; **R** = vocal **R**esonance]. Added sounds that disappear when the patient coughs are not significant.

Vocal resonance

The tests for vocal resonance and whispering pectoriloquy are shown in Figs 9.39 and 9.40.

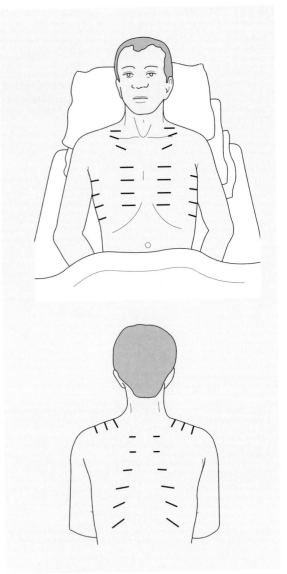

Fig. 9.33 Sites for percussion. (From *Macleod's Clinical Examination*, 10th ed. Edited by J.F. Munro, I.W. Campbell. New York, Churchill Livingstone, 2000, p. 135.)

Summary

Once you have finished your examination, sum up the positive findings in a clear and concise manner. Figure 9.41 shows some possible findings on examination for a patient with COPD. Figure 9.42 is a summary of the signs found on examination of the respiratory system as a whole.

Percussion		
Test performed	**Sign observed**	**Differential diagnosis**
place your nondominant hand on the chest wall, palm downwards, with fingers slightly separated; the second phalanx of the middle finger should be in an intercostal space directly over the area to be percussed; strike this finger with the terminal phalanx of the middle finger of the other hand	increased resonance (resonance depends on the thickness of the chest wall and the amount of air in the structures underlying it)	increased air in lung: • emphysema • large bullae • pneumothoraces • asthma
to achieve a good percussion note, the striking finger should be partially flexed and struck at right angles to the other finger; the striking movement must be a flick of the wrist on percussion you will hear a percussion note and feel vibrations percuss from top to bottom including axilla; to check for disease in the lung apices, percuss directly onto the clavicles; do not percuss more heavily than you need and always compare both sides, front and back	dullness (solid lung tissue does not reflect sound as readily as aerated lung); if a dull area exists, map out its limits by percussing from the resonant to the dull area	consolidation: • fibrosis • collapse • pleural thickening • tuberculosis • extensive carcinoma
dullness occurs as you percuss over the liver; note that the right diaphragm is higher than the left diaphragm	stony dullness	fluid present: • pleural effusion

Fig. 9.34 Tests, signs, and differential diagnosis when doing percussion of the thorax.

Auscultation of the thorax	
Sign observed	**Differential diagnosis**
vesicular breath sounds	breath sounds are produced in the larger airways where flow is turbulent; sounds are transmitted through smaller airways to the chest wall; vesicular breath sounds are normal
	if vesicular breath sounds are reduced or absent: • airway obstruction • asthma • chronic obstructive pulmonary disease • tumor
bronchial breath sounds (described in relation to timing; a gap exists between inspiration and expiration, which are of equal duration; harsh clear breath sounds)	normal, if heard at the tip of the scapula; otherwise caused by: • consolidation • pneumonia • lung abscess
	if inaudible: • severe emphysema • bullae • pneumothorax • pleural effusion

Fig. 9.35 Tests, signs, and differential diagnosis in auscultation of the thorax.

Wheeze and stridor	
Sign observed	**Differential diagnosis**
prolonged musical sound	none: the amount of wheeze is not a good indicator of the degree of airway obstruction
polyphonic sound (many musical notes), mainly in expiration	small airway obstruction: narrowing caused by combination of smooth muscle contraction; inflammation within airways; increased bronchial secretions
monophonic sound	large airway obstruction: a worrying finding, suggesting a single narrowing (e.g. tumor)
loud inspiratory sound	large airway narrowing (larynx, trachea, main bronchi): • laryngotracheobronchitis • epiglottitis • laryngitis

Fig. 9.36 Signs and differential diagnosis in stridor and wheeze.

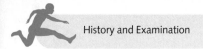

Fig. 9.37 Tests, signs, and differential diagnosis in crackles.

Crackles		
Test performed	**Sign observed**	**Differential diagnosis**
listen to the patient breathing crackles may be mimicked by rolling hair on your temple between two fingers; timing during the respiratory cycle is of huge significance	nonmusical, short, uninterrupted sounds heard during inspiration	crackles represent equalization of intraluminal pressure as collapsed small airways open during inspiration
	early inspiratory crackles	diffuse airflow limitation chronic obstructive pulmonary disease pulmonary edema
	late inspiratory crackles	conditions that largely involve alveoli: • fibrosis • fibrosing alveolitis • bronchiectasis

Pleural rub		
Test performed	**Sign observed**	**Differential diagnosis**
listen to the patient breathing	leathery creaking sound associated with each breath inspiratory and expiratory sound that is not shifted by cough; reoccurs at the same time in each respiratory cycle	caused by inflamed surfaces of pleura rubbing together: • pneumonia • pulmonary embolism • emphysema • pleurisy

Fig. 9.38 Tests, signs, and differential diagnosis in pleural rub.

Whispering pectoriloquy		
Test performed	**Sign observed**	**Differential diagnosis**
place the stethoscope on to the chest and ask the patient to repeatedly whisper '99' or '1, 2, 3'	words are clear and seem to be spoken right into the listener's ears (whispering pectoriloquy)	whispered speech cannot usually be heard over healthy lung; solid lung tissue conducts sound better than normally aerated lung, indicating consolidation, cavitation, tuberculosis, or pneumonia

Fig. 9.40 Tests, signs, and differential diagnosis in whispering pectoriloquy.

Vocal resonance		
Test performed	**Sign observed**	**Differential diagnosis**
auscultatory equivalent to vocal fremitus; place the stethoscope on to the chest and ask the patient to repeatedly say '99' or '1, 2, 3'	normal lung attenuates high-frequency notes; normally, booming low-pitched sounds are heard	as for vocal fremitus

Fig. 9.39 Tests, signs, and differential diagnosis in vocal resonance.

Signs of COPD	
on inspection	central cyanosis
	barrel chest
	use of accessory muscles
	intercostal indrawing
	pursed-lip breathing
	flapping tremor
	tachypnea
on palpation	tachycardia
	tracheal tug
	reduced expansion
on percussion	hyperresonant lung fields
on auscultation	wheeze
	prolongation of expiration

Fig. 9.41 Signs found on examination of a patient with COPD.

Signs found on examination of the respiratory system

	Consolidation	Pneumothorax	Pleural effusion	Lobar collapse	Pleural thickening
Chest radiograph	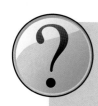				
Mediastinal shift	none	none (simple), away (tension)	none or away	towards	none
Chest wall excursion	normal or decreased	normal or decreased	decreased	decreased	decreased
Percussion note	normal or decreased	increased	decreased (stony)	decreased	decreased
Breath sounds	increased (bronchial)	decreased	decreased	decreased	decreased
Added sounds	crackles	click (occasional)	rub (occasional)	none	none
Tactile vocal fremitus or vocal resonance	increased	decreased	decreased	decreased	decreased

Fig. 9.42 Summary table of signs found on examination of the respiratory system.

- Why is the family and social history so important in respiratory medicine?
- What features of a patient's past medical history might be relevant?
- Give an example of an open-ended and a closed-ended question. How is each type used?
- Give a brief framework for a consultation.
- Why is the initial observation of the patient important?
- Describe the visible effects of long-term steroid use.
- List the causes of tachypnea.
- List the different patterns of breathing and their significance.
- Describe the common causes of clubbing and how to look for clubbing.
- Describe the significance of unilateral muscle wasting of the hand.
- Describe the relevance of tracheal position in tension pneumothorax.
- Name the common scars seen on the thorax and the possible operations that the patient may have undergone.
- List the surface markings of the lungs for percussion.
- Describe the relationship between added sounds and disease.
- How does lung disease alter examination findings?

10. Tests and Imaging

Introduction

There are a large number of tests in respiratory medicine, ranging from basic bedside tests to more invasive procedures such as bronchoscopy. As you read this chapter, you should bear in mind that some of the investigations below are performed only rarely in specialized pulmonary laboratories while others are performed by patients at home every day. You should have a thorough knowledge of the tests that are most commonly performed, including:

- Arterial blood gas analysis
- Sputum examination
- Pulmonary function tests
- Bronchoscopy
- Chest x-rays.

Routine tests

Hematology

In the associated figures, you will find some of the commonly performed hematologic tests:

- Complete blood count (Fig. 10.1)
- White blood cell count with differential (Fig. 10.2)
- Other hematologic tests (Fig. 10.3).

Clinical chemistry

The commonly performed biochemical tests are shown in Fig. 10.4.

If malignancy is suspected, you should also perform liver function tests and test alkaline phosphatase as an indicator of metastases. In addition, endocrine tests should be performed for paraneoplastic manifestations.

Tests of blood gases
Arterial blood gas analysis

Blood gas analysis of an arterial blood sample is mandatory in all acute pulmonary conditions. The analysis should always be repeated soon after starting oxygen therapy to assess response to treatment.

A heparinized sample of arterial blood is tested using a standard automated machine, which measures:

- P_aO_2
- P_aCO_2
- Oxygen saturation.

Blood pH, standard bicarbonate and base excess are either given on the standard readout or can be calculated.

The patient's results are compared with the normal ranges (Fig. 10.5) and assessed in two parts:

- Degree of arterial oxygenation—is the patient hypoxic?
- Acid–base balance disturbances.

Before accurate interpretation of the results, a detailed history of the patient, including a detailed drug history, is needed.

Pulse oximetry

This is a simple, noninvasive method of monitoring the percentage of hemoglobin that is saturated with oxygen. The patient wears a probe on their finger or ear lobe, and this is linked to a unit which displays the readings. The unit can be set to sound an alarm when saturation drops below a certain level (usually 90%). The pulse oximeter works by calculating the absorption of light by hemoglobin, which alters depending on whether it is saturated or desaturated with oxygen. A number of factors may lead to inaccurate oximeter readings. These include:

- Poor peripheral perfusion
- Carbon monoxide poisoning
- Skin pigmentation
- Nail varnish
- Dirty hands.

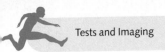

Complete blood count			
		diagnostic inference	
test	**normal values**	**increased values**	**decreased values**
hemoglobin (g/dl)	male: 12–18 female: 12–16	may indicate polycythemia (see below under red blood cells)	decreased in anemia (look at MCV for further information); a normal MCV (i.e., normocytic anemia) is common in chronic disease
mean corpuscular volume (fl)	80–100	macrocytosis (e.g., B12 or folate deficiency)	microcytosis (common in iron deficiency anemia and thalassemia)
red blood cells (10^9/ml)	male: 4.6–6.2 female: 4.2–5.4	polycythemia, may be secondary to chronic lung disease, smoking, altitude	anemia

Fig. 10.1 Tests performed and diagnostic inference for complete blood count. Normal values may vary between laboratories.

Differential white blood cell count			
		Diagnostic inference	
Cell type	**Normal values**	**Increased values**	**Decreased values**
white blood cell	4000–10 000/µl	bacterial infections malignancy pregnancy	viral infections drugs systemic lupus erythematosus overwhelming bacterial infection
neutrophil	47–77%	bacterial infections malignancy pregnancy steroid therapy	viral infections drugs systemic lupus erythematosus overwhelming bacterial infection
eosinophil	0.3–7%	allergic reactions asthma sarcoidosis pneumonia eosinophilic granulomatosus	steroid therapy
monocyte	0.5–10%	tuberculosis	chronic infection
lymphocyte	16–43%	infection cytomegalovirus infection toxoplasmosis tuberculosis	tuberculosis

Fig. 10.2 Tests performed and diagnostic inference for differential white blood cell count. Normal values may vary between laboratories.

Microbiology

Microbiologic examination is possible with samples of sputum, bronchial aspirate, pleural aspirate, throat swabs, and blood. The aim of examination is to identify bacteria, viruses, or fungi.

Tests to request are microscopy, culture, and drug sensitivity. The microbiologic findings should be interpreted in view of the whole clinical picture.

Bacteriology
Sputum

Testing of sputum for the presence of bacteria is the most common microbiologic test performed in

Other hematological tests

Test performed	Normal values	Diagnostic inference	
		Increased values	Decreased values
C-reactive protein (CRP)	Normal <4 mg/L Changes more rapidly than erythrocyte sedimentation rate	Acute infection; inflammation; same as erythrocyte sedimentation rate	Levels often normal in malignancy
Anti-streptolysin O (ASO) titer	Normal <200 IU/mL	Confirms recent streptococcal infection	

Fig. 10.3 Other hematologic tests and their diagnostic inference. Normal values may vary between laboratories.

Biochemical blood tests

Test performed	Normal values	Diagnostic inference	
		Increased values	Decreased values
potassium	3.5–5.0 mmol/L		adrenocorticotropic hormone (ACTH) secreting tumor β-agonists
angiotensin converting enzyme (ACE)	8–52 U/L	sarcoidosis	
calcium	2.12–2.65 mmol/L 9–10.5 mg/dL	malignancy sarcoidosis squamous cell carcinoma of the lung	
glucose (fasting)	3.5–5.5 mmol/L less than 100 mg/dL	adrenocorticotropic hormone (ACTH) secreting tumor long-term steroid use pancreatic dysfunction diabetes	

Fig. 10.4 Biochemical tests and their diagnostic inference. Normal values may vary between laboratories.

Arterial blood gases

Test performed	Normal values	Diagnostic inference	
		Increased values	Decreased values
pH	7.35–7.45	alkalosis hyperventilation	acidosis CO_2 retention
P_aO_2	>80 mmHg		hypoxic
P_aCO_2	35–45 mmHg	respiratory acidosis (if pH decreased)	respiratory alkalosis (if pH increased)
base excess	±2 mmol/L	metabolic alkalosis	metabolic acidosis
standardized bicarbonate	22–25 mmol/L	metabolic alkalosis	metabolic acidosis

Fig. 10.5 Tests performed and diagnostic inference for arterial blood gases.

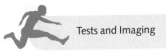
respiratory medicine. Obtain the sample, preferably of induced sputum, before antibiotic treatment is started. Collect into a sterile container, inspect the sample, and send to the laboratory.

Request Gram stain, Ziehl–Neelson stain, and anaerobic cultures. Culture on Lowenstein–Jensen medium to detect tuberculosis. A sputum sample is valuable in diagnosing suspected pneumonia, tuberculosis, and aspergillosis, or if the patient presents with an unusual clinical picture.

Failure to isolate an organism from the sputum is not uncommon.

Resistance to commonly used antibiotics is often found in bacteria responsible for respiratory tract infections; therefore, antibiotic sensitivity testing is vital.

Blood culture
A blood culture should always be performed in patients with fever and lower respiratory tract infection. Collect two or three cultures over 24 hours.

Blood cultures identify systemic bacterial and fungal infections. Results may be positive while sputum culture is negative.

Upper respiratory specimens
Microscopy is generally unhelpful because of the abundant commensals of the upper respiratory tract, which contaminate samples.

Throat specimens can be collected using Dacron or calcium alginate swab. The tonsils, posterior pharynx and any ulcerated areas are sampled. Avoid contact with tongue and saliva, as this can inhibit identification of group A streptococci.

A sinus specimen is collected with a needle and syringe. The specimen is cultured for aerobic and anaerobic bacteria. Common pathogens of sinuses are *Streptococcus pneumoniae*, *Haemophilus influenzae*, *Mycoplasma catarrhalis*, *Staphylococcus aureus*, and anaerobes.

Coxiella bunetti, *Mycoplasma pneumoniae*, and *Legionella* spp. are difficult to culture; therefore, results of serology must be used.

Lower respiratory specimens
Techniques used to collect samples include expectoration, cough induction with saline, bronchoscopy, bronchial alveolar lavage, transtracheal aspiration, and direct aspiration through the chest wall. Some of these techniques are considered below under the more invasive procedures.

Viral testing
Because of the small size of viral particles, light microscopy provides little information: it is able to visualize viral inclusions and cytopathic effects of viral infection.

Viral serology
Viral serology is the most important group of tests in virology. Serologic diagnoses are obtained when viruses are difficult to isolate and grow in cell culture.

Specimens should be collected early in the acute phase because viral shedding for respiratory viruses lasts 3–7 days; however, symptoms commonly persist for longer. A repeated sample should be collected 10 days later.

Specimens should be tested serologically only after the second sample has been received. The laboratory measures antibody type and titer in response to the viral infection: a four-fold increase in titer (rising titer) taken over 10 days is significant.

Viral serology also identifies the virus and its strain or serotype and is able to evaluate the course of infection.

Cell culture
Specimens for cell cultures are obtained from nasal washings, throat swabs, nasal swabs, and sputum. Viruses cannot be cultured without living cells.

Fungal testing
Fungal infections may be serious, especially in the immunocompromised patient, where they can cause systemic infection; invasive fungal infections require blood culture. Repeated specimens from the site need to be taken to rule out contaminants in cultures.

Common fungal infections are *Candida* and *Aspergillus* spp. Microscopic identification may be difficult for *Aspergillus* because it is common in the environment. Culture is rarely helpful in identifying *Aspergillus*; the *Aspergillus precipitans* test is of more use.

More invasive procedures

Bronchoscopy
Bronchoscopy allows the visualization of the trachea and larger bronchi and can be used to sample tissues

via brushings, lavage, or biopsy. Two types of bronchoscope are used:
- Flexible fiberoptic bronchoscope
- Rigid bronchoscope (under general anesthetic).

In practice, the flexible bronchoscope is used in most instances. Patients may be lightly sedated to reduce anxiety and suppress the cough mechanism. Topical lidocaine (lignocaine) is used to anesthetize the pharynx and vocal cords.

The main indications for bronchoscopy are:
- Diagnosis of lung cancer (e.g., after an abnormal chest x-ray or hemoptysis)
- Staging of lung cancer
- Diagnosis of diffuse lung disease
- Diagnosis of infections (especially in immunocompromised hosts).

Bronchoalveolar lavage (BAL)
Sterile saline is infused down the flexible bronchoscope and then aspirated. This technique is commonly used to look for evidence of neoplasms or opportunistic infections in immunocompromised patients.

Transbronchial biopsy
Transbronchial biopsy provides samples from outside the airways, e.g. of alveolar tissue. The technique is performed using biopsy forceps attached to a flexible bronchoscope. The bronchoscopist cannot directly visualize the biopsy site and may be assisted by fluoroscopic imaging. Complications include pneumothorax or hemorrhage.

Percutaneous fine needle aspiration
This technique is used to sample peripheral lesions under the guidance of radiography.

Open and thoracoscopic lung biopsy
In some cases of diffuse lung disease, or when a lesion cannot easily be reached, more extensive lung biopsy is required for diagnosis. Open lung biopsy is performed through a thoracotomy with the patient under general anesthesia. However, video-assisted thorascopic techniques are increasingly used as a less-invasive alternative.

Histopathology

Histopathology is the investigation and diagnosis of disease from the examination of tissues.

Histopathologic examination of biopsy material
The histopathologic examination is a vital test in cases of suspected malignancy, allowing a definitive diagnosis to be made. Biopsy material is obtained from the techniques described above, in addition to:
- Pleural biopsy
- Lymph node biopsy

Histologic features of malignant neoplasms are:
- Loss of cellular differentiation
- Abundant cells undergoing mitosis, many of which are abnormal
- High nuclear:cytoplasm ratio
- Cells or nuclei varying in shape and size.

Other uses of histopathology include diagnosing interstitial lung diseases such as cryptogenic fibrosing alveolitis.

Cytologic examination of sputum
Cytologic examination is useful in diagnosing bronchial carcinoma and has the advantage of being a noninvasive, quick test; however, it is dependent upon adequate sputum production. Sputum is obtained by:
- Induction–inhalation of nebulized hypertonic saline
- Transtracheal aspiration
- Bronchoscopy
- Bronchial washings.

Exfoliated cells (in the sputum, pleural fluid, bronchial brushings/washings, or fine-needle aspirate of lymph nodes and lesions) are examined, primarily for signs of malignancy.

Tests of pulmonary function

Tests of pulmonary function are used in:
- Diagnosis of lung disease
- Monitoring disease progression
- Assessing patient response to treatment.

205

Pulmonary function tests can seem confusing, but there are just three basic questions that most tests aim to answer:
1. Are the airways narrowed (PEFR, FEV_1, FEV_1:FVC, flow volume loops)?
2. Are the lungs a normal size (TLC, RV, and FRC)?
3. Is gas uptake normal ($D_{L(CO)}$ and $D_{L(CO)}$/VA)?

So, as a minimum, make sure you have a good understanding of peak flow monitoring and spirometry and know how you would measure RV, FRC, and gas transfer.

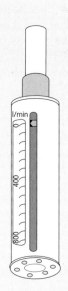

Fig. 10.6 Peak flow meter.

Tests of ventilation

Ventilation can be impaired in two basic ways:
- The airways become narrowed (obstructive disorders)
- Expansion of the lungs is reduced (restrictive disorders).

These two types of disorder have characteristic patterns of lung function (see Chapter 4) which can be measured using the tests below.

Forced expiration

Peak expiratory flow rate (PEFR) is a simple and cheap test that uses a peak flow meter (Fig. 10.6) to measure the maximum expiratory rate in the first 10 ms of expiration. Peak flow meters can be issued on prescription and used at home by patients to monitor their lung function.

Before measuring PEFR (Fig. 10.7), the practitioner should instruct the patient to:
- Take a full inspiration to maximum lung capacity
- Seal the lips tightly around the mouthpiece
- Blow out forcefully into the peak flow meter, which is held horizontally.

The best of three measurements is recorded and plotted on the appropriate graph. At least two recordings per day are required to obtain an accurate pattern. Normal PEFR is 400–650L/min in healthy adults.

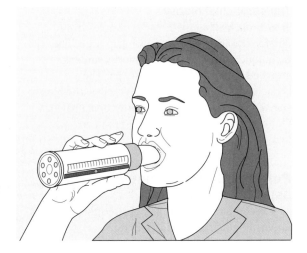

Fig. 10.7 Patient performing peak expiratory flow rate test.

PEFR is reduced in conditions that cause airway obstruction:
- Asthma, in which there is wide diurnal variation in PEFR known as "morning dipping" (Fig. 10.8)
- Chronic obstructive pulmonary disease
- Upper airway tumors.

Other causes of reduced PEFR include expiratory muscle weakness, inadequate effort, and poor technique. PEFR is not a good measure of air flow limitation because it measures only initial expiration; it is best used to monitor progression of disease and response to treatment.

Visit a respiratory therapist and ask for a demonstration of PEFR tests.

Forced expiratory volume and forced vital capacity

The forced expiratory volume in one second (FEV_1) and the forced vital capacity (FVC) are measured using a spirometer. The spirometer works by converting volumes of inspiration and expiration into a single line trace. The subject is connected by a mouthpiece to a sealed chamber (Fig. 10.9). Each time the subject breathes, the volume inspired or expired is converted into the vertical position of a float. The position of the float is recorded on a rotating drum by means of a pen attachment.

Electronic devices are becoming increasingly available.

FEV_1 and FVC

FEV_1 and FVC are related to height, age, and sex of the patient.

FEV_1 is the volume of air expelled in the first second of a forced expiration, starting from full inspiration. FVC is a measure of total lung volume exhaled. The patient is asked to exhale with maximal effort after a full inspiration.

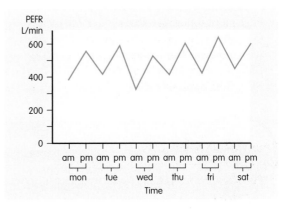

Fig. 10.8 Typical peak expiratory flow rate graph for an asthmatic patient.

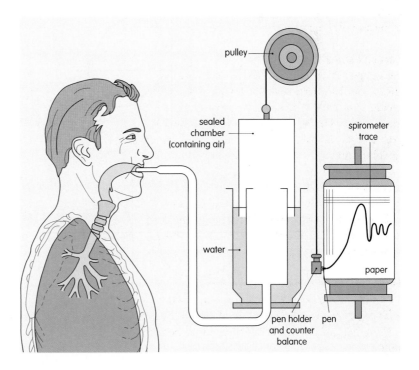

Fig. 10.9 Spirometry. The measurement of lung volume by displacement of a float within a sealed chamber is recorded on a paper roll by a pen.

207

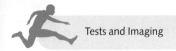

FEV₁:FVC ratio

The FEV_1:FVC ratio is a more useful measurement than FEV_1 or FVC alone. FEV_1 is 80% of FVC in normal subjects. The FEV_1:FVC ratio is an excellent measure of airway limitation and allows us to differentiate obstructive from restrictive lung disease.

In restrictive disease:
• Both FEV_1 and FVC are reduced, often in proportion to each other
• FEV_1:FVC ratio is normal or increased (>80%).

Whereas in obstructive diseases:
• High intrathoracic pressures generated by forced expiration cause premature closure of the airways with trapping of air in the chest
• FEV_1 is reduced much more than FVC
• FEV_1:FVC ratio is reduced (<80%).

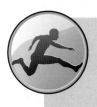

Patterns of lung function are often tested in exams. Chapter 4 contains more details about patterns of obstructive and restrictive diseases.

Flow–volume loops

Flow–volume loops are graphs constructed from maximal expiratory and inspiratory maneuvers performed on a spirometer. The loop shape can identify the type and distribution of airway obstruction. After a small amount of gas has been exhaled, flow is limited by:
• Elastic recoil force of the lung
• Resistance of airways upstream of collapse.

Flow–volume loops are useful in diagnosing upper airway obstruction (Fig. 10.10). In restrictive diseases:
• Maximum flow rate is reduced
• Total volume exhaled is reduced
• Flow rate is high during latter part of expiration because of increased lung recoil.

In obstructive diseases:
• Flow rate is low in relation to lung volume
• Expiration ends prematurely because of early airway closure
• Scooped-out appearance is often seen after point of maximum flow.

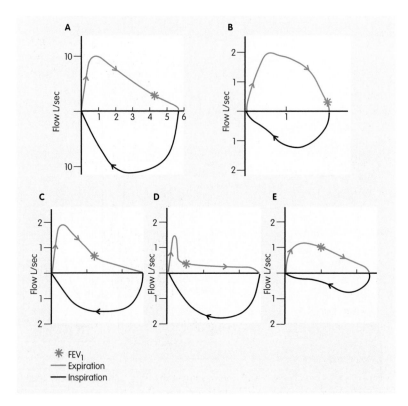

Fig. 10.10 Typical flow–volume loops. (A) Normal; (B) restrictive defect (phrenic palsy); (C) volume-dependent obstruction (e.g., asthma); (D) pressure-dependent obstruction (e.g., severe emphysema); (E) rigid obstruction (e.g., tracheal stenosis).

Tests of lung volumes

The amount of gas in the lungs can be thought of as being split into subdivisions (Fig. 4.3), with disease processes altering these volumes in specific ways. In measuring tidal volume and vital capacity, we use spirometry; alternative techniques are needed for the other volumes.

Residual volume (RV) and functional residual capacity (FRC)

One important lung volume, residual volume (RV), cannot be measured in simple spirometry, because gas remains in the lungs at the end of each breath (otherwise the lungs would collapse). Without a measure for RV, we cannot calculate functional residual capacity (FRC) or total lung capacity (TLC).

> Remember that FRC is the volume of gas remaining in the lung at the end of a quiet expiration. RV is the volume remaining at the end of a maximal expiration. Look back at the subdivisions of lung volumes on p. 47 (Fig. 4.3) if you are unsure as to how FRC, RV, and TLC relate to each other.

RV is a useful measure in assessing obstructive disease. In a healthy subject, residual volume is approximately 30% of total lung capacity. In obstructive diseases, the lungs are hyperinflated with "air trapping" so that RV is greatly increased and the ratio of RV:TLC is also increased. There are three methods of measuring RV: helium dilution, plethysmography, and nitrogen washout.

Helium dilution

The patient is connected to a spirometer containing a mixture of 10% helium in air. Helium is used because it is an insoluble, inert gas that does not cross the alveolar–capillary membrane. At the end of an expiration, the patient begins to breathe from the closed spirometer; after several breaths, the helium concentration in the spirometer and lung becomes equal.

The helium concentration is known at the start of the test and is measured when equilibrium has occurred. The dilution of helium is related to total lung capacity. Residual volume can be calculated by subtracting vital capacity from total lung capacity.

The helium dilution method measures only gas that is in communication with the airways.

Body plethysmography

Plethysmography determines changes in lung volume by recording changes in pressure. The patient sits in a large air-tight box and breathes through a mouthpiece (Fig. 10.11). At the end of a normal expiration, a shutter closes the mouthpiece and the patient is asked to make respiratory efforts. As the patient tries to inhale, box pressure increases. Using Boyle's law, lung volume can be calculated.

This method measures all intrathoracic gas including cysts, bullae, and pneumothoraces. In contrast to the helium dilution method, body plethysmography defines the extent of noncommunicating airspace within the lung; this is important in subjects with chronic obstructive pulmonary disease (e.g., emphysema).

Nitrogen washout

Following a normal expiration, the patient breathes 100% oxygen. This "washes out" the nitrogen in the lungs. The gas exhaled subsequently is collected and

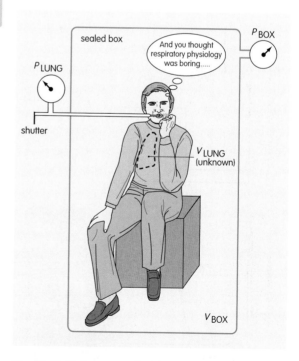

Fig. 10.11 Plethysmography. This assumes pressure at the mouth is the pressure within the lung.

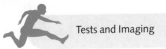

its total volume and the concentration of nitrogen are measured. The concentration of nitrogen in the lung before washout is 80%. The concentration of nitrogen left in the lung can be measured by a nitrogen meter at the lips measuring end expiration gas. Assuming no net change in the amount of nitrogen (it does not participate in gas exchange) it is possible to estimate the FRC.

Anatomic dead space

The volume of anatomic dead space (i.e., areas of the airway not involved in gaseous exchange) is usually about 150ml, or 2ml/kg of body weight. In a healthy person, the physiologic and anatomic dead spaces are nearly equal; however, in patients with alveolar disease and nonfunctioning alveoli (e.g., in emphysema), physiologic dead space may be up to ten times that of the anatomic deadspace.

Fowler's dead space

Fowler's dead space method uses the single-breath nitrogen test to measure anatomic dead space.

The patient makes a single inhalation of 100% O_2. On expiration, the nitrogen concentration rises as the dead space gas (100% O_2) is washed out by alveolar gas (a mixture of nitrogen and oxygen). If there were

no mixing of alveolar and dead space gas during expiration there would be a stepwise increase in nitrogen concentration when alveolar gas is exhaled (Fig. 10.12A). In reality, mixing does occur which means that the nitrogen concentration increases slowly, then rises sharply. As pure alveolar gas is expired, nitrogen concentration reaches a plateau (the alveolar plateau). Nitrogen concentration is plotted against expired volume; dead space is the volume at which the two areas under the plot are equal (Fig. 10.12B).

Tests of diffusion

Oxygen and carbon dioxide pass by diffusion between the alveoli and pulmonary capillary blood. The diffusing capacity of carbon monoxide ($D_{L(CO)}$ known as the Transfer Factor or T_LCO in Europe) measures the ability of gas to diffuse from inspired air to capillary blood, and also reflects the uptake of oxygen from the alveolus into the red blood cells. Carbon monoxide is used because:

- It is highly soluble
- It combines rapidly with hemoglobin.

The single-breath test is the test most commonly used to determine diffusing capacity.

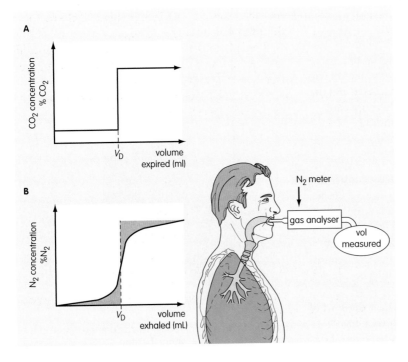

Fig. 10.12 Measurement of anatomic dead space. (A) Using Fowler's method, it would be expected that the gas expired from those areas not undergoing gas exchange (anatomic dead space) would contain no nitrogen and thus a stepwise change would occur to the nitrogen concentration of expired gas. The volume at which this occurs would be equal to the anatomic dead space volume. (B) On a graph showing the real-world results, a dotted line has been drawn to approximate the step change in nitrogen concentration.

Single-breath test

The patient takes a single breath from residual volume to total lung capacity. The inhaled gas contains 0.28% carbon monoxide and 13.5% helium. The patient is instructed to hold his or her breath for 10 seconds before expiring. The concentration of helium and carbon monoxide in the final part of the expired gas mixture is measured and the diffusing capacity of carbon monoxide is calculated. You need to know the hemoglobin level before the test.

In the normal lung, $D_L CO$ accurately measures the diffusing capacity of the lungs whereas, in diseased lung, diffusing capacity also depends on:

- Area and thickness of alveolar membrane
- Ventilation:perfusion relationship.

Diffusing capacity

Diffusing capacity ($D_L CO$) is defined as the amount of carbon monoxide transferred per minute, corrected for the concentration gradient of carbon monoxide across the alveolar capillary membrane (Fig. 10.13).

$D_{L(CO)}$ is reduced in conditions where there are:

- Fewer alveolar capillaries
- Ventilation:perfusion mismatches
- Reduced accessible lung volumes.

Gas transfer is a relatively sensitive but nonspecific test, useful at detecting early disease in lung parenchyma; $D_L CO/VA$ ratio is a better test. The $D_L CO$ is corrected for alveolar volume (VA) and is useful in distinguishing causes of low $D_L CO$ due to loss of lung volume:

- $D_L CO$ and $D_L CO/VA$ are low in emphysema and fibrosing alveolitis
- $D_L CO$ is low, but $D_L CO/VA$ is normal in pleural effusions and consolidation.

Tests of blood flow

Pulmonary blood flow can be measured by two

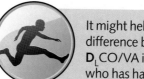

It might help to think of the difference between $D_L CO$ and $D_L CO/VA$ in terms of a patient who has had a lung removed. Clearly, lung volumes are reduced and therefore so is $D_L CO$. But $D_L CO/VA$ corrects for the lost volume, and if the remaining lung is normal, $D_L CO/VA$ is also completely normal.

methods: the Fick method and the indicator dilution technique.

Fick method

The amount of oxygen taken up by the blood passing through the lungs is related to pulmonary blood flow and the difference in oxygen content between arterial and mixed venous blood. Oxygen consumption is measured by collecting expired gas in a large spirometer and measuring its oxygen concentration.

Indicator dilution technique

Dye is injected into the venous circulation; the concentration and time of appearance of the dye in the arterial blood are recorded.

Similarly, in the thermal solution method ice-cold saline is injected into the venous system (usually the right heart). The change in temperature in blood is measured in the pulmonary artery over time and is the basis for calculation of blood flow.

Conditions that affect diffusing capacity	
Decreased $D_{L(CO)}$	Increased $D_{L(CO)}$
anemia	polycythemia
loss of functioning alveolar-capillary bed: emphysema, restrictive lung disease	increased alveolar capillary blood volume: left heart failure
poor ventilation of alveoli with inspiration; severe asthmatic attack, emphysema with poor effort	increased airway resistance asthma, cystic-fibrosis
	pulmonary hemorrhage

Fig. 10.13 Conditions that affect diffusing capacity.

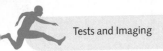

Testing patterns of ventilation
Ventilation:perfusion relationships
Ventilation:perfusion relationships are measured by means of isotope scans; these are described in the section on imaging below.

Inequality of ventilation
In diseases such as asthma or COPD the lungs may be unevenly ventilated. Inequality of ventilation is measured using the single-breath nitrogen test, similar to the method for measuring anatomic dead space described above.

Four phases are recognized in the single-breath nitrogen test, according to the composition of exhaled breath:
1. Pure deadspace.
2. Mixture of deadspace and alveolar gas.
3. Pure alveolar gas.
4. Toward the end of expiration, an abrupt increase in nitrogen concentration is seen.

The third phase, the alveolar plateau, is almost flat in healthy subjects. In patients with lung disease, alveolar nitrogen concentration continues to rise during expiration because of:
- Uneven dilution of the alveolar nitrogen by inspired oxygen
- The poorly ventilated alveoli (i.e., those containing more nitrogen) emptying last.

The change in nitrogen percentage concentration occurring between 750ml and 1250ml of expired volume is used as an index of uneven ventilation.

Testing lung mechanics
Lung compliance
Compliance is a measure of distensibility. It is defined as the volume change per unit of pressure across the lung. Lung compliance increases in emphysema, as the lung architecture is destroyed. In contrast, pulmonary fibrosis stiffens alveolar walls and decreases compliance (Fig. 10.14).

Lung compliance is measured by introducing a balloon into the esophagus to estimate intrapleural pressure. A lung of high compliance expands to a greater extent than one of low compliance when both are exposed to the same transpulmonary pressure.

To measure compliance:
- The patient breathes out from total lung capacity into a spirometer in steps

Causes of altered lung compliance	
Reduced compliance	Increased compliance
pulmonary venous pressure increased	old age
alveolar edema	emphysema
fibrosis	bronchoalveolar drugs
airway closure	

Fig. 10.14 Causes of altered lung compliance.

- Esophageal pressure is measured simultaneously
- The lung is given time to stabilize for a few seconds after each step, so that equalization of pressure is achieved at a number of lung volumes throughout inspiration and expiration
- A pressure–volume curve is obtained, which displays the elastic behavior of the lung.

Airway resistance
A large proportion of the resistance to air flow is offered by the upper respiratory tract. Airway resistance is defined as the pressure difference between the alveolus and mouth required to produce airflow of 1 L/s.

A number of disease states increase airway resistance, including:
- Asthma
- COPD
- Endobronchial obstruction (e.g., tumor or foreign body).

Airway resistance can be measured by plethysmography. The patient is seated in a constant pressure within the body plethysmograph and instructed to pant. The pressure within the plethysmograph changes: during inspiration the volume increases whereas during expiration it decreases. The greater the airway resistance, the greater are the pressure swings in the chest and plethysmograph.

In practice, estimates of airway resistance are much more commonly used than plethysmography. PEFR and FEV_1 are both useful estimates of resistance, based on the relationship between resistance and airflow.

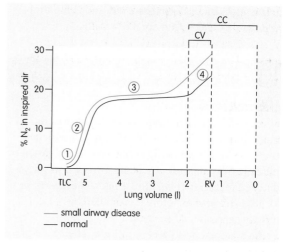

— small airway disease
— normal

Fig. 10.15 Closing volume. Airways in lower lung zones close at low lung volumes, and only those alveoli at the top of the lungs continue to empty. Because concentration of nitrogen in alveoli of upper zones is higher, the slope of the curve abruptly increases (phase 4). Phase 4 begins at larger lung volumes in individuals with even minor degrees of airway obstruction, increasing closing volume. CV = closing volume; CC = closing capacity; TLC = total lung capacity. (Courtesy of The Ciba Collection of Medical Illustrations, illustrated by Frank H. Netter, 1979.)

Closing volume

As lung volumes decrease on expiration there is a point at which smaller airways begin to close; this is known as the closing volume of the lungs (Fig. 10.15). Closing volume is usually expressed as a percentage of vital capacity. In young subjects, closing volume is approximately 10% of vital capacity and increases with age, being approximately 40% of vital capacity at 65 years of age.

In diseases such as asthma or COPD, the smaller airways close earlier, i.e., at a higher lung volume. An increase in closing volume against predicted values is a sensitive measure of early lung disease and may even show changes caused by cigarette smoking before the patient is symptomatic.

The test uses the single-breath nitrogen method, as described above, but in this case it is phase 4 that is of most interest. The start of phase 4 indicates the lung volume above residual volume at which closure of lung airways first occurs. Phase 4 is caused by preferential emptying of the apex of the lung after the lower zone airways have closed.

Exercise testing

Exercise testing is primarily used to:
- Diagnose unexplained breathlessness which is minimal at rest
- Assess the extent of lung disease, by stressing the system
- Determine the level of impairment in disability testing
- Assist in differential diagnosis (e.g., when it is not known whether a patient is limited by cardiac or lung disease)
- Test the effects of therapy on exercise capacity

Exercise testing is absolutely contraindicated for patients with various serious cardiovascular conditions, thrombotic or embolic disease, uncontrolled or untreated asthma, pulmonary edema or respiratory failure.

There are a number of established tests, including the treadmill or exercise stress test, which is commonly performed on a cycle ergometer.

This is performed in a laboratory and stresses the patient to a predetermined level based on heart rate. A number of tests are made as the patient exercises, including:
- ECG
- Arterial bloodgases
- Pulse oximetry
- Volume of gas exhaled
- Concentration of oxygen and carbon dioxide in exhaled gas.

The volume of gas exhaled per minute (V_E L/min), oxygen consumption (VO_2 L/min) and carbon dioxide output (VCO_2 L/min) are then calculated. The test indicates whether exercise tolerance is limited by the cardiovascular or respiratory system

213

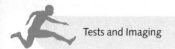
and assesses increases in heart rate and ventilation against a known oxygen uptake.

Imaging of the respiratory system

Ultrasound

Ultrasound uses high frequency sound waves to image internal structures. In respiratory medicine the technique is primarily used in the investigation of pleural effusions and empyemas. Ultrasound can detect an effusion that is not seen on chest x-ray or localize an effusion before it is drained by thoracocentesis.

A variation on this technique, Doppler ultrasound, is a noninvasive method for detecting deep vein thrombosis. It is used in investigating patients with suspected pulmonary thromboembolism. The technique examines blood flow and can detect thrombus in the veins above the popliteal fossa.

Plain film x-ray

The plain film x-ray is of paramount importance in the evaluation of pulmonary disease. The standard radiographic examinations of the chest are described below.

Posteroanterior erect radiograph (PA chest)

In the PA erect radiograph, x-rays travel from the posterior of the patient to the film, which is held against the front of the patient (Fig. 10.16). The scapula can be rotated out of the way, and accurate assessment of cardiac size is possible. The radiograph is performed in the erect position because:

- Gas passes upwards, making the detection of pneumothorax easier
- Fluid passes downwards, making pleural effusions easier to diagnose
- Blood vessels in mediastinum and lung are represented accurately.

Lateral radiograph

Lateral views help to localize lesions seen in PA views; they also give good views of the mediastinum and thoracic vertebrae (Fig. 10.17). Valuable information can be obtained by comparison with older films, if available.

In women of reproductive age, radiography should be performed within 28 days of last menstruation.

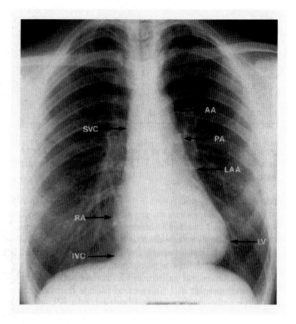

Fig. 10.16 Normal posteroanterior chest radiograph. The lungs are equally transradiant, the pulmonary vascular pattern is symmetrical. AA = aortic arch; SVC = superior vena cava; PA = pulmonary artery; LAA = left atrial appendage; RA = right atrium; LV = left ventricle; IVC = inferior vena cava. (Courtesy of Dr D. Sutton and Dr J.W.R. Young.)

Reporting a chest x-ray

Always view chest radiographs on a viewing box and follow a set routine for reporting plain films. If possible, compare with the patient's previous films.

Follow a set pattern for reading chest x-rays—that way you will not miss anything.

Clinical data

Take down the following details:
- Patient's name
- Age and sex
- Clinical problem
- Date of radiography.

Technical qualities

Note that radiographs contain right- or left-side markers.

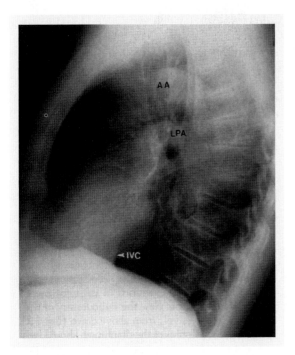

Fig. 10.17 Normal lateral chest radiograph. AA = aortic arch; LPA = left pulmonary artery; IVC = inferior vena cava. (Courtesy of Dr D. Sutton and Dr J.W.R. Young.)

With good penetration of x-rays, you should just be able to see the vertebral bodies through the cardiac shadow. In overpenetration, the lung fields appear too black. Conversely, in underpenetration, the lung fields appear too white.

Note the projection (AP, PA, or lateral; erect or supine). To deduce whether the patient was straight or rotated, compare the sternal ends of both clavicles.

With adequate inspiration, you should be able to count six ribs anterior to the diaphragm. Make sure that the whole lung field is included.

Heart and mediastinum
When examining the cardiac shadow, observe the position, size, and shape of the heart. Are the cardiac borders clearly visible?

Note whether the trachea is central or deviated to either side. Identify blood vessels and each hilum.

Other
Note the following points:
- Diaphragm—visible behind the heart. Costophrenic angles acute and sharp

- Lungs—divide the lungs into zones (upper, middle, and lower); compare like with like
- Bones—ribs, clavicles, sternum, thoracic vertebrae
- Finally, recheck the apices, behind the heart, and hilar and retrodiaphragmatic regions.

Lateral radiograph
On a lateral radiograph, note the following:
- Diaphragm—right hemidiaphragm seen passing through the heart border
- Lungs—divide lungs into area in front, behind, and above the heart
- Retrosternal space—an anterior mass will cause this space to be white
- Fissures—horizontal fissure (faint white line that passes from midpoint of hilum to anterior chest wall); oblique fissure (passes from T4/5 through hilum to the anterior third of the diaphragm)
- Hilum
- Bones—check vertebral bodies for shape, size, and density; check sternum.

Interpreting abnormalities
Once you have completed your overall review of the film, return to any areas of abnormal lucency or opacity and assess them according to:
- Number—single or multiple
- Position and distribution (lobar, etc.)
- Size, shape and contour
- Texture (homogenous, calcified, etc.).

The radiologic features of common lung conditions are described below.

Collapse
Atelectasis (collapse) is loss of volume of a lung, lobe, or segment for any cause. The most important mechanism is obstruction of a major bronchus by tumor, foreign body, or bronchial plug.

PA and lateral radiographs are required. Compare with old films where available. The silhouette sign can help localize the lesion (Fig. 10.18).

The lateral borders of the mediastinum are silhouetted against the air-filled lung that lies underneath. This silhouette is lost if there is consolidation in the underlying lung.

Signs of lobar collapse

Signs of lobar collapse are:
- Decreased lung volume
- Displacement of pulmonary fissures
- Compensatory hyperinflation of remaining part of the ipsilateral lung
- Elevation of hemidiaphragm on ipsilateral side
- Mediastinal and hilar displacement. Trachea pulled to side of collapse
- Radiopacity (white lung)
- Absence of air bronchogram.

Some signs are specific to lobe involvement.

In upper lobe collapse of the right lung, a PA film is most valuable in making diagnoses; the collapsed lobe lies adjacent to mediastinum (Fig. 10.19A).

In the left lung, a lateral film is most valuable in making diagnoses; the lobe collapses superiomedially and anteriorly (Fig. 10.19B).

Lower lobe collapse causes rotation and visualization of the oblique fissure on PA film.

A lateral film is most valuable in diagnosing middle lobe collapse. Thin, wedge-shaped opacity between horizontal and oblique fissures is seen.

Consolidation

Consolidation is seen as an area of white lung and represents fluid or cellular matter where there would normally be air (Figs 10.20 and 10.21). There are many causes of consolidation including:
- Pneumonia
- Pulmonary edema.

The silhouette sign	
Nonaerated area of lung	**Border that is obscured**
right upper lobe	right border of ascending aorta
right middle lobe	right heart border
right lower lobe	right diaphragm
left upper lobe	aortic knuckle and upper left cardiac border
lingula of left lung	left heart border
left lower lobe	left diaphragm

Fig. 10.18 The silhouette sign.

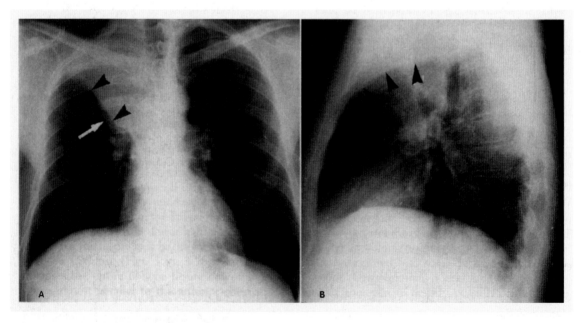

Fig. 10.19 (A and B) Right upper lobe collapse. The horizontal and oblique fissures (black arrowheads) are displaced. There is a mass (white arrow) at the right hilum. (Courtesy of Dr D. Sutton and Dr J.W.R. Young.)

Fig. 10.20 Radiologic distribution of alveolar processes.

Radiologic distribution of alveolar processes		
	Bat-wing pattern	
Segmental pattern	**Acute**	**Chronic**
pneumonia	pulmonary edema	atypical pneumonia
pulmonary infarct	pneumonia	lymphoma
segmental collapse	pulmonary hemorrhage	sarcoidosis
alveolar cell carcinoma		pulmonary alveolar proteinosis
		alveolar cell carcinoma

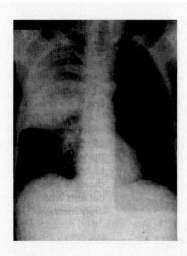

Fig. 10.21 Consolidation of the right upper lobe. (Courtesy of Professor C.D. Forbes and Dr W.F. Jackson.)

In contrast to collapse:
• The shadowing is typically heterogeneous (i.e., not uniform)
• The border is ill-defined
• Fissures retain their normal position.

There are two patterns of distribution:
• Segmental or lobar distribution
• Bat's-wing distribution.

Peripheral lung fields may be spared (e.g., in pulmonary edema). Air bronchograms may be seen; these are air-filled bronchi delineated by surrounding consolidated lung.

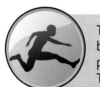

The presence of air bronchograms can be a useful pointer to the correct diagnosis. They are mostly seen in infection, when consolidated alveoli are lying adjacent to air-filled small and medium bronchioles.

Interstitial patterns

Three types of interstitial pattern exist (linear, nodular, and honeycomb), and overlap may occur.

Linear pattern

A linear pattern is seen as a network of fine lines running throughout the lungs. These lines represent thickened connective tissue and are termed Kerley A and B lines:
• A Upper lobes—long, thin lines
• B Lower lobes—short, thin horizontal lines 1–2 cm in length.

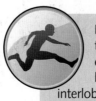

Kerley B lines can help to limit the possible diagnoses. They are caused by increased fluid between alveoli, in the interlobular septa. They are seen in pulmonary edema and malignant lymphatic infiltration.

217

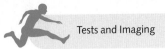

 Tests and Imaging

Nodular pattern

This pattern is seen as numerous well-defined small nodules (1–5mm) evenly distributed throughout the lung. Causes include miliary tuberculosis and chickenpox pneumonia.

Honeycomb pattern

A honeycomb pattern indicates extensive destruction of lung tissue, with lung parenchyma replaced by thin-walled cysts. Pneumothorax may be present. Normal pulmonary vasculature is absent. Pulmonary fibrosis leads to a honeycomb pattern.

Pulmonary nodules
Solitary nodules

The finding of a solitary pulmonary nodule on a plain chest radiograph is not an uncommon event. The nodule, which is commonly referred to as a coin lesion, is usually well circumscribed, less than 6cm in diameter, lying within the lung. The rest of the lung appears normal and the patient is often asymptomatic.

A solitary nodule on a chest x-ray may be an artifact or it may be due to:
- Malignant tumor—bronchial carcinoma or secondary deposits
- Infection—tuberculosis (Fig. 10.22) or pneumonia
- Benign tumor—hamartoma.

If the patient is older than 35 years of age, then malignancy should be at the top of the list of possible differential diagnoses. If the lesion is static for a long period of time, as determined by reviewing previous radiographs, then it is likely to be a benign lesion. However, a slow-growing nodule in an elderly patient is likely to be malignant.

It is important to take into account clinical history and compare with a past chest radiograph if available. You should be able to distinguish carcinoma from other causes:
- Size of lesion—if lesion is >4cm diameter, be suspicious of malignancy
- Margin—an ill-defined margin suggests malignancy
- Cavitation indicates infection or malignancy
- Calcification—unlikely to be malignancy
- Presence of air bronchogram—sign of consolidation, not malignancy.

Multiple nodules

Metastases are usually seen as well-defined nodules varying in size, which are more common at the periphery of lower lobes (Fig. 10.23); cavitation may be present. Abscesses are cavitated with thick and irregular wall. Cysts are often large.

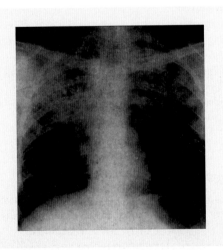

Fig. 10.22 Tuberculosis in a Greek immigrant. This film shows multiple areas of shadowing, especially in the upper lobes, and several lesions have started to cavitate. (Courtesy of Professor C.D. Forbes and Dr W.F. Jackson.)

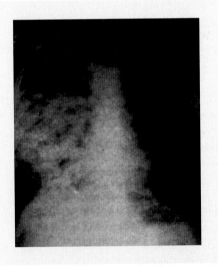

Fig. 10.23 Snowstorm mottling in both lung fields. In this case, the underlying diagnosis was testicular seminoma, with disseminated hematogenous metastases. (Courtesy of Professor C.D. Forbes and Dr W.F. Jackson.)

218

Fig. 10.24 Unilateral and bilateral causes of hilar enlargement.

Causes of hilar enlargement		
Unilateral enlargement	**Bilateral enlargement**	
	Enlarged lymph nodes	**Enlarged vessels**
bronchial carcinoma	lymphomas	left-to-right cardiac shunts
metastatic malignancy	sarcoidosis	pulmonary arterial hypertension
lymphomas	cystic fibrosis	chronic obstructive pulmonary disease
primary tuberculosis	infectious mononucleosis	left heart failure
sarcoidosis	leukemia	pulmonary embolism
pulmonary embolus		
pulmonary valve stenosis		

Mediastinal masses		
Anterior masses	**Middle masses**	**Posterior masses**
retrosternal thyroid	bronchial carcinoma	neurogenic tumor
thymic mass	lymphoma	paravertebral abscess
dermoid cyst	sarcoidosis	esophageal lesions
lymphomas	primary tuberculosis	aortic aneurysm
aortic aneurysm	bronchogenic cyst	

Fig. 10.25 Mediastinal masses.

Other nodules include:
- Rheumatoid nodules
- Wegener's granulomatosis
- Multiple arteriovenous malformations.

Hilar masses
Normal hilar complex includes:
- Proximal pulmonary arteries and bifurcations
- Bronchus
- Pulmonary veins
- Lymph nodes, not seen unless enlarged.

Hilar size varies from person to person, so enlargement is difficult to diagnose (Fig. 10.24). Radiologic features of the hilum are:
- Concave lateral margin
- Equal radiopacity
- Left hilum lies higher than right.

PA films are most valuable in assessing hilar shadow, but you must always consult the lateral film. Technical qualities of the film need to be adequately assessed before conclusions can be made because patient rotation commonly mimics hilar enlargement.

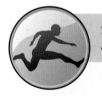 Sarcoidosis commonly presents as bilateral lymphadenopathy.

Mediastinal masses
A mediastinal mass typically has a sharp, concave margin, visible due to the silhouette sign. Lateral films may be particularly useful. Mediastinal masses are frequently asymptomatic and are grouped according to their anatomical position (Fig. 10.25). Computerized tomography (CT) is advised where there is a doubt as to the nature of the lesion.

Anterior mediastinal masses

Characteristics of anterior mediastinal masses are:
- Hilar structures still visible
- Mass merges with the cardiac border
- A mass passing into the neck is not seen above the clavicles
- Small anterior mediastinal masses are difficult to see on PA films.

Middle mediastinal masses

A middle mediastinal mass merges with hila and cardiac border
- The majority are caused by enlarged lymph nodes.

Posterior mediastinal masses

In posterior mediastinal masses the cardiac border and hila are seen but the posterior aorta is obscured. Vertebral changes may be present.

Pleural lesions
Pneumothorax

Pneumothorax is usually obvious on normal inspiratory PA films. Look carefully at upper zones, because air accumulates first here; you will see an area devoid of lung markings (black lung), with the lung edge outlined by air in the pleural space. Small pneumothoraces can be identified on the expiratory film and may be missed in the supine film.

Tension pneumothorax

Tension pneumothorax is seen as a displacement of the mediastinum and trachea to the contralateral side, depressed ipsilateral diaphragm, and increased space between the ribs.

> Tension pneumothorax is a medical emergency. Review an expiratory film if possible and bear in mind the patient's clinical state. If breathlessness is progressive and you suspect a tension pneumothorax, start treatment without waiting for a chest x-ray.

Pleural effusions

PA erect radiography is performed. Classically, there is a radiopaque mass at the base of the lung and blunting of the costophrenic angle, with the pleural meniscus higher laterally than medially. Large effusions can displace the mediastinum contralaterally.

A horizontal upper border implies that a pneumothorax is also present. An effusion has a more homogeneous texture than consolidation and air bronchograms are absent.

Mesothelioma

Mesothelioma is a malignant tumor of the pleura, which may present as discrete pleural deposits or as a localized lesion.

Thickened pleura is observed with irregular medial margin on radiography; in 50% of cases, pleural plaques are elsewhere. Pleural effusions are common, usually containing blood (Fig. 10.26). Rib destruction is uncommon.

Vascular patterns
Normal vascular pattern

Lung markings are vascular in nature. Arteries branch vertically to upper and lower lobes. On erect films, upper lobe vessels are smaller than the lower lobe vessels. It is difficult to see vessels in the peripheral one-third of lung fields.

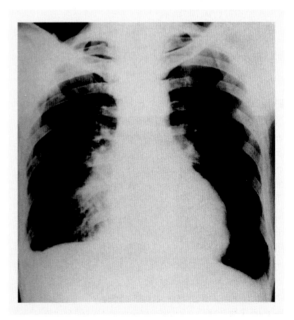

Fig. 10.26 Small pleural effusions. Both costophrenic angles are blunted. (Courtesy of Dr D. Sutton and Dr J.W.R. Young.)

Pulmonary venous hypertension

On erect films, upper lobe vessels are larger than the lower lobe vessels. Pulmonary venous hypertension is associated with edema and pleural effusions.

Pulmonary arterial hypertension

Pulmonary arterial hypertension is seen as bilateral hilar enlargement associated with long-standing pulmonary disease.

Ventilation:perfusion scans

Ventilation:perfusion scans are primarily used to detect pulmonary emboli. The principle is that a pulmonary embolus produces a defect on the perfusion scan (a "filling defect") which is not matched by a defect on the ventilation scan (i.e., there is an area of the lung that is ventilated but not perfused).

Ventilation scans

Ventilation is detected by inhalation of a gas or aerosol labeled with the radioisotope, Xe^{133}. The patient breathes and rebreathes the gas until it comes into equilibrium with other gases in the lung.

Perfusion scans

Radioactive particles larger than the diameter of the pulmonary capillaries are injected intravenously, where they remain for several hours. Tc^{99m}-labeled macroaggregated albumin (MAA) is used. A gamma camera is then used to detect the position of the MAAs. The pattern indicates the distribution of pulmonary blood flow.

Diagnosis of pulmonary embolism

Abnormalities in the perfusion scan are checked against a plain chest x-ray; defects on the perfusion scan are not diagnostic if they correspond to radiographic changes. Scans are classified based on the probability of a pulmonary embolism as:
1. Normal—commonly reported as "low-probability."
2. High probability.
3. Nondiagnostic.

Nondiagnostic scans include those where patients have obstructive diseases such as asthma or COPD which lead to perfusion and ventilation defects; pulmonary embolus cannot be diagnosed if such a pattern is obtained—other tests (see below) are then indicated.

Pulmonary angiography

Pulmonary angiography is the gold standard test for diagnosing pulmonary embolus. Indications are:
- When a ventilation:perfusion scan is inconclusive for pulmonary embolus, but the patient is acutely ill
- Before surgery or thrombolysis for pulmonary embolism.

The test is performed by injection of contrast media through a catheter introduced in the main pulmonary artery using the Seldinger technique. Obstructed vessels or filling defects can be seen clearly and emboli show as filling defects. Despite the accuracy of the test, in practice pulmonary angiography is not often performed because it is invasive and time-consuming. Where ventilation:perfusion scans are inconclusive, and the patient is not acutely ill, it is more common to proceed to lower limb venography or Doppler ultrasound. When angiography is performed, a less invasive test involving computerized tomography (CTPA) is increasingly preferred.

Computerized tomography

Computerized tomography (CT) is the imaging modality of choice for mediastinal and many pulmonary conditions. CT scans provide detailed cross-sectional images of the thorax. The images can be electronically modified to display different tissues (e.g., by using a bone setting compared with a soft-tissue setting).

The patient passes through a rotating gantry which has x-ray tubes on one side and a set of detectors on the other. Information from the detectors is analyzed and displayed as a two-dimensional image on visual display units, then recorded.

CT gives a dose of radiation approximately 100 times that of a standard plain film chest radiograph.

Applications of computerized tomography

Detection of pulmonary nodules

CT can evaluate the presence of metastases in a patient with known malignancy; however, it cannot distinguish between benign and malignant masses.

Mediastinal masses

CT is a useful technique in searching for lymphadenopathy in a person with primary lung carcinoma.

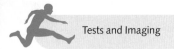

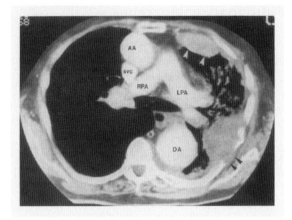

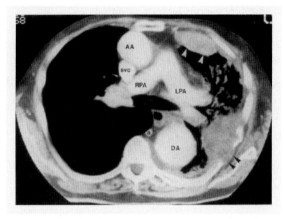

Fig. 10.27 CT scan of a pleural mass. Enhanced CT scan at level of bifurcation of main pulmonary artery. The left lung is surrounded by pleural masses (arrowheads), and the posterior mass is invading the chest wall. The vascular anatomy of the mediastinum is well shown. a = azygos vein; RPA = right pulmonary artery; LPA = left pulmonary artery; AA = ascending aorta; SVC = superior vena cava; DA = descending aorta. (Courtesy of Dr D. Sutton and Dr J.W.R. Young.)

Fig. 10.28 Technical differences between CT and high-resolution CT (HRCT).

Carcinoma of the lung
CT can evaluate the size of a lung carcinoma, and detect mediastinal extension and staging.

Pleural lesions
CT is effective at detecting small pleural effusions and identifying pleural plaques (Fig. 10.27).

Vascular lesions
Contrast studies allow imaging of vascular lesions (e.g. aortic aneurysms).

High-resolution computerized tomography
High-resolution CT is useful in imaging diffuse lung disease: thinner sections of 1–2mm show greater lung detail (Fig. 10.28).

Applications of high-resolution computerized tomography
Bronchiectasis
High-resolution CT has replaced bronchography. In dilated bronchi, the technique can show:
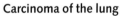
- Collapse
- Scarring
- Consolidation.

Interstitial lung disease
High-resolution CT is more specific than plain film radiography. Disorders that have specific appearances on high-resolution CT include sarcoidosis, occupational lung disease, and interstitial pneumonia.

High-resolution CT can be used for biopsy guidance.

Atypical infections
High-resolution CT provides diagnosis earlier than using plain chest radiography and is useful in monitoring disease and response to treatment. It also provides good delineation of disease activity and destruction.

High-resolution CT is used in imaging of patients with AIDS (e.g., PCP).

Diagnosis of lymphangitis carcinomatosa
High resolution CT can be used in the diagnosis of lymphangitis carcinomatosa.

Magnetic resonance imaging (MRI)
MRI uses the magnetic properties of the hydrogen atom to produce images. MRI gives excellent imaging of soft tissues and the heart, but has limited use in the respiratory system. Flowing blood does not provide a signal for MRI imaging, and vascular structures appear as hollow tubes. MRI imaging can be used to differentiate masses around the aorta or in the hilar regions. It has the advantage of not using ionizing radiation.

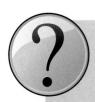

- Summarize the basic hematologic tests performed.
- What key information does arterial blood gas analysis give us?
- What tests can be performed on a sputum sample?
- What is the main use of the histopathology laboratory in diagnosing respiratory disease?
- Describe how to accurately perform a PEFR test.
- List the uses and limitations of the PEFR test.
- How do you test for airway narrowing?
- What is the importance of spirometry in differentiating obstructive from restrictive disorders?
- Describe the differences between obstructive and restrictive lung disease.
- Interpret and draw abnormal flow–volume loops.
- Discuss the implications of an abnormal diffusing capacity test result.
- How can airway compliance and resistance be calculated?
- When is exercise testing used?
- What are the main uses for ultrasound in respiratory medicine?
- Describe how to read a PA plain film chest radiograph.
- What are the differences between interstitial and alveoli appearances?
- What is the silhouette sign? What are its uses?
- What is an air bronchogram? What are its uses?
- Describe the differences between collapse and consolidation on chest radiographs.
- What are the uses and limitations of CT and MRI imaging in respiratory imaging?

Index

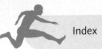

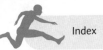

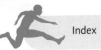

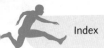

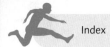

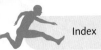

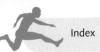

CRASH COURSE
Respiratory System

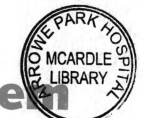